Advances in Artificial Intelligence for Healthcare Applications

Advances in Artificial Intelligence for Healthcare Applications comprehensively covers the theoretical foundations, applications, and research potential of artificial intelligence in the healthcare domain.

Features:

- Discusses advanced concepts such as biomedical large language models, and natural language processing applications.
- Covers machine vision applications for robotics in healthcare, challenges, and trends in rehabilitation devices in healthcare, and robotic interactions and control for wearable devices.
- Presents the Internet of Things-based disease monitoring systems, Internet of nano-things for healthcare applications, and wearable Medical Internet of Things devices for accessible healthcare services.
- Explains the use of artificial intelligence in bone and brain imaging, molecular imaging using artificial intelligence, and medical image segmentation.
- Illustrates the importance of using generative artificial intelligence for clinical documentation, and medical imaging applications using generative artificial intelligence.

The text is primarily written for senior undergraduates, graduate students, and academic researchers in the fields of electrical engineering, electronics and communications engineering, computer science and engineering, and biomedical engineering.

Future Generation Information Systems

Series editor- Bharat Bhushan

With the evolution of future generation computing systems, it becomes necessary to occasionally take stock, analyze the development of its core theoretical ideas, and adapt to radical innovations. This series will provide a platform to reflect the theoretical progress, and forge emerging theoretical avenues for the future generation information systems. The theoretical progress in the Information Systems field (IS) and the development of associated next-generation theories is the need of the hour. This is because Information Technology (IT) has become increasingly infused, interconnected, and intelligent in almost all context.

Industry 6.0: Technology, Practices, Challenges, and Applications
Kishor Kumar Reddy C, Srinath Doss, Lavanya Pamulaparty, Kari J Lippert and Ruchi Doshi

Convergence of Deep Learning and Artificial Intelligence in Internet of Things
Ajay Rana, Arun Rana, Sachin Dhawan, Sharad Sharma and Ahmed A. Elngar

Next Generation Communication Networks for Industrial Internet of Things Systems
Sundresan Perumal, Mujahid Tabassum, Moolchand Sharma and Saju Mohanan

Artificial Intelligence and Optimizing Techniques for Smart Information System Generations
Edited by: Aleem Ali, Rajdeep Chakraborty and Nawaf R. Alharbe

Advances in Artificial Intelligence for Healthcare Applications
Edited by: Anoop V.S, Suhasini Verma and Usharani Hareesh Govindarajan

Advances in Artificial Intelligence for Healthcare Applications

Edited by
V.S. Anoop
Suhasini Verma
Usharani Hareesh Govindarajan

CRC Press
Taylor & Francis Group
Boca Raton London New York

CRC Press is an imprint of the
Taylor & Francis Group, an **informa** business

Designed cover image by Owen Beard on Unsplash

First edition published 2025
by CRC Press
2385 NW Executive Center Drive, Suite 320, Boca Raton FL 33431

and by CRC Press
4 Park Square, Milton Park, Abingdon, Oxon, OX14 4RN

CRC Press is an imprint of Taylor & Francis Group, LLC

ISBN: 978-1-032-82187-0 (hbk)
ISBN: 978-1-032-82190-0 (pbk)
ISBN: 978-1-003-50338-5 (ebk)

DOI: 10.1201/9781003503385

Typeset in Times
by SPi Technologies India Pvt Ltd (Straive)

Contents

Preface...viii
Editors...ix
List of Contributors...xi

Chapter 1 Revolutionizing Healthcare: Exploring Robotics' Role and Impact in the Recent Years..1

N. Sai Kusum Sarayu and V. M. Manikandan

Chapter 2 Enhancing Healthcare Through Medical IoT: Current Trends and Future Directions...19

Z. Tanveer Baig, M. N. Rajesh and Apurva Puttaswamy

Chapter 3 Exploring the Potential of Smart Healthcare Wearable Devices and Its Future: A Study on Consumer Adoption and Attitude............32

Usha Yadav and Sheetal Soni

Chapter 4 OralMedIE: Fine-tuning Biomedical Language Model for Clinical Information Extraction for Oral Medicine and Radiology....................45

V. S. Anoop and R. Ardra

Chapter 5 Generative AI for Healthcare Security: Addressing Privacy Challenges through Anomaly Detection in Healthcare Communications...60

Arul Kumar Natarajan, Kamal Upreti, Pravin R. Kshirsagar and Tan Kuan Tak

Chapter 6 Navigating the Ethereal: Ethical Frameworks in AI for Healthcare...72

Bodhibrata Nag, Mahesh Devnani and Ranjan Pal

Chapter 7 Case Study on Explainable Artificial Intelligence in Healthcare Diagnostics...86

Muskan Jalan, Malhar Desai, Sunik Malik and Gurpreet Kaur Grewal

Chapter 8 Robust CNN based on LIME for Glaucoma Classification 99

Sonali Dash and V. Keerthi Kiran

Chapter 9 Tumor Detection and Classification of Oral Squamous Cell Carcinoma on Histopathological Images utilizing Personalized Transfer Learning Approaches 121

Singaraju Ramya and R. I. Minu

Chapter 10 Artificial Intelligence (AI)-Enabled Diabetic Retinopathy Detection Techniques 140

Ravi Bhushan Dixit and Chandan Kumar Jha

Chapter 11 Artificial Intelligence and Machine Learning in Radiology: Benefits, Drawbacks and Prospects 156

Aditya Shah, Anagha Brahmajosyula, Varnika Gupta and Bhag Chand Jain

Chapter 12 Unlocking Effective Applications of Artificial Intelligence for Healthcare Management Systems 170

Shreyan Saha and Esha Saha

Chapter 13 Transformative Synergy: Revolutionizing Healthcare Accounting Information Systems with AI 184

Hrishikesh Desai

Chapter 14 Canadian Rural Medicare 2047: Envisioning Equal Access Through Digitalization 199

Lionel Huntley Henderson and John Wilson

Chapter 15 Revolutionizing Patient Access Through AI in Healthcare 208

Herat Joshi, Jahanvi Bansal and Parag Shukla

Chapter 16 Transformation of Insurance Sector in the Era of Artificial Intelligence 228

Suhasini Verma, Jeevesh Sharma, V. S. Anoop and Shweta Goyal

Chapter 17 "Prevention is Better Than Cure": Relevance of mHealth in Prevention Health Care Industry in India 241

S. Vijayalakshmi, Ravi Kiran Erra and Kanika Shetty

Chapter 18 AI in Medicine: Addressing Advancements, Personhood Status and Liability Concerns for AI-Related Errors 264

Ditipriya Dutta Chowdhury and Sangeeta Roy Maitra

Chapter 19 Adoption and Implementation Challenges of Artificial Intelligence in Healthcare Settings 276

John T. Abraham, Swapna K. Cherian, Blessing T. John and Angel T. John

Index 291

Preface

Artificial Intelligence (AI), the study of making machines intelligent, is growing by leaps and bounds, and it is challenging to find sectors that do not have at least one AI use case. This is true for any sector, such as agriculture, healthcare, education, and space science. The proliferation of information and communication technologies in all walks of life has caused a significant amount of data to be generated at an enormous speed. These data can be used to train or teach computers, enabling them to make decisions independently without explicit programming. The advancements in deep learning have made it possible to train computers with large amounts of data where traditional machine-learning models may fail to converge. Healthcare is one of the prominent areas being disrupted by the power of Artificial Intelligence. The traditional healthcare data analytics and rule-based decision-making processes have been entirely replaced by powerful deep learning models and algorithms that can automatically identify features from the data. During the early stages of development, artificial intelligence-based systems were only accessible and affordable to a limited number of healthcare professionals. The democratization of healthcare is now enabling more healthcare stakeholders to adopt artificial intelligence-based models into clinical practice and decision-making processes that bring better healthcare outcomes. The scope of this proposed edited book is to discuss the theoretical foundations, the emergence, and the application areas of artificial intelligence in the healthcare domain in an easy-to-understand manner that would be highly helpful for researchers, academicians, and industry professionals. This edited book will also set the trend to evolve new concepts and ideas and share issues and challenges faced during the research with probable solutions applied to AI for healthcare, which may be integrated with other computing techniques such as IoT and Blockchain. This proposed book presents the evolution of AI in healthcare, from fundamental theories to present forms, and explains the concepts of artificial intelligence in healthcare, specifically, AI-assisted drug discovery, NLP for intelligent healthcare, AI for precision medicine, AI for virtual nursing, Epidemiology, and also covers a variety of applications with real-world case studies in these areas.

Editors

Dr. V. S. Anoop completed his Doctor of Philosophy (Ph.D.) and Master of Philosophy (M.Phil.) in Computer Science with a specialization in Artificial Intelligence, from the Cochin University of Science and Technology (CUSAT). He completed his Integrated Master of Computer Applications from the School of Computer and Information Sciences, and a Post Graduate Diploma in Higher Education from the School of Education, Indira Gandhi National Open University, New Delhi. Anoop is currently working as an Assistant Professor of Information Systems and Analytics at Thiagarajar School of Management (Autonomous), Madurai, India. In his previous role, he worked as a Research Officer with the School of Digital Sciences, Kerala University of Digital Sciences, Innovation and Technology, Thiruvananthapuram, India. He has also obtained his postdoctoral fellowship with the Smith School of Business at Queen's University, Canada. He has worked in various roles such as Research Scientist, Assistant Professor, Data Scientist, and Visiting Faculty. Anoop's primary research interests are Applied Natural Language Processing and Text Mining. He has several publications, including edited books, book chapters, articles in international journals, and conference proceedings. He is also a recipient of the prestigious Mozilla Responsible Computing Challenge Grant jointly awarded by the Mozilla Foundation and United States Agency for International Development.

Dr. Suhasini Verma is an Associate Professor at the Department of Business Administration, Faculty of Management and Commerce, Manipal University Jaipur. Dr. Verma holds a master's degree in economics and management and cleared UGC-NET in Management. She is an alumnus of the Indian Institute of Management, Ahmedabad. She has 15 years of research and teaching experience in finance, FinTech, and economics. She has presented several research papers in international and national seminars and published research papers and book chapters in reputed journals and books. She has edited books in the domain of Cybersecurity. She is a recipient of the honorable mention award in Case Writing Competition organized by ISB Hyderabad and Ivey Business. Her research interests include FinTech, Corporate Governance, and Corporate Social Responsibility. She is currently guiding four research scholars, while one of her scholars has been awarded a Ph.D. degree.

Dr. Usharani Hareesh Govindarajan is a Tenured Assistant Professor of Information Management and Systems at the Business School, University of Shanghai for Science and Technology, Shanghai, China. He received his Doctoral degree in Industrial Engineering from Tsing Hua University (Hsinchu), a master's in engineering in Computer Science, and a master's in science in informatics from the University of Delhi, India. Prior to joining the University of Shanghai for Science and Technology, Hareesh was an Assistant Research Professor (on contract) at the Shanghai Jiao Tong University, where he was the principal recipient of the 2019 international talent induction plan from the China Science Foundation. Additionally, before joining the Ph.D. degree, Hareesh had several years of work experience.

His work experience as a research and development Engineer for the Nokia Siemens Networks (a joint venture between Nokia of Finland and Siemens of Germany) and Verizon Wireless in America has helped him understand the iterative development of technologies in Europe and America. Further, he is currently a part of various industrial-academic initiatives across China, India, and France and has published research papers in leading international journals such as IEEE Transactions on Engineering Management, Complexity, IEEE Engineering Management Review, Advanced Engineering Informatics, World Patent Information, etc.

Contributors

John T. Abraham
Bharata Mata College
Kerala, India

Swapna K. Cherian
MSM College
Kerala, India

Ditipriya Dutta Chowdhury
Burdwan University
West Bengal, India

Jahanvi Bansal
GSFC University
Vadodara, India

Anagha Brahmajosyula
Kempegowda Institute of Medical Sciences
Bangalore, Karnataka, India

Sonali Dash
Chandigarh University
Chandigarh, India

Hrishikesh Desai
Arkansas State University
USA

Malhar Desai
Lovely Professional University
Phagwara, Punjab, India

Mahesh Devnani
Post Graduate Institute of Medical Education and Research
Chandigarh

Ravi Bhushan Dixit
Indian Institute of Information Technology
Bhagalpur, India

Ravi Kiran Erra
RV University
Bengaluru, Karnataka, India

Shweta Goyal
Manipal University Jaipur
India

Gurpreet Kaur Grewal
Lovely Professional University
Phagwara, Punjab, India

Varnika Gupta
Lala Lajpat Rai Memorial Medical College
Meerut, Uttar Pradesh

Lionel Huntley Henderson
British Management University
Tashkent, Uzbekistan

Bhag Chand Jain
Sawai Man Singh Medical College
Jaipur, Rajasthan, India

Muskan Jalan
Lovely Professional University
Phagwara, Punjab, India

Chandan Kumar Jha
Indian Institute of Information Technology
Bhagalpur, India

Angel T. John
Mar Baselios Engineering College
Kerala, India

Blessing T. John
Mount Zion Medical College
Kerala, India

Herat Joshi
Great River Health Systems
Burlington, Iowa, USA

V. Keerthi Kiran
Raghu Engineering College,
Visakhapatnam, Andhra Pradesh, India

Pravin R. Kshirsagar
J D College of Engineering & Management
Nagpur, Maharashtra, India

M.N. Rajesh
Jio Platforms Limited
Bangalore, Karnataka India

Sangeeta Roy Maitra
Government Centre of Legal Education
Hooghly Mohsin College Campus
West Bengal, India

Sunik Malik
RT-PCR (Covid-19) Laboratory
Civil Hospital
S.B.S Nagar, Punjab, India

V. M. Manikandan
SRM University - AP
Andhra Pradesh, India

R. I. Minu
SRM Institute of Science and Technology
Kattankulathur, Chennai, India

Bodhibrata Nag
Indian Institute of Management Calcutta

Arul Kumar Natarajan
Samarkand International University of Technology
Samarkand, Uzbekistan

Ranjan Pal
Massachusetts Institute of Technology

Apurva Puttaswamy
Sambhram University
Jizzax, Jizzax Region, Uzbekistan

Singaraju Ramya
SRM Institute of Science and Technology
Kattankulathur, Chennai, India

S. Vijayalakshmi
RV University
Bengaluru, Karnataka, India

Esha Saha
Indian Institute of Technology (Indian School of Mines) Dhanbad
Jharkhand, India

Shreyan Saha
Indian Institute of Technology (Indian School of Mines) Dhanbad
Dhanbad, Jharkhand, India

N. Sai Kusum Sarayu
SRM University - AP
Andhra Pradesh, India

Aditya Shah
Shri Jagannath Pahadiya Medical College
Bharatpur, Rajasthan, India

Jeevesh Sharma
Manipal University Jaipur
India

Kanika Shetty
RV University
Bengaluru, Karnataka, India

Parag Shukla
The Maharaja Sayajirao University of Baroda
Vadodara, India

Sheetal Soni
National Institute of Fashion Technology
Jodhpur, Rajasthan, India

Tan Kuan Tak
Singapore Institute of Technology
Punggol, Singapore

Kamal Upreti
Christ (Deemed to be University)
Delhi NCR, India

V. S. Anoop
Thiagarajar School of Management (Autonomous)
Madurai, Tamil Nadu, India

Suhasini Verma
Manipal University Jaipur
India

John Wilson
Webster University
Shanghai, China

Usha Yadav
National Institute of Fashion Technology
Bengaluru, Karnataka, India

Z. Tanveer Baig
Amity University in Tashkent
Uzbekistan

Ardra R.
Kerala University of Digital Sciences, Innovation and Technology
Kerala, India.

1 Revolutionizing Healthcare
Exploring Robotics' Role and Impact in the Recent Years

N. Sai Kusum Sarayu and V. M. Manikandan

1.1 INTRODUCTION

AI has revolutionized healthcare robotics, enabling robots to perform complex tasks in nursing, surgery, and therapy with high precision (Denecke & Baudoin, 2022). In nursing, robots assist with routine care and patient monitoring, freeing up nurses for more critical tasks. In surgery, AI-driven systems improve minimally invasive procedures, enhancing precision and reducing recovery times. Additionally, robots offer personalized treatments in physical and cognitive therapies with real-time feedback.

Beyond these applications, AI improves diagnostics, predictive analytics, and personalized medicine by analyzing vast amounts of medical data to refine diagnoses and treatments (Babarinde et al., 2023). During the COVID-19 pandemic, robots played a pivotal role in disinfection, delivering medications, and supporting remote monitoring, easing the burden on healthcare workers and reducing virus transmission risks (Azer & Oran, 2023).

As healthcare robotics evolve, ethical considerations like patient safety, privacy, robotic autonomy, and job displacement must be addressed (Elendu et al., 2023). This chapter explores the history, roles, and applications of healthcare robots across various sectors.

1.2 WHAT IS ROBOTICS

Robotics is a diverse discipline comprising mechanics, computer science, and electronics. This field's objective is to design and create machines that can reciprocate human behavior. The greatest technological achievement to date has been regarded as the integration of robots and artificial intelligence. Robots gain the ability to sense their surroundings and decide for themselves using current information. This interdisciplinary collaboration, as shown in Figure 1.1, enables the development of sophisticated robotic systems that can accurately and efficiently carry out challenging tasks.

DOI: 10.1201/9781003503385-1

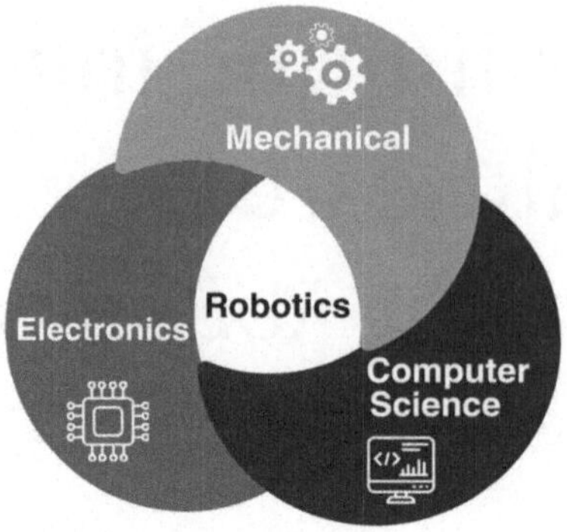

FIGURE 1.1 Robotics as a multidisciplinary field.

1.3 HISTORY OF ROBOTS IN HEALTHCARE

The concept of surgical robotics dates back over 50 years, but practical use began in the late 1980s with ROBODOC, an orthopedic image-guided system developed by Integrated Surgical Systems, U.S. AI can enhance surgical outcomes by delivering real-time information and feedback to surgeons, improving surgical planning and decision-making processes, and minimizing the risk of complications during procedures (Nawrat, 2023).

The first surgical robot PUMA 560 shown in Figure 1.2 was built in 1985; it is a robotic arm modified to perform a stereotactic brain biopsy with an accuracy of 0.05mm. This served as a prototype for Neuromate.

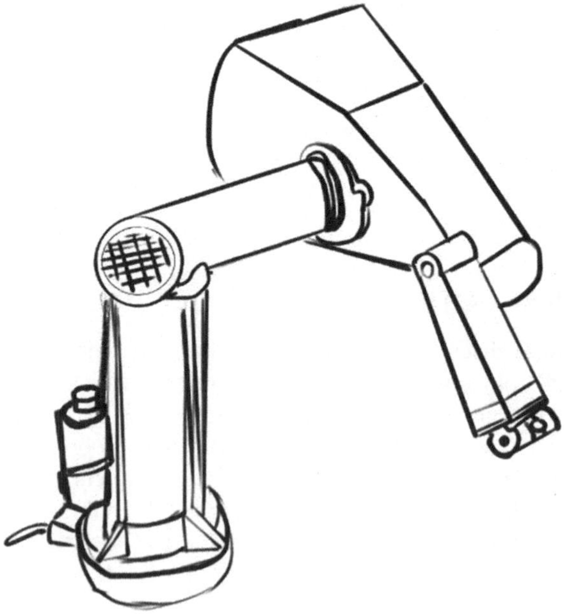

FIGURE 1.2 PUMA 560.

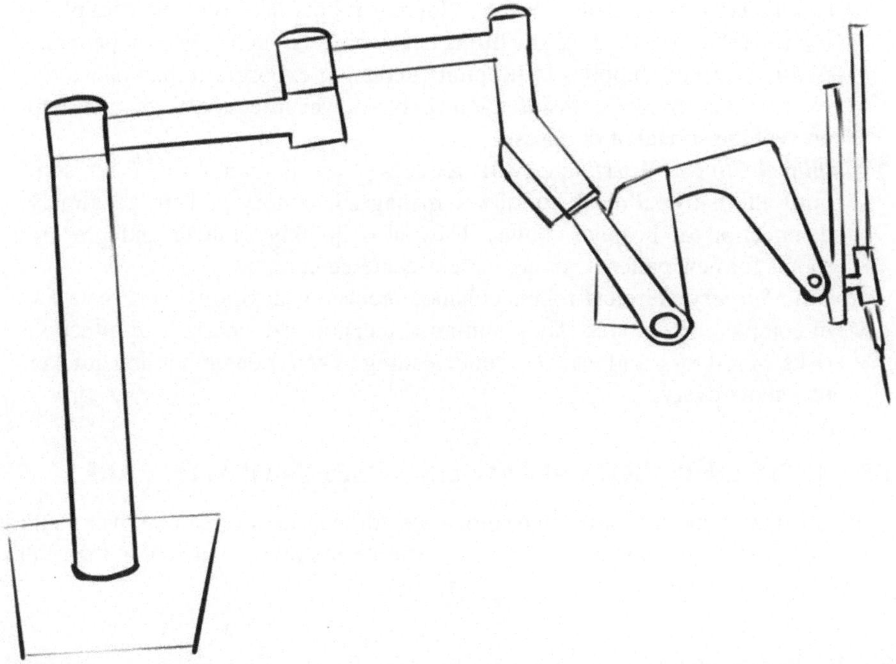

FIGURE 1.3 da Vinci Robot.

But it was not until the 1980s that these mechanical robots came into practical use in surgeries, though the technology was not fully developed until the 1990s. The famous robotic system in Figure 1.3 is the da Vinci Surgical System developed 24 years ago in 2000. It offers a less invasive surgical procedure. It is used in a variety of medical conditions, including cardiology, neurology, gynecology, pediatrics, and general surgery. Approximately 75% of prostate cancer surgeries in the U.S. are performed using this robotic system.

1.4 WHY ROBOTICS IN HEALTHCARE

As generations advance, the integration of robots in healthcare has significantly increased, providing numerous benefits to both providers and patients. These robots enhance personal care, promote greener treatments, and create a safer environment for everyone involved. They streamline logistics and disinfection processes, allowing healthcare professionals more time to engage with patients and transforming surgical practices. During the COVID-19 pandemic, the adoption of robots expanded to minimize infection risks, enhancing operational efficiencies and adding value in various ways. High-quality medical robots can perform straightforward procedures, monitor chronic health conditions, assist with medication management, and provide social interaction support for the elderly. The extensive benefits (Elendu et al., 2023) of robots demonstrate their essential role in the healthcare sector. Some of the key advantages include:

Occupational Environmental Safety: Nursing robots help prevent workplace injuries (Darko et al., 2023) by lifting heavy objects, such as beds or patients. AMRs transport supplies in hospitals, reducing exposure to pathogens for workers. Cleaning and disinfection robots, lower infection risks, and help prevent the spread of diseases.

Simplified Clinical Workflows: AMR reduces physical strain on workers, supports alternative clinical workflows, manages inventory, and ensures timely disinfection of hospital rooms. They also quickly sanitize and prepare rooms for new patients, aiding patient-centered care.

Robotic Surgery: Surgical robots enhance precision, flexibility, and accuracy in complex procedures. They minimize incision size and reduce infection risks, blood loss, and recovery time, leading to better outcomes and quicker patient recovery.

1.5 TYPES OF ROBOTS AND THEIR ROLES IN HEALTH CARE

There are many types of robots in healthcare, with their uses spreading over medical assistance. The following are a few types of robots and their efficiency in the healthcare industry.

1.5.1 Robot Nurses

Nurses are considered the backbone of the medical institution system, and their roles are essential inpatient care. Recognizing the importance of their contribution, technological advancements have introduced nursing robots to supplement their efforts. Table 1.1 shows some of the pioneering inventions of AI robot nurses, including their main services. The first nurse robot is the "HelpMate" robot, developed by Joseph Engelberger's company, HelpMate Robotics Inc., and introduced in 1986. It was

TABLE 1.1
AI Robotic Nurses and Their Main Services

Robot Names	Year of Invention	Description of Robots
Grace	2021	A humanoid robot that serves as a doctor's assistant uses sensors, including a thermal camera, to detect patient temperature and pulse, aiding in diagnosis and treatment.
Asha	2020	A multitasking humanoid robot capable of human-like interactions, from checking body temperature and inquiring about patients' well-being to offering them a drink of water, streamlines patient care with efficiency and compassion.
Moxi	2017	A robot that autonomously navigates healthcare environments, interacts with patients, and fulfills duties like delivering supplies and collecting linens.
ROBEAR	2015	A bear robot designed to lift patients from standing or ground position, transfer them to a wheelchair, and provide essential patient mobility support.

designed to assist hospital staff by transporting medical supplies, medications, and other items, thereby reducing the workload on nurses and other healthcare professionals. These robotic nurses act as associates to the human nurses with the resource of efficiently performing smooth, time-ingesting, and each day's responsibilities. By delegating those responsibilities to nursing robots, healthcare professionals can redirect their attention toward extra specialized and critical elements of affected care.

1.5.2 Ambulance Drones

In today's fast-paced international environment, the risk of medical emergencies is high, and timely assistance is critical for survival. To address this issue, drone ambulances can significantly reduce response times by utilizing airspace rather than congested highways, where poor road conditions and traffic can delay traditional ambulances. Drones can transport essential medical equipment, such as defibrillators, as illustrated in Figure 1.4.

Ambulance drones, a type of unmanned aerial vehicle (UAV), are employed by medical teams to swiftly deliver critical supplies during emergencies. For instance, in cases of heart attacks or allergic reactions, every second counts, and local medical teams may take precious minutes to arrive. Ambulance drones can bridge this gap by delivering life-saving technologies, including pharmaceuticals and CPR kits, directly to the scene (Frith & Amiri, 2022). The benefits of these drones in healthcare are highlighted in Table 1.2.

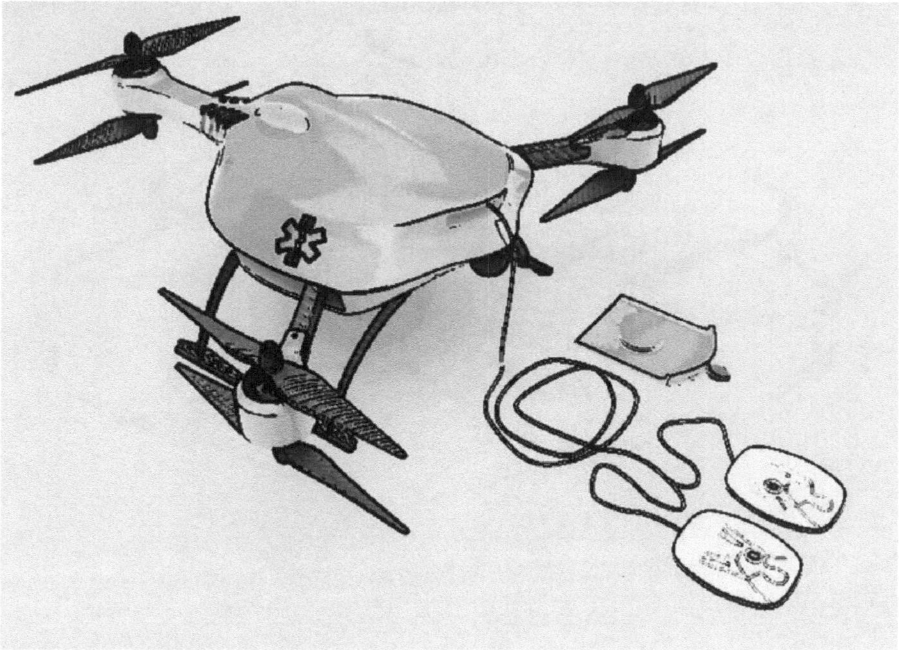

FIGURE 1.4 Drone defibrillator.

TABLE 1.2
Advantages of Ambulance Drones

- **Accelerate Response Times:** Ambulance drones bypass traffic to deliver medical supplies quickly, enabling immediate treatment and potentially saving lives.
- **Reach Difficult Places:** Drones provide critical resources to remote locations, improving survival chances before traditional help arrives.
- **Expand Operations:** Drones lower costs for ambulance services, reducing staff needs and allowing hospitals to extend services to nearby communities.
- **Improve Disaster Response:** Drones aid in surveillance, victim location, and on-site medical assistance, essential for adapting to emergencies like COVID-19.

Additionally, some companies are exploring the use of drones for patient transport. A notable example is EHang's eVTOL, which was utilized for emergency aerial responses during the COVID-19 pandemic in China, as shown in Figure 1.5. Overall, drones are emerging as a transformative technology in medical response, offering significant advantages in emergency care delivery.

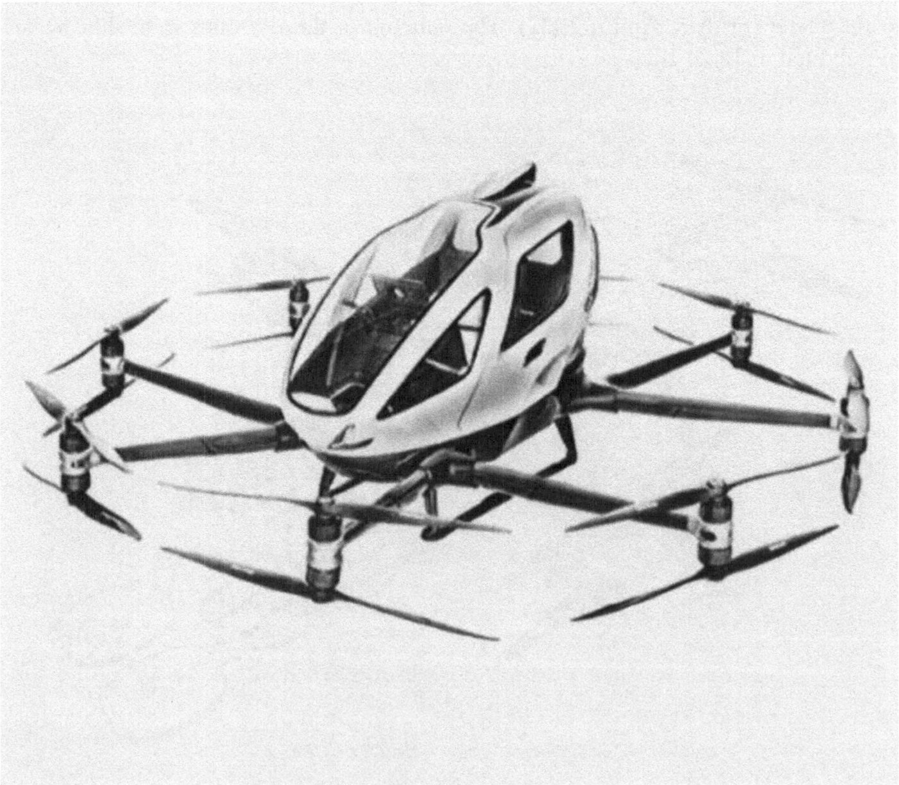

FIGURE 1.5 Ehang's eVTol autonomous drone.

1.5.3 Surgical Robots

The concept of a surgical robot dates back to 1967, but it took nearly 30 years to develop a fully practical system. The da Vinci Surgical System (Figure 1.3) is now widely used globally for minimally invasive surgeries, allowing precise control beyond human capability.

Robotic techniques enable doctors to perform complex procedures with greater precision, flexibility, and control, often through small incisions but occasionally in open surgeries.

Surgical robots are employed in fields like urology, gynecology, and orthopedics for procedures such as laparoscopy and thoracoscopy, using small incisions to access deep anatomical areas (Knudsen et al., 2024). Early "stereotactic robots" were used for precision brain biopsies, including SCARA in Figure 1.6, AcroBot, and ROBODOC. The second generation enhanced endoscopic procedures, with examples like PROBOT, Zeus, and da Vinci being referred to as "endoscopic robots" (Dagnino & Kundrat, 2024).

These systems consist of robotic arms for handling instruments, a high-definition 3D camera, and a surgeon's console for precise control, improving accuracy in complex surgeries. For patients, robot surgical treatment gives numerous capacity advantages over traditional open surgical procedures, as showcased in below Table 1.3.

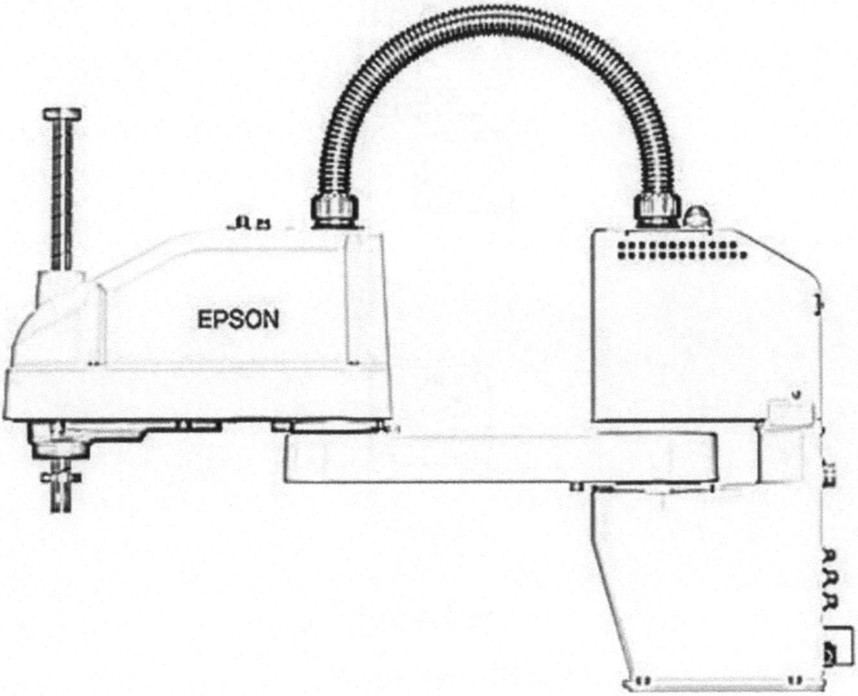

FIGURE 1.6 SCARA Robot.

TABLE 1.3
Advantages of Robotic Surgery for Patients

- Less pain and use of pain medicinal drug
- Less blood loss and less scarring
- Less hazard of contamination
- Shorter healing time and clinic stays
- Increased rate of success in the case of complex surgery

1.5.4 Teleassistance/Telesurgical Robots

Remote healthcare facilities often face shortages of scientific services due to limited resources and staffing. Remote technologies aim to bridge these gaps by connecting facilities with specialists, facilitating patient referrals, and enabling global health-care delivery. Telesurgery, a key innovation, allows specialists to perform surgeries remotely (Mohan et al., 2021), improving access to care in underserved areas and enhancing surgical accuracy. Haptic sensors and tele-manipulators enable remote

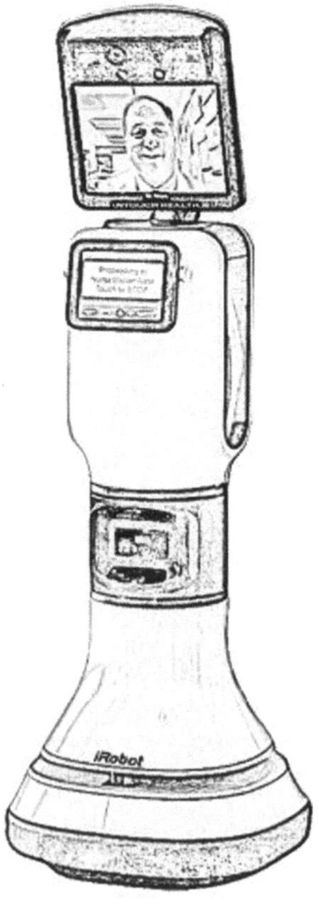

FIGURE 1.7 RP-VITA.

control during surgeries, with real-time visual signals sent to surgeons. Early systems, such as a 3 DOF robotic platform, were used for remote ultrasonography, though they lacked dynamic movement capabilities.

A notable teleassistance robot is RP-VITA as shown in Figure 1.7, which uses sensors, cameras, and mapping technology to autonomously navigate hospital environments.

It enables real-time communication between doctors and patients through high-definition video and audio, while transmitting vital data for remote assessments. This technology promotes collaboration between on-site and remote specialists, improving access to timely, quality care and ensuring patient privacy during telemedicine sessions.

1.5.5 Disinfecting Robots

In the rapidly advancing healthcare industry, maintaining high standards of hygiene and sanitation is critical. While traditional disinfection methods have been effective, they come with limitations. Disinfection robots are emerging as a game-changer in addressing these gaps, using advanced techniques like UV light (Mehta et al., 2023) to eliminate infection-causing microorganisms that are often invisible on surfaces. UV light disrupts the DNA and RNA of these organisms, preventing their reproduction. A real-world example of the benefits of these robots is Massachusetts General Hospital (MGH), which has been using UV-light-powered disinfection robots since 2017. As a result, MGH has seen a 40% reduction in hospital-acquired infections (HAIs). This success highlights the vital role these robots play in patient safety and infection control. Along with UV-based methods, chemical disinfectants are also used. Notable disinfection robots in healthcare include Nimbus shown in Figure 1.8, LightStrike, and

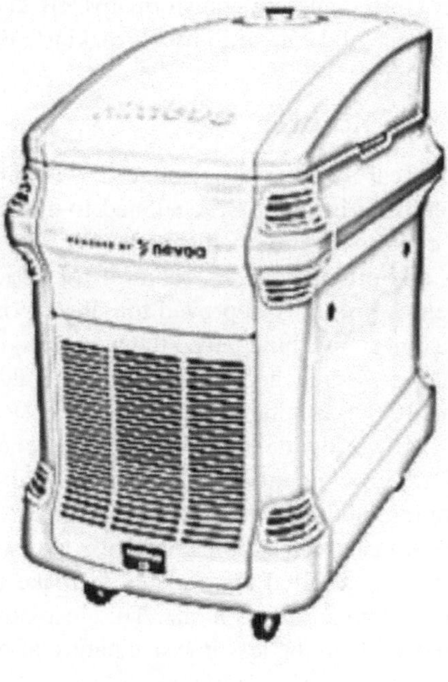

FIGURE 1.8 Nimbus.

TABLE 1.4
Differences between Nimbus, LightStrike, and XAG Drones

Feature	Nimbus	LightStrike	XAG Drones
Functionality	Developed by Blue Ocean Robotics, Nimbus uses UV-C light for 360-degree autonomous disinfection.	Made by Xenex, it uses pulsed xenon UV light for quick disinfection.	Developed by XAG, these drones use spraying technology to cover large areas.
Effectiveness	Highly effective against bacteria and viruses, with easy autonomous operation.	Effective against a broad range of pathogens, but requires manual positioning.	Efficient for large areas, but requires drone operation skills.
Cost and Maintenance	High cost and moderate maintenance, requiring minimal training due to its autonomous nature.	High cost and maintenance, with moderate training needed for operation.	Moderate to high cost and maintenance, needing pilot training.

XAG Drones. All these robots are developed to disinfect the microorganisms, yet there are a few differences between them, which are stated in Table 1.4.

1.6 REAL-LIFE ROBOT HEROES

In this section, we delve into the real-life existence of clinical robots and their pivotal characteristic in improving medical disciplines. Specifically, we illuminate the groundbreaking advancements executed with India's first surgical robot, the SSi Mantra, unveiling its development, programs, and transformative effect on healthcare practices inside the area. Here are some of the medical robots making a difference in healthcare.

1.6.1 da Vinci Surgical Robot

In 2000, the da Vinci Surgical System was introduced as the first commercially available robotic surgical platform in the U.S., designed to enhance surgeons' abilities and offer a less invasive alternative to open surgery. With its multi-armed design, it reduces surgical errors and provides precise control for various procedures. In the U.S., the da Vinci system is primarily approved for single-port urological surgeries. Its success in urologic surgery in China paved the way for broader use in other specialties. A major milestone was reached on December 21, 2021, when Prof. Zhang and his team completed 10,000 robotic-assisted surgeries (RAS), making them the first in Asia and the second worldwide to achieve this (Gu et al., 2023). This accomplishment underscores the growing success of RAS in minimally invasive surgery, marking significant progress in the field.

The da Vinci system enhances a surgeon's precision by using magnified 3D high-definition vision and wrist-controlled instruments to make tiny, delicate incisions that would be difficult for human hands alone. This leads to greater control and a faster recovery for patients due to the less invasive nature of the procedure. The system has three key components:

1. *Surgeon Console*: Where the surgeon controls the instruments while viewing the anatomy in 3D.
2. *Patient Cart*: Positioned beside the patient, holding the camera and instruments controlled by the surgeon.
3. *Vision Cart*: Ensures communication between components and supports the 3D vision system.

da Vinci procedures are used to treat a range of conditions across various specialties, including cardiac, urologic, gynecologic, pediatric, and general surgical procedures as illustrated in Figure 1.9.

1.6.2 The Xenex Germ-Zapping Robot

Apart from minimizing surgical errors, HAIs are another significant issue in healthcare that can be addressed with the usage of robots. HAIs frequently occur because it is not feasible for hospitals to achieve 100% sterility in room sanitation. Consequently, patients with compromised immune systems are more vulnerable to bacterial infections. As COVID-19 spread globally, the demand for disinfecting robots surged.

To address this issue, the Xenex an automated and transportable robot shown in Figure 1.10, is used to disinfect entire clinic rooms in minutes. Xenex, based in Houston, was created in 2009 and commercially released in 2013. This robot uses ultraviolet (UV) light to target pathogens, effectively destroying the germs that cause HAIs (Mackenzie, 2020). Ultraviolet (UV) radiation has proven effective in killing various bacteria, including spore-forming organisms, by destroying their nucleic acids (Beal et al., 2016). Lakeland Surgical & Diagnostic Centre (the first ambulatory surgical center in Florida) is the first to apply this disinfection robot as a part of its rigorous contamination program. The robot disinfects diagnostic center ORs, procedures, and treatment rooms.

The robot is placed in the empty room after it has been cleaned. It then emits a 5-minute cycle of pulsed xenon UV light, which is significantly more intense than

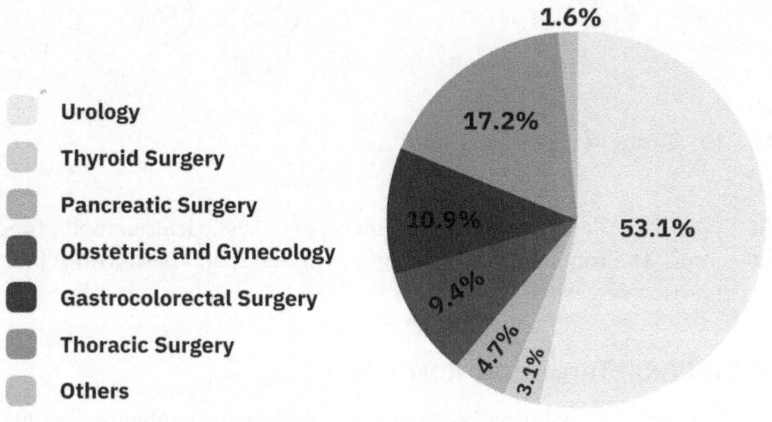

FIGURE 1.9 da Vinci Statistics in 2021.

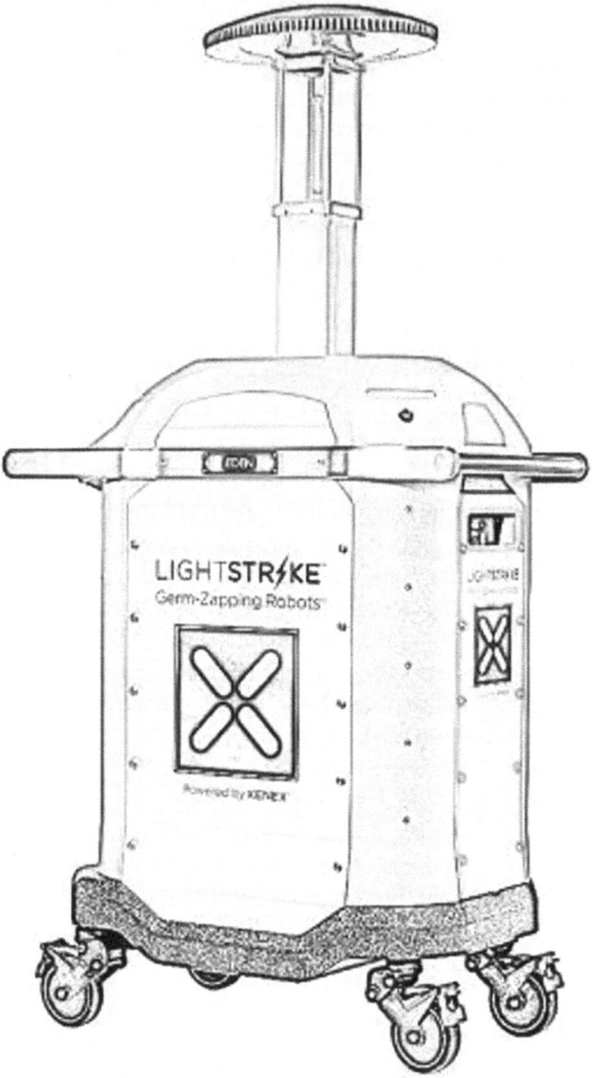

FIGURE 1.10 Xenex Robot.

sunlight. In just 2 or 3 cycles, the light eradicates viruses, bacteria, mold, fungi, and bacterial spores. The robot effectively sanitizes surfaces and hard-to-reach areas by targeting microscopic germs.

1.6.3 The PARO Therapeutic Robot

PARO is an interactive baby harbor seal robot designed to enhance the quality of life for patients recovering from surgery or coping with dementia and mental health issues. Drawing inspiration from veterinary medicine, it serves as a therapeutic companion, offering emotional support without the need for live animals. Made of leather and equipped with sensors, PARO promotes well-being by engaging patients during treatment, helping to combat psychological distress, and alleviating feelings of hopelessness, especially in socially isolated individuals (Granier et al., 2023). PARO provides psychological comfort, motivation, and physiological support in symptom management, and enhances social interaction among patients and staff. Acting autonomously, PARO responds to its environment, mimicking feelings during interactions. Key features include:

- Artificial Fur: Antibacterial and easily cleaned with sanitizing wipes.
- Light Sensor: PARO becomes sleepy at night.
- Vocal Response: Responds to touch and voice with a “coo” sound.
- Microphone: Listens to voices and remembers the patient’s chosen name.

Research shows that interactions with PARO have therapeutic effects, uplifting mood and alleviating depression. Isolated elderly individuals reported feeling happier and more willing to discuss past pets. Figure 1.11 illustrates PARO’s effectiveness,

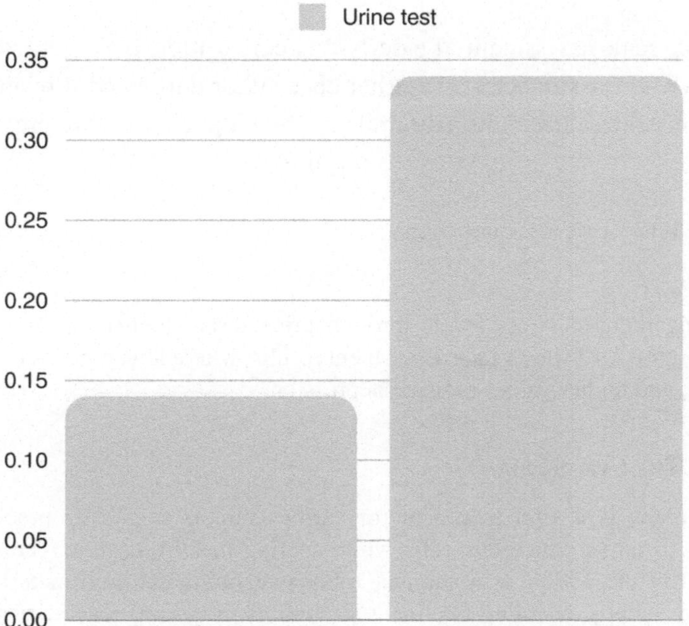

Urine test in an elderly-day center. Stress was reduced by the introduction of PARO. Higher values showcase lower stress.

FIGURE 1.11 Urine test.

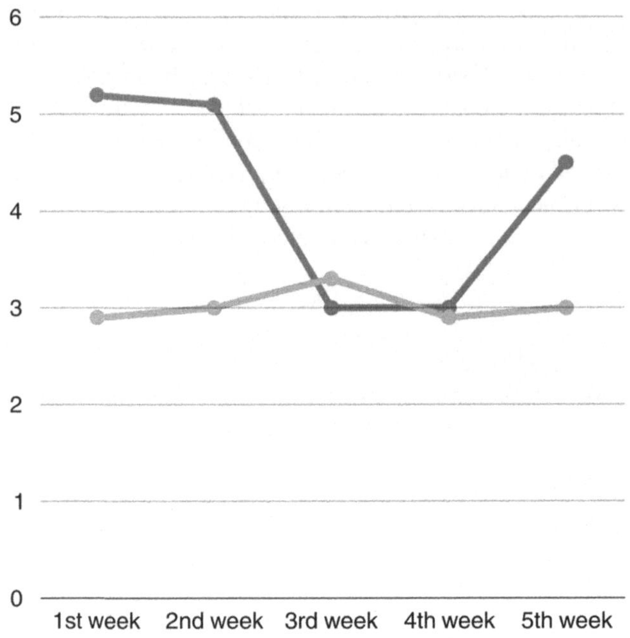

Fig Face scale assessment at elderly-day care center. Before introduction of PARO, the subjects were either cheerful or depressed. Lower value demonstrates cheerful state (smiley) while higher values depressive state (crying)

FIGURE 1.12 Face assessment test.

indicating reduced stress levels through urine tests—higher values denote lower stress. Figure 1.12 shows face assessment results, where lower values reflect a cheerful state, and higher values indicate depression.

1.6.4 The CyberKnife

Radiotherapy is a vital treatment for various tumors, requiring precise radiation delivery to target cancerous cells while sparing healthy tissues. The CyberKnife, invented in the 1990s, is a surgical robot that offers sub-millimeter precision in radiation therapy, enabling treatment for tumors in hard-to-reach areas such as the prostate, head, neck, and liver. This non-invasive system minimizes radiation exposure to sensitive organs by employing a lightweight linear accelerator mounted on a robotic arm to deliver high-energy X-rays. The CyberKnife can adjust to multiple angles to target the tumor without requiring patient repositioning (Karkar & Chaudhari, 2023). It utilizes two therapy types: Stereotactic Radiosurgery (SRS)

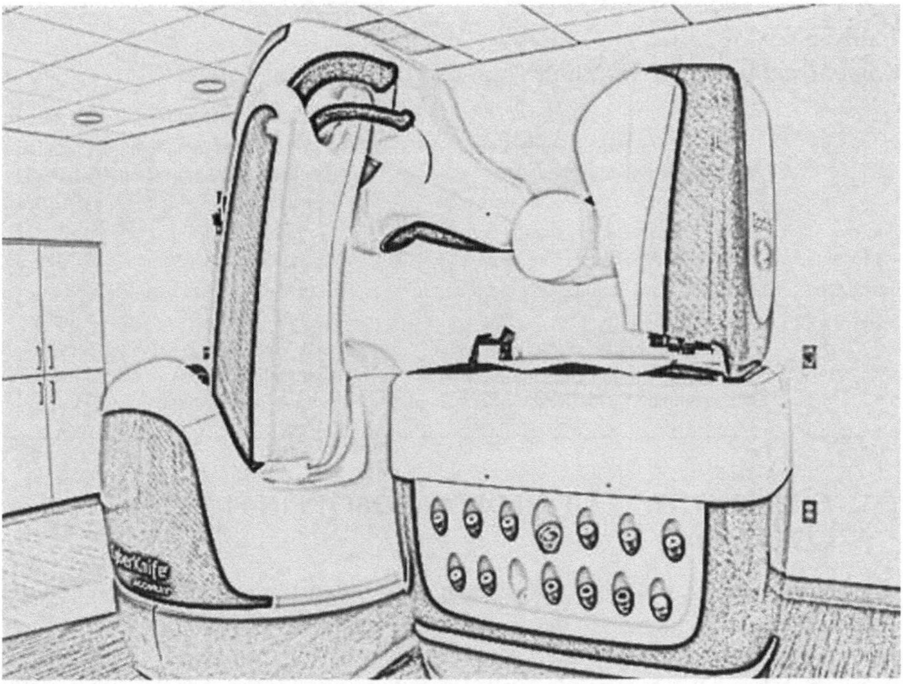

FIGURE 1.13 CyberKnife.

and Stereotactic Body Radiation Therapy (SBRT). As illustrated in Figure 1.13, the CyberKnife System employs advanced technologies to accurately track tumor movement, ensuring radiation is delivered to the tumor's current location through real-time motion synchronization. Before administering the radiation beam, the CyberKnife identifies the tumor's exact position and adjusts accordingly, enhancing the precision of the treatment.

1.6.5 SSi Mantra

SSi Mantra is India's primary robotic surgical device, commercially launched at the Rajiv Gandhi Cancer Institute in New Delhi in July 2022. It is evaluated against global devices for its wide range of surgical applications, from throat to gynecological procedures, and its cost-effectiveness. SSi Mantra is robust, safe, and efficient for all urological surgeries (Singh et al., 2023). Within six months of its launch, the robot successfully completed 100 surgeries, demonstrating its capability to perform complex procedures with precision. Priced at one-third the cost of its international competitor, the da Vinci system, SSi Mantra has made robotic surgeries more accessible. A detailed comparison between SSi Mantra and the da Vinci system is provided in Table 1.5.

TABLE 1.5
Comparison between SSi Mantra and da Vinci Surgical Robots

Feature	SSi Mantra	da Vinci
Key Feature	The key features include high precision, compact design	The key features include high precision, 3D high vision, EndoWrist instruments
Control Mechanism	Console-based with hand controls typically with 3–4 arms	Console-based with master controls typically with 4 arms
Instrument Controls	SSi Mantra includes advanced haptic feedback	The da Vinci system uses EndoWrist instruments with 7 degrees of freedom
Cost	The SSi Mantra typically comes at a lower initial and ongoing cost compared with the da Vinci system	The da Vinci system is known for its high cost with its extensive capabilities and support infrastructure

1.7 CONTRIBUTION OF MEDICAL ROBOTS IN FIGHTING COVID-19

Medical robotics is a clinical subject that took off in the early 1990s. While the implementation is expensive, the benefits are significant, especially in situations where human limitations become a barrier, such as during the COVID-19 crisis. The outbreak of the COVID-19 pandemic has had numerous adverse effects on the health of healthcare workers. With robots playing their roles as the front liners in the medical field, the spread of COVID-19 has been lowered (Raje et al., 2021) as direct contact between humans and COVID-19 is reduced. A few contributions of the robots during COVID-19 include:

1. *Temperature Tracking*: Robots with thermal cameras were used to check body temperatures at medical centers, reducing COVID-19 transmission and minimizing direct contact between patients and healthcare workers.
2. *COVID-19 Testing*: A fully automated swab robot developed by Danish engineers (Chen et al., 2022) facilitated faster testing and reduced contact between patients and healthcare staff, addressing the risk of infection among workers.
3. *Sanitization and Sterilization*: Robots performed regular cleaning and disinfection in hospitals and COVID-19 facilities, lowering staff exposure to pathogens and maintaining hygiene without disrupting staff schedules.

1.8 BIO-INSPIRED MEDICAL TECHNOLOGIES

In the dynamic landscape of modern medicine, nature serves as a valuable source of inspiration. Evolution has crafted a vast array of ingenious solutions to complex challenges, from the precision of spider silk to the efficiency of dragonfly flight. These natural designs have significantly influenced innovations in clinical robotics. For instance, continuum robots, inspired by the flexibility of elephant trunks shown in Figure 1.14, enable minimally invasive surgical procedures by navigating

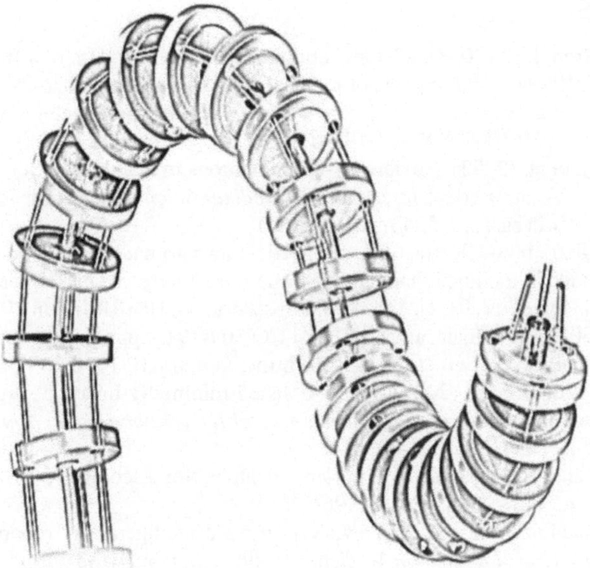

FIGURE 1.14 Continuum Robots.

tight spaces and delicately handling objects. Microrobots, modeled after the movements of bacteria and sperm cells, are enhancing targeted drug delivery systems with remarkable precision in the bloodstream.

Notable examples of bio-inspired robots include:

OctopusGripper: This gentle robot gripper takes ideas from the dexterity of octopus tentacles (Qian et al., 2021) and is designed for delicate managing tasks in surgical settings.

SkinSens: A bio-stimulated synthetic skin with tactile sensors similar to human contact, used in robot prosthetics or exoskeletons to offer users an experience of touch and enhance their control over the gadgets.

RehabRex: An exoskeleton for rehabilitation stimulated by way of the biomechanics of human movement (Shi et al., 2019), assisting sufferers with mobility impairments in walking and performing other activities during the recovery process.

1.9 ROBOTICS AND THE FUTURE OF HEALTHCARE

Emerging in the 1980s, the first medical robots used robotic arms to assist in surgery. Since then, advancements in AI, computer vision, and data analysis have expanded their roles across various healthcare fields. Today, robots support surgical procedures, assist in preventing infectious virus spread, and perform tasks like drug transportation and laundry. For instance, giant teddy bear-like nursing robots help care for elderly patients, and nanorobots hold promise for revolutionizing cancer treatments.

REFERENCES

Azer, Ö. A., & Oran, İ. B. (2023). AI applications in health sector: Use of artificial intelligence in COVID-19 crisis and impacts of medical robots on global economy. In K. T. Çalıyurt (Ed.), *Corporate sustainability in times of virus crises* (pp. [specific pages]). Springer. https://doi.org/10.1007/978-981-19-9079-3_11

Babarinde, A. O., et al. (2023). Review of AI applications in healthcare: Comparative insights from the USA and Africa. *International Medical Science Research Journal*, *3*(3), 92–107. https://doi.org/10.51594/imsrj.v3i3.641

Beal, A., et al. (2016). First UK trial of Xenex PX-UV, an automated ultraviolet room decontamination device in a clinical haematology and bone marrow transplantation unit. *Journal of Hospital Infection*, *93*(2), 164–168. https://doi.org/10.1016/j.jhin.2016.03.016

Chen, Y., et al. (2022). A collaborative robot for COVID-19 oropharyngeal swabbing. *Robotics and Autonomous Systems*, *148*, 103917. https://doi.org/10.1016/j.robot.2021.103917

Dagnino, G., & Kundrat, D. (2024). Robot-assisted minimally invasive surgery: Trends and future directions. *International Journal of Intelligent Robotics and Applications*. https://doi.org/10.1007/s41315-024-00341-2

Darko, E. M., et al. (2023). Robotics in nursing: Protocol for a scoping review. *JMIR Research Protocols*, *12*. https://doi.org/10.2196/50626

Denecke, K., & Baudoin, C. R. (2022). A review of artificial intelligence and robotics in transformed health ecosystems. *Frontiers in Medicine*, *9*. https://doi.org/10.3389/fmed.2022.795957

Elendu, C., et al. (2023). Ethical implications of AI and robotics in healthcare: A review. *Medicine*, *102*(50), e36671. https://doi.org/10.1097/MD.0000000000036671

Frith, K. H., & Amiri, A. (2022). Drones could offer solutions for emergency responses and healthcare in remote areas. *Nursing Education Perspectives*, *43*(3), 203–204. https://doi.org/10.1097/01.NEP.0000000000000977

Granier, K., et al. (2023). Getting the seal of approval: A critical literature review of the evidence for the use of the PARO robotic companion seal with older adults with cognitive impairment in long-term care. *Journal of Aging and Long-Term Care*, *6*(2), 57–79. https://doi.org/10.51819/jaltc.2023.1243669

Gu, L., et al. (2023). Robotic surgery in China. *The Innovation*, *4*(5). https://doi.org/10.1016/j.xinn.2023.100499

Karkar, D., & Chaudhari, P. (2023). Cyberknife treatment for different types of tumor. *Journal of Pharmaceutical Research*, *8*(2), 248–252.

Knudsen, et al. (2024). Clinical applications of artificial intelligence in robotic surgery. *Journal of Robotic Surgery*, *18*(1), 102. https://doi.org/10.1007/s11701-024-01867-0

Mackenzie, D. (2020). Ultraviolet light fights new virus. *Engineering (Beijing, China)*, *6*(8), 851–853. https://doi.org/10.1016/j.eng.2020.06.009

Mehta, I., et al. (2023). UV disinfection robots: A review. *Robotics and Autonomous Systems*, *161*, 104332. https://doi.org/10.1016/j.robot.2022.104332

Mohan, A., et al. (2021). Telesurgery and robotics: An improved and efficient era. *Cureus*, *13*, e14124. https://doi.org/10.7759/cureus.14124

Nawrat, Z. (2023). Introduction to AI-driven surgical robots. *Artificial Intelligence Surgery*, *3*, 90–97. https://doi.org/10.20517/ais.2023.14

Qian, C., et al. (2021). Octopus-inspired microgripper for deformation-controlled biological sample manipulation. *IEEE Transactions on Neural Networks and Learning Systems*, *33*(5), 1857–1866. https://doi.org/10.1109/TNNLS.2021.3070631

Raje, S., et al. (2021). [Retracted] Applications of healthcare robots in combating the COVID-19 pandemic. *Applied Bionics and Biomechanics*, *2021*(1). https://doi.org/10.1155/2021/7099510

Shi, et al. (2019). Biologically inspired and rehabilitation robotics. *Applied Bionics and Biomechanics*, 1–2. https://doi.org/10.1155/2019/2428707

Singh, A., et al. (2023). MP68-12: Our early clinical experience with Mantra multi arm surgical robotic system (SS Innovations Group Company) in major uro-oncological surgeries. *The Journal of Urology*, *209*(Suppl 4), e957. https://doi.org/10.1097/JU.0000000000003331.12

2 Enhancing Healthcare Through Medical IoT

Current Trends and Future Directions

Z. Tanveer Baig, M. N. Rajesh and Apurva Puttaswamy

2.1 INTRODUCTION

The Internet of Things (IoT) is an idea which refers to platforms which consist of interconnected devices which are web-enabled, have software applications, have various sensors, processors, and other hardware to capture, communicate, analyse, and manage data as well as allowing them to connect with other devices and provide services to achieve a specific purpose through the Internet. The IoT devices operate with physical devices and sensors, along with the wireless networking technology, with cloud computing and built with innovative data analytics tools (Parihar et al. 2024). The IoT vital operating techniques include, wherein the physical devices remain connected with wire or connected wirelessly to each other. These devices gather the data over sensors using external datasets or through the use of information networks. The

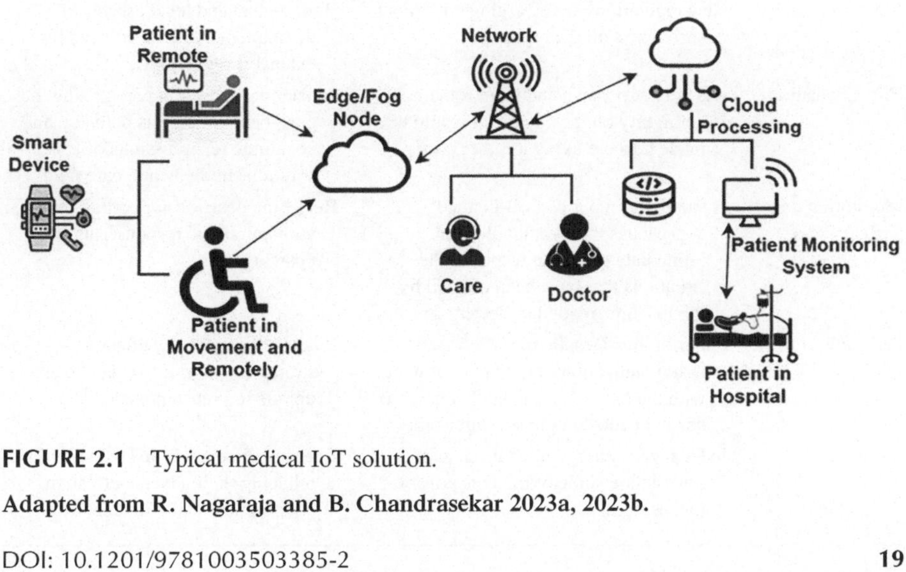

FIGURE 2.1 Typical medical IoT solution.

Adapted from R. Nagaraja and B. Chandrasekar 2023a, 2023b.

DOI: 10.1201/9781003503385-2

data gathered is warehoused in the cloud or transitional network or inside the device. The data is then managed, by means of an ML Algorithm. Introduction to Medical IoT.

The Medical Internet of Things (MIoT) stands fundamentally the IoT adopted precisely in the healthcare domain. MIoT is a network of interconnected devices as well as software applications, along with the sensors which collect and analyse medical data specifically. These devices gather and communicate patient's health data, that would be analysed for numerous purposes including diagnosis of diseases and anomalies, early disease detection remote monitoring of patients or telemedicine consultations, and treatment for healthcare anomalies through which MIoT has the potential to transform healthcare by improving treatment outcomes comprehensively. Figure 2.1 represents a typical Medical IoT Solution. Table 2.1 discusses the various research gaps.

TABLE 2.1
Research Identified through Different Literature and Compared with Effectiveness in Monitoring

Research Gap	Current Sate	Needs in specific
Interoperability	Medical devices	Standard protocols with interoperability and seamless.
Privacy and security in data	Prone to more cyber attacks	More robust security techniques.
Scalability with infrastructure	issues arising from the scalability of IoT solutions due large health systems of federations.	Solutions and architectures design for large-scale implementation which include bandwidth, storage and processing.
Integration of data and analysis	In Incorporating data from IoT devices in via the healthcare system.	Sophisticated data fusion strategies and methods for handling and analysing the information arising from the IoT.
User acceptance	Resistance from the side of healthcare practitioners and clients due to ignorance and lack of training.	Clear communications, good training, and visual materials or and good design.
Ethical Issues	New regulations are emerging with much variation with the region.	Both ethical and legal aspects of the matter should be covered by extensive regulations.
Cost Evaluation	it is very expensive and there remains ambiguity on the gains that would be made hence making it rather costly.	Academic studies on recognizing the cost–benefit analysis potential and economic repercussions of IoT solutions in the health care field.
Monitoring on Real Time	A smaller number of well-defined approaches that would allow an immediate real-time response to situations that have been defined by the IoT information collected.	Real-time decision support systems with automatic responses as an upswing.
Personalization	opportunities Despite the individualization of patient treatment with the help of IoT data, this potential has not been completely unlocked.	Studies to propose healthcare strategies that use IoT data to create unique reference points.
Sustainability	IoT gadgets, energy utilization, and e-waste are some of the concerns of IoT devices.	Energy efficiency of IoT systems and reducing their adverse effect on environment and climate.

2.2 RESEARCH GAPS IN MEDICAL INTERNET OF THINGS (IoT)

Addressing the above research gaps helps significantly in Medical IoT, which improves healthcare, patient outcomes and secures patient's data from third parties.

2.3 THE KEY MEDICAL IoT FUNCTIONALITY

Devices and Applications: A core aspect of MIoT is the physical devices used. These can range from wearable sensors that track vital signs to ingestible capsules that monitor internal conditions, smart implants and connected medical equipment. A comprehensive study was done by Li, et al. (2024) and some of the notable examples of MIoT applications can be Remote Patient Monitoring Systems, Implantable Glucose Monitoring Systems, Activity Trackers During Specialized and Focused Treatment, Heart Rate and Condition Monitors with Reporting, Medical Condition Alert Systems, Ingestible Sensors for patients, Patient Medication.

Data Collection and Analysis: MIoT systems generate a large amount of patient data. When the IoT Data (Li, et al. 2024) is adequately analysed using advanced Machine Learning or Deep Learning Algorithms, the real-time insights generated could provide vital judgement for healthcare providers. Figure 2.2 shows a basic MIoT Data Collection and Analysis flow (Krishnan and Singh 2022). It consists of the collection of data from various sensors, data is processed through the microcontrollers and is fed to the decision support system, which could be based on Artificial Intelligence or Machine Learning and is assessed if the Data is normal or abnormal data. This assessment is notified to the end user.

Remote Patient Monitoring: MIoT allows for continuous health monitoring outside of a traditional hospital setting. This can be particularly beneficial in early identification of health problems as well allow for timely intervention, as well to monitor and treat when there is chronic conditions or post-surgical care needed.

Telemedicine and MIoT: MIoT provides the foundation for telemedicine consultations, where patients can connect with healthcare providers remotely. A detailed study of the Telemedicine and its usage (Garcia et al. 2024) is discussed. It is to be noted that Telemedicine is on the rise, but adoption varies across specialities. Experts are emphasizing elements like visual inspection, observation, and listening as crucial aspects of a telemedicine exam (Wang et al. 2023). Additionally, physician-guided self-examinations by patients might be suitable replacements for traditional exams in certain cases. Figure 2.2 shows the data technique and its communication tool.

Security: Security while using sensitive medical information. MIoT systems need to be secure against hacking and data breaches. Medial IoT devices incorporate vigorous security procedures for example encryption as well as authentication mechanisms along with adherence to regulatory standards such as HIPAA so as to safeguard patient details from unlawful access. Various security and privacy aspects with MIoT (Krishnan and Singh 2022) are discussed. Categories of security breach can be at

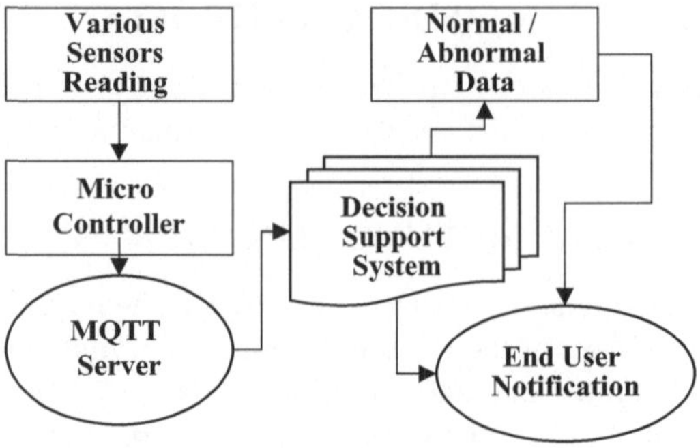

FIGURE 2.2 Data collection and analysis.

data level, sensor level, server level. The increasing use of medical devices associated with the internet (medical IoT) as well as data-driven medical apps raises privacy concerns (Krishnan and Singh 2022) These devices collect, store, and analyse a lot of sensitive patient data. On top of security risks, there are privacy issues like data breaches, unauthorized access to corporate medical data, and confusion about who owns and is accountable for this data. Even patient location information can be leaked. Medical service providers capture User Data as well as Medical Device Information for example the device type information as well as measurement context as well as frequency as well as vital sign readings as well as historical usage patterns which is User Private information and needs to be kept secure.

2.4 CURRENT STATE OF MEDICAL IoT: TECHNOLOGIES AND APPLICATIONS MEDICAL IoT

The IoT is revolutionizing healthcare through a range of connected devices as well as associated systems. This growing trend offers significant advantages for both patients as well as health care providers. When we speak of Patients, the Wearable devices and mobile medical apps allow them to easily track their health data, authorizing them to take a more energetic part in their welfare. When we speak about Providers, the Hospitals can leverage IoT to locate equipment, staff, and even patients in real-time, improving efficiency and safety. Some of the Key Technologies that are driving the Medical IoT as shown in Figure 2.3.

Networks: Healthcare IoT relies on a robust communication network to function effectively. This network needs to handle both short-range communication between devices (like wearables and smartphones) and long-range communication for connecting to healthcare providers. For short-range connections, technologies such as Bluetooth Low Energy (BLE) as well as Near Field Communication (NFC) are well-suited for low-power medical sensors.

Cloud Computing: Cloud computing (Singh et al. 2022) plays a key role in healthcare IoT, offering on-demand access to computing resources like storage,

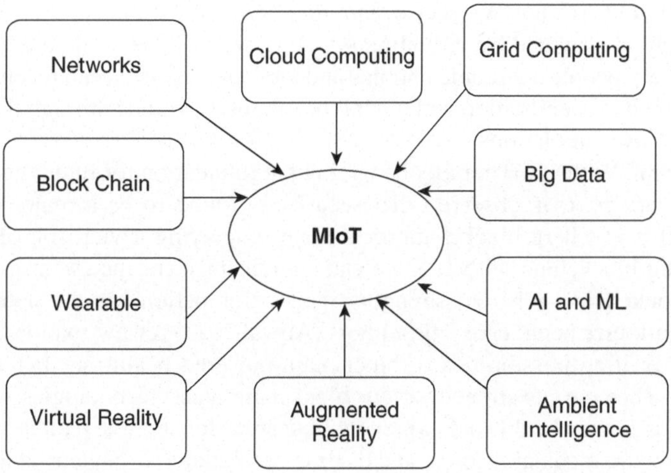

FIGURE 2.3 Showing the Key Technologies that are driving the Medical IoT.

Source: Nagaraja and Chandrasekar 2023a, 2023b.

networks, and applications. Unlike traditional IT infrastructure, cloud computing is flexible and cost-effective, with users only paying for what they use.

Grid Computing: Grid computing emerges as a promising tool for healthcare IoT. Advancements in low-power wireless communication and non-invasive sensors allow for continuous health monitoring of mobile patients using wearable devices. These tiny gadgets may be able to track vital signs like blood pressure, temperature, and even the electrical activity of the heart and muscles, even with their limited processing capability and memory (Hammad et al. 2023).

Wearables: The health of the population as a whole and patient participation on an individual basis can both be significantly enhanced by wearable medical equipment. Wearables fall into three categories: gamification, targeted healthcare communities, and connected information.

Big Data: New issues are being created by the explosion of data coming from wearables and sensors in the healthcare IoT space. Due to its size (Singh et al. 2022), diversity, and frequent messiness, analysing this data will take a lot of time and computing resources.

AI / ML: Artificial Intelligence and Machine Learning (Diwakar et al. 2023) are adopted in various Medical Data Processing such as Clinical Imaging, Conclusion of sicknesses, Clinical preliminary examination, Shrewd electronic well-being records, Heart illness forecast, Diagnosis model coronavirus (Veeraiah et al. 2023) Healthcare has always demanded the highest standards of accuracy and compliance. This makes it a critical area for innovation. The emergence of IoT provides exciting possibilities aimed at the medical field, potentially solving some of its longstanding challenges (Tehlan et al. 2023).

Virtual Reality (VR): A precise and immersive environment for exposure therapy is provided by virtual reality ecosystem (Rane et al. 2023), which also help people overcome phobias and anxieties. Patients can receive assistance with rehabilitation and mental health interventions through the use of immersive simulations.

Blockchain: With MIoT rapidly becoming the foundation for future healthcare applications, it is observed that security is found to be a major concern and this is where blockchain technology is playing a vital role. By integrating blockchain with IoT, we can significantly enhance security thanks to blockchain's inherent strengths. This combination has the potential to revolutionize healthcare. The authors (Auwal 2023) review, explore and discuss exciting possibilities of blockchain-powered healthcare IoT applications. They have examined various blockchain types, technologies, and their applications in healthcare, which include areas like remote patient monitoring, secure medical records, and disease prediction (Al-Nbhany et al. 2024) Al-Nbhany. Examples and Impact of Medical IoT on Healthcare Delivery Case studies (Lawal 2023) indicate that IoT enhances healthcare in several ways such as Chronic disease management, Rural healthcare, Emergency response, Preventive healthcare, and Scalable telemedicine.

2.5 THE POWER OF DATA: LEVERAGING AI AND ANALYTICS IN MEDICAL IoT

Artificial Intelligence (AI): The fusion of AI as well as big data through fog computing as well as IoT technologies has significantly advanced medical systems. In Lung Cancer detection using radiomics features and ML-based approach (Nagaraja et al. 2023), using CT Images, the Radiomics built model has five stages. It begins with the CT images augmentation, followed by the second step of image segmentation. The third stage involves feature extraction using the PyRadiomics library, followed by the fourth stage of feature selection and reduction. Finally, in the last stage, these features are analysed using ML classifier models to forecast outcomes, as shown in Figure 2.4.

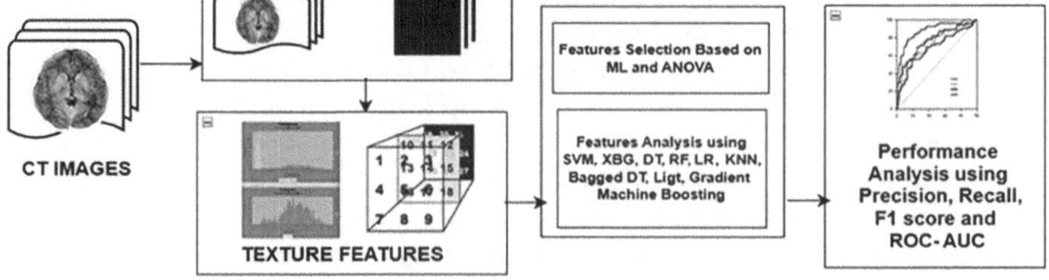

FIGURE 2.4 Architecture of a typical ML trained created Classification Model (Nagaraja and Chandrasekar 2023a, 2023b).

2.6 THE DATA COLLECTION IN MEDICAL IoT DEVICES AND ITS ANALYSIS

Significant technologies related to big data that are relevant to medical systems include data fusion mechanisms, data migration, data replacement, and security. Below is a detailed summary of all the important topics covered:

a. **Big Data Fusion Mechanism:** A strong data fusion mechanism is essential in the background of medical systems because of the variety of data sources, including imaging data, device parameters, medical records, and patient information. The goal of the fusion mechanism is to extract useful information from both structured and unstructured heterogeneous data sources.
b. **Data Migration Technologies:** As healthcare systems get more multifaceted, moving huge quantities of patient data between them becomes crucial. Big data migration technology, via a layered storage approach, simplifies this process. It comprises three steps: extract, convert, and load (ECL).

2.7 THE DATA ANALYSIS USING AI FOR BETTER DIAGNOSTICS AND TREATMENT

AI (Diwakar et al. 2023) is a contemporary approach that's become intensely rooted in information technology. It involves creating algorithms that give machines the ability to learn as well as work effectively on responsibilities that typically require human know-how. This is accomplished through the usage of a variety of techniques, including machine learning (ML) as well as deep learning (DL) as well as conventional neural networks (CNN) as well as fuzzy logic along with speech recognition. Concurrently, Internet of Medical Things (IoMT) has emerged as a state-of-the-art bio-analytical tool integrating the unified biomedical equipment by means of software applications to improve human welfare.

AI, ML, DL and Radiomics approaches are vastly used to understand the anomalies and staging of the cancer (Nagaraja and Chandrasekar 2023a, 2023b). Using DL Algorithms such as ResNet-50 (Nagaraja and Chandrasekar 2023a, 2023b). as well as RegNetY-320 (El-Hamed et al. 2024) which were trained to understand the staging of cancer using MR images and the trained models were used to classify the stages of the cancer. Various DL models were also trained and used for the classification of cancer.

2.8 CASE STUDIES: SUCCESSFUL IMPLEMENTATIONS OF MEDICAL IoT

Medical IoT is getting accepted as a way for quicker alert and treatment, as a prioritized personalized medical support. The components of a typical patient Monitoring system are indicated in the Figure 2.5.

The focus on the non-intrusive and novel approach to diabetes detection: moving towards Wearable Tech in identifying type-II diabetes using readily available body

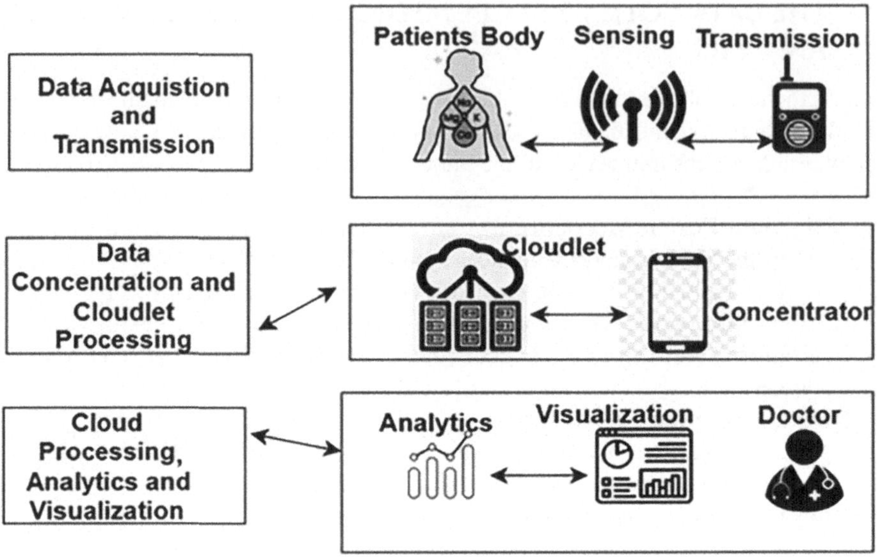

FIGURE 2.5 Components adopted for System Monitoring The Patient [35].

signals. The system utilizes three sensors to gather health data: temperature, pulse, and (unspecified) biological measurement. Users wear these sensors for data collection. The gathered data is then communicated securely to a cloud platform for investigation. This analysis includes calculating Body Mass Index (BMI). Based on the results, the system provides feedback on the user's health status. If the system identifies potential health risks, it recommends preventive measures. Cancer Detection using ML Algorithm on the radiomics features extracted from CT Images Interestingly (Nagaraja et al. 2023). The entire process is shown in Figure 2.6a.

2.8.1 WheelChair Medical IoT

People with limited mobility rely heavily on wheelchairs (Arefin et al. 2024) for daily activities. Wheelchairs provide not only physical support (somatic assistance) but also a sense of independence and control (psychological assistance). Researchers are exploring HMI-based intelligent wheelchairs using EEG and ECG based, Sip and Puff based, Voice based, Tongue interfaces, Touchscreen based interfaces and Facial movement-based interfaces. For the cardiac abnormality patient or subject, the researcher proposed adopting a microcontroller-built heart rate abnormality detecting system attached to the patient and connected to a regular wheelchair along with the communicating systems so as to be used as M IoT device to detect any cardiovascular abnormality and track patient position as well alert the caretakers as in the Figure 2.6b. Various Joy Stick-based Control of the Wheelchairs such as joysticks: Control through Electroencephalogram or Electrocardiogram signals, Control through Head or Chin, Tongue control, Face or Gaze or through Mobile phone Apps network could then be used to guide the wheelchair user and steer it in the right

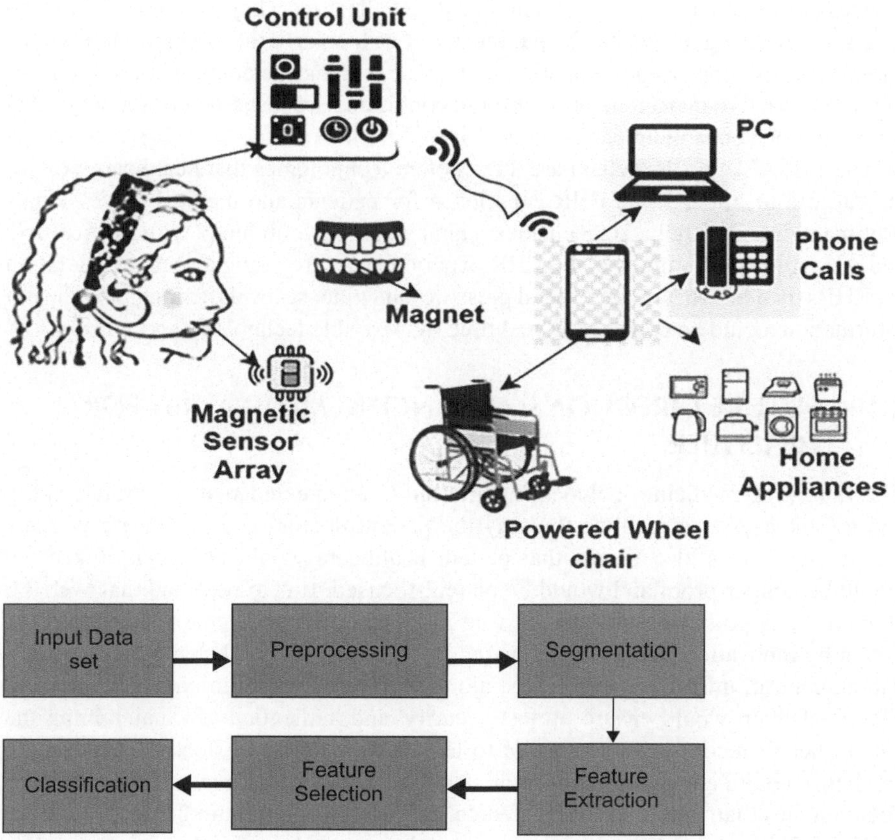

FIGURE 2.6 (a) A typical computer vision-based diagnosis system. (b) Block diagram for collection of data.

direction, track the wheelchair's location and offer additional assistance Scientists are exploring the possibility of equipping wheelchairs with navigation and tracking systems, obstacle management and avoidance systems Opportunities, Challenges and Considerations: Security, Privacy, and Interoperability of Implementing Medical IoT Solutions.

2.9 HEALTHCARE PROVIDER ADOPTION AND IMPLEMENTATION STRATEGIES FOR MEDICAL IoT

The contemporary progress in IoT technology (Arefin et al. 2024), united with the unambiguous authenticities uncovered by the contagion, is generating a faultless storm for prevalent acceptance in medicine. Two major factors—increasing user comfort and smarter devices with richer data—are driving this shift. The pandemic's emphasis on digital health solutions and remote monitoring has made people who were previously sceptical of IoT more receptive to its potential advantages. IoT devices are developing into more than just data collectors. They can now analyse the data and offer insights that can be put into practice thanks to the integration of AI and cloud services. Improved medication adherence, enhanced remote patient monitoring, and proactive management of chronic conditions are just a few of the ways that this evolution is changing patient care.

The IoT, AI, and Blockchain are three potent technologies that healthcare providers can use to improve the EHR experience for patients and medical professionals (Pulimamidi and Buddha 2023). Blockchain technology combined with medical IoT and AI significantly improves the EHR experience by providing a secure foundation for EHRs. Patients' heart rates, blood pressure, and glucose levels, among other health information, could be collected in real time by wearable technology and sensors.

2.10 FUTURE DIRECTIONS: ADVANCING MEDICAL IoT FOR HEALTHIER

The Future of medicine includes integration of augmented reality, virtual reality and the metaverse to revolute the way the patient doctors and healthcare workers are involved. This also means that patient healthcare would be decentralized yet would be tamper-proof and would be patient-focused. It is to be noted that Web 3.0 technology is poised to play a vital role in pushing Telemedicine for better reach driven by innovation. Metaverse powered by AR, VR and blockchain would offer a patient-centric, immersive experience along with huma touch to each consultation. The blockchain would ensure utmost security, and authenticity in maintaining the patient health records, yet accessible to legitimate patients or doctors. Blockchain can help to build a legally monetizable health record management system. The Key Technologies that would drive the Medical IoT is shown in Figure 2.7.

The IoT is changing healthcare along with several digital technologies that are being used to improve healthcare, including telemedicine, wearable sensors, virtual rehabilitation, and intelligent fabrics. Through the use of other technologies, such as video interactions, telemedicine enables individuals with health issues to consult doctors remotely. In addition to saving time and money, this can make healthcare more accessible to those living in rural areas. Wearable sensors can be used to track blood pressure, blood sugar levels, and vital signs like heart rate. Physicians could use this information to inform their treatment choices. Patients can receive at-home assistance in recovering from illnesses or injuries with virtual rehabilitation. In addition to saving money and time, this can encourage patients to continue with their therapy. Self-configuring virtual structures are being realized through the use of intelligent fabrics. Healthcare facility design could be enhanced by the application of this technology.

In addition, the paper highlights the necessity of incorporating ethical principles to direct clinical practice and biomedical research by emphasizing their integration into all aspects of the design, implementation, and administration lifecycle of digital medicine technologies. In order to effectively address ethical challenges, the researchers (Kumar et al. 2024) identify a few process adaptations. With the use of digital medicine, developers need a comprehensive plan that addresses potential issues throughout a device's lifecycle. This plan should have three key components: Deep Education in

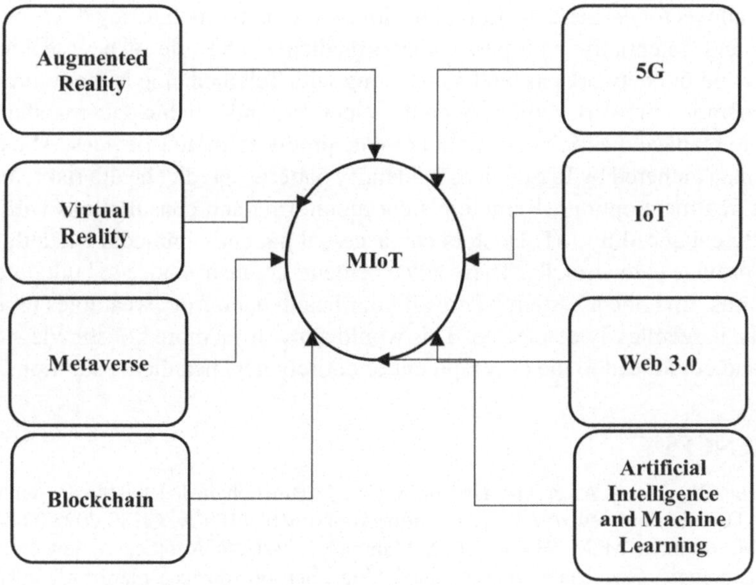

FIGURE 2.7 Showing the Key Technologies that would drive the Medical IoT.

Ethics, Designing Ethical Behaviour, and Continuous Ethical Monitoring. Developers involved in digital medicine need extensive training in ethical considerations. This training should go beyond basic principles and delve into the specific ethical challenges posed by digital health technologies. Digital medicine devices should be programmed to behave ethically. This could involve features that ensure patient privacy, prevent bias in algorithms, and prioritize patient well-being in decision-making. The ethical implications of a digital medicine device shouldn't be a one-time consideration. A broader framework for ongoing ethical investigation is needed.

2.11 CONCLUSION

To summarize firstly IoT is already being used in healthcare, but there's a lot more to come. Secondly, advancements in sensor technology, data collection, and AI will drive future innovation. Thirdly, smart sensors will allow for more accurate monitoring and analysis of health data. Fourthly, improved data collection will reduce errors and make healthcare more efficient. Fifthly, AI integration will speed up complex procedures and improve decision-making and lastly better connectivity through AI will promote preventive care as well as improve patient results. The potential of a powerful combination of the IoT and advanced technologies in revolutionizing healthcare. Power of IoT in healthcare is derived from huge number of advanced IoT technologies along with high speed and accuracy. Imagine a vast network of medical devices, wearables as well as sensors as well as implants, all connected to the internet. This creates a constant stream of real-time data about a patient's health. With so much data, researchers can analyse it faster and more precisely.

This allows for earlier detection of health issues, better monitoring of chronic conditions, and potentially even personalized medicine. The role of new technologies with 5G and 6G networks as well as AI along with Telemedicine is the future. These next-generation networks will provide the super-fast and reliable data transfer speeds needed to manage the massive amount of data produced by IoT devices. AI can analyse the data gathered by IoT devices to identify patterns, predict health risks, and even suggest treatment options. Remote patient monitoring and consultations will be significantly enhanced by IoT. Doctors can access a patient's immediate health info as well as provide care virtually. These advancements create a chance to build integrated ecosystems. Imagine a system where all your health data, from wearables to medical implants, is seamlessly connected. This would allow for a more holistic view of your health and could lead to the development of entirely new healthcare solutions.

REFERENCES

Al-Nbhany, W., Zahary, A., & Al-Shargabi, A. (2024). Blockchain-IoT healthcare applications and trends: A review. *IEEE Access*. https://doi.org/10.1109/ACCESS.2023.3349187

Arefin, M., Rahman, M. M., Hasan, M., & Mahmud, M. (2024). A topical review on enabling technologies for the internet of medical things: Sensors, devices, platforms, and applications. *Micromachines*, *15*, 479. https://doi.org/10.3390/mi15040479

Auwal, A. M. (2023). IoT integration in telemedicine: Investigating the role of internet of things devices in facilitating remote patient monitoring and data transmission. https://doi.org/10.21203/rs.3.rs-3419693/v1

Diwakar, M., Singh, P., & Ravi, V. (2023). Medical data analysis meets artificial intelligence (AI) and internet of medical things (IoMT). *Bioengineering*, *10*, 1370. https://doi.org/10.3390/bioengineering10121370

El-Hamed, O., Abd El-Samie, F., Badawy, W., & Abd El-atty, S. (2024). Blockchain for IoT and medical data management. https://doi.org/10.21203/rs.3.rs-3976623/v1

Garcia, J., et al. (2024). A narrative review of telemedicine and its adoption across specialties. *mHealth*, *10*, 19. https://doi.org/10.21037/mhealth-23-28

Hammad, M. M., Banat, S., Baker, Q. B., Al-Refai, M., & Abudhais, B. (2023). A comprehensive study of cloud, fog, and edge computing technologies for healthcare IoT systems. https://doi.org/10.22541/au.169178406.62298915/v1

Krishnan, D., & Singh, S. (2022). Medical IoT: Opportunities, issues in security and privacy a comprehensive review. In *Opportunities and Challenges in Digital Healthcare Innovation* (pp. 91–112). https://doi.org/10.1201/9781003239895-6

Kumar, D., Pawar, P., Gonaygunta, H., Nadella, G., Meduri, K., & Singh, S. (2024). Machine learning's role in personalized medicine & treatment optimization. *World Journal of Advanced Research and Reviews*, *2*, 1675–1686. https://doi.org/10.30574/wjarr.2024.21.2.0641

Lawal, R. (2023). Transformative potential of IoT on smart healthcare and remote patient monitoring in Nigeria: A literature review. *MSc Internet of Things with Data Analytics A Literature*. https://doi.org/10.13140/RG.2.2.24453.52966

Li, C., Wang, J., Wang, S., & Zhang, Y. (2024). A review of IoT applications in healthcare. *Neurocomputing*, *565*, 127017. https://doi.org/10.1016/j.neucom.2023.127017

Nagaraja, R., & Chandrasekar, B. (2023a). Multi-class classification of PCa MR images based on UCLA score using deep learning ResNet-50 model. *Journal of Biomechanical Science and Engineering*, *1*, 48–67. https://doi.org/10.17605/OSF.IO/4R7W8

Nagaraja, R., & Chandrasekar, B. (2023b). Multi-class classification of prostate cancer MR images based on UCLA score using RegNetY-320 model. *ARPN Journal of Engineering and Applied Sciences*, *18*(2), 90–101.

Nagaraja, R., Tanni, N., & Baig, Z. (2023). Lung cancer detecting using radiomics features and machine learning algorithm. https://doi.org/10.1109/ICTACS59847.2023.10389900

Parihar, A., Prajapati, J. B., Prajapati, B. G., Trambadiya, B., Thakkar, A., & Engineer, P. (2024). Role of IoT in healthcare: Applications, security & privacy concerns. *Intelligent Pharmacy*. https://doi.org/10.1016/j.ipha.2024.01.003

Pulimamidi, R., & Buddha, G. (2023). The future of healthcare: Artificial intelligence's role in smart hospitals and wearable health devices. *Tuijin Jishu/Journal of Propulsion Technology*, *s44*, 2498–2504. https://doi.org/10.17613/f53e-ea13

Rane, N., Choudhary, S., & Rane, J. (2023). Healthcare metaverse: Applications, challenges, and future development. *SSRN Electronic Journal*. https://doi.org/10.2139/ssrn.4637901

Singh, N., Sasirekha, S. P., Dhakne, A., Thrinath, B. V. S., Ramya, D., & Thiagarajan, R. (2022). IoT enabled hybrid model with learning ability for e-health care systems. *Measurement: Sensors*, *24*, 100567. https://doi.org/10.1016/j.measen.2022.100567

Tehlan, A., Moharana, A., Chintapalli, G., Mary, A. P., & Behera, S. (2023). Role of artificial intelligence and machine learning for enabling IoT-enabled healthcare systems. https://doi.org/10.9734/bpi/ratmcs/v2/5880C

Veeraiah, V., et al. (2023). Diagnosing of disease using machine learning in healthcare by internet of things. *International Journal of Intelligent Systems and Applications in Engineering*, *11*, 954–973.

Wang, L., Fabiano, A., Venkatesh, A., Patel, N., & Hollander, J. (2023). Telehealth clinical appropriateness and quality. *Telemedicine Reports*, *4*, 87–92. https://doi.org/10.1089/tmr.2023.0019

3 Exploring the Potential of Smart Healthcare Wearable Devices and Its Future

A Study on Consumer Adoption and Attitude

Usha Yadav and Sheetal Soni

3.1 INTRODUCTION

With the growing interest in fitness, health, well-being, and illness prevention, as well as the trend toward personalised and individual-controlled healthcare, wearable devices are becoming a more and more attractive platform for healthcare services (Lee & Lee, 2018). These cutting-edge devices, embedded with advanced sensors and technology, offer a spectrum of functionalities aimed at empowering users to monitor vital health metrics, manage chronic conditions, and facilitate seamless interaction with healthcare services in real-time. People are increasingly recognising the versatility and potential of smart healthcare wearables, from fitness trackers that meticulously monitor physical activity to continuous glucose monitors that aid in diabetes management, as pivotal components in the evolution of healthcare delivery.

Amidst the expanding interest in smart healthcare wearable devices, understanding the intricacies of consumer adoption and attitudes towards these technologies emerges as a crucial requirement. While the promise of these devices is undeniable, their widespread adoption remains contingent upon various factors, ranging from perceived usefulness and ease of use to design aesthetics and social influence (Yoon et al., 2020). Data security and privacy are another serious consideration, as these devices' capacity to track, preserve, and transmit medical records is scrupulous (Perez & Zeadally, 2018). Delving into the nuances of consumer behaviour and preferences is paramount for unravelling the particulars of adoption dynamics and outlining the opportunities for the seamless integration of wearable health technologies into mainstream healthcare practices. This comprehensive study aims to delve into the multifaceted realm of smart healthcare wearable devices and explore the intricacies of consumer adoption and attitudes towards these transformative technologies.

DOI: 10.1201/9781003503385-3

It aims to find out what makes people adopt them and what problems and opportunities are ahead (Lee & Lee, 2018; Park, 2020).

This study aims to fill the gaps in existing research about people's adoption of smart healthcare wearables. Detailed attention is required for issues like privacy, keeping data safe, and building trust. Strong rules and protections are crucial as these devices become more common in healthcare to ensure their responsible use. This study sets out to explore the world of smart healthcare wearables with curiosity, thoroughness, and a clear purpose. The *core contribution* of the study is to provide a thorough synthesis of current research on smart healthcare wearable devices, identifying existing gaps and suggesting areas for further study, and examining the primary factors that affect consumer adoption of smart healthcare wearables, such as technological proficiency, perceived usefulness, and user attitudes. The study integrates both empirical research and qualitative analysis to provide a comprehensive understanding of consumer perspectives and behaviours towards wearable health technologies. Investigate the potential challenges and opportunities that arise from integrating smart healthcare wearables into the healthcare sector. This study adds new insights into how technological proficiency shapes consumer opinions and highlights the critical role of perceived usefulness in the acceptance of smart healthcare wearables. Sections 3.2 and 3.3 provide a comprehensive overview of the background and related concepts, including the integration of technology and the investment perspective in smart healthcare wearable devices. Sections 3.4 and 3.5 provide a detailed explanation of the literature study conducted in the relevant field, including a tabular comparison and an assessment of the research gaps. Sections 3.6 to 3.11 outline the methodology adopted, participants, measures, analysis, and result discussion. Section 3.12 concludes the entire chapter's work.

3.2 INTEGRATION WITH TECHNOLOGY

Smart healthcare wearables represent a paradigm shift in the way individuals monitor their health and well-being, leveraging cutting-edge technologies to deliver personalised insights, facilitate proactive health management, and enhance overall quality of life. At the core of these cutting-edge gadgets lies a blend of technologies, such as artificial intelligence (AI), the Internet of Things (IoT), big data analysis, and blockchain, all contributing significantly to unleashing the potential of wearable health technologies. Incorporating technology into healthcare service development can boost productivity and maximise the use of available resources (Keikhosrokiani et al., 2018).

Artificial Intelligence is essential for the operation of healthcare wearables, allowing them to interpret and analyse volumes of data gathered from various sensors in real-time. Machine learning algorithms power features such as activity monitoring, sleep tracking, and heart rate analysis, empowering wearables to provide users with health insights and practical recommendations. Additionally, predictive analytics driven by AI can predict health risks.

The *Internet of Things* plays a role in facilitating connectivity and interoperability among healthcare wearables, facilitating seamless communication between devices, users, and healthcare providers. IoT sensors embedded within wearable devices collect a myriad of physiological data, transmitting this information to centralised platforms or mobile applications in real-time. IoT apps can save vital time in an emergency by quickly alerting and informing carers of an older person (Manas et al., 2018).

Big Data Analytics: The proliferation of wearable health devices has generated vast amounts of health-related data. Big Data analytics techniques are instrumental in harnessing the potential of this wealth of data, extracting actionable insights, and driving evidence-based decision-making in healthcare. Through advanced analytics algorithms, wearables can analyse trends, identify patterns, and correlate various health metrics to provide personalised recommendations tailored to individual users' needs. Furthermore, aggregated Big Data from wearable devices can fuel population health management initiatives, enabling public health agencies and policymakers to identify health trends, allocate resources efficiently, and implement targeted interventions to improve community health outcomes.

Blockchain technology: It has the potential to tackle issues concerning data security, privacy, and interoperability within the field of healthcare wearables. By using decentralised tamper ledgers, blockchain platforms can maintain the authenticity and confidentiality of health information while allowing secure sharing and access controls. Furthermore, blockchain-based smart contracts can support traceable transactions, promoting data exchange and encouraging data sharing among various parties, such as users, healthcare providers, and researchers.

3.3 LITERATURE REVIEW

The integration of smart healthcare wearable devices into daily life has garnered significant attention due to its potential to revolutionise healthcare practices. This review of the literature intends to offer a thorough overview of the present status of research on wearable smart healthcare devices, with a particular emphasis on consumer acceptance and attitude. Table 3.1 compares the most recent research papers in the same field.

In this research (Abdo & Almuraqab, 2021), the purpose of this study is to better understand the factors that affect consumers' decisions to purchase smartwatches. A model based on the Technology Acceptance Model (TAM) was developed and tested to accomplish this. Using SmartPLS software, the partial least squares method is applied to the data analysis. The findings demonstrated that the primary motivators behind people's adoption of smartwatches are their visibility, social influence, and perceived simplicity of usage. The study also discovered that cost and intention to use have a big impact on customers' purchase decisions. Numerous types of research have been conducted utilising several TAMs, including the theory of responded action (TRA), TAM, UTAUT2, and theory of planned behaviour (TPB), to understand the adoption of these devices better (Talukder et al., 2020). The use of wearable technology has grown rapidly and is now crucial in sectors like healthcare. The goal of the study is to identify the many themes and patterns that appear frequently in wearable technology literature (Ferreira et al., 2021). However, research in this area

TABLE 3.1
Tabular Comparison amongst Latest Research Papers

Title	Methodology	Size	Key Findings	Significance
Addressing privacy concerns with wearable health monitoring technology (Sivakumar et al., 2024)	Cross-sectional design in Quantitative study to assess privacy concern and user behaviour	300	Resolve the concerns raised by 60% of users by putting strong data protection mechanisms in place and adhering to current privacy regulations.	A comprehensive strategy to empower knowledgeable decisions on wearable health data.
Characteristics and Attitudes of Wearable Device Users and Nonusers in a Large Health Care System (Venn et al., 2024)	Multivariable logistic regression was employed to determine the variables connected to gadget use.	11000	Consumer wearable device use is widespread, and the majority of users value wearable health data.	Relationships between the use of wearable technology and long-term clinical outcomes offer a framework for assessing mobile health-based treatment options.
Adoption model of healthcare wearable devices (Huarng et al., 2022)	Surveyed by questionnaire, and path analysis was used to examine causality.	335	Consumers are more likely to use wearable medical devices if they offer strong data privacy, are easy to use, and provide reliable health information. On the other hand, the high costs associated with these devices and services can discourage people from using them.	The determinants of an individual's readiness to adopt a wearable medical device include financial limitation, the confidentiality of data, perceived ease of use (PEOU), inclination to adopt (IA), and perceived usefulness (PU).
Promoting smart wearable devices in the health-AI market: the role of health consciousness and privacy protection (Zhu et al., 2023)	Structural equation modelling was used, and multi-group analysis was done to test the hypotheses.	250	The utilisation of smart wearable devices is negatively impacted by consumers' privacy concerns, while it is positively impacted by consumers' health consciousness.	A model is developed that takes privacy and health considerations into account to explain how customers utilise smart wearables.
Exploring the factors affecting behavioural intention to adopt wearable devices (Misra et al., 2023)	Structural equation modelling was performed.	139	The influence of connectivity and healthcare on TTF is substantial. The behavioural intention to acquire a smartwatch is influenced by the TTF model and the TAM model. However, the study's findings showed that perceived privacy did not affect BI.	Worked on variables like healthcare, fashionability, and ease of use that have possibilities for affecting the adoption of wearable devices.

remains scattered, lacking a clear method to study and understand the use of these technologies and their future impact. Using bibliometric analysis and a methodical literature assessment, they identified five themes. The analysis shows that although the research spans multiple disciplines, there is a lack of integration between detailed and broader perspectives. This has led to disconnected terms, overlapping research questions, studies with inappropriate results, and confusion among different theories. Cheung et al. (2019) aims to fill that gap by testing a theoretical model that examines how consumers' health beliefs, the accuracy of health information, and privacy protection affect the perceived usefulness of wearable healthcare technology. This study also examines the relationship between consumer ingenuity, perceived utility, and reference group influence on wearable healthcare technology adoption intentions. According to Chandrasekaran et al. (2020) the primary goal of this study was to investigate the use of wearable healthcare devices and identify the key factors predicting their use among US adults. It examines how often people use wearable healthcare devices, how frequently they do so, and their willingness to share health data from these devices with healthcare providers. They are mostly used by younger, healthier, wealthier, and more educated people, excluding other groups.

3.4 RESEARCH GAP

There are several identified research gaps in the field of smart healthcare wearable devices. Some studies have explored short-term effects, such as adoption intention or immediate behaviour change, but there is a gap in understanding the long-term efficacy and sustainability of smart healthcare wearable devices in promoting health outcomes. There is a need for research that examines the adoption and usage patterns of smart healthcare wearable devices among a broader range of demographic groups, including individuals from different socio-economic backgrounds, cultural contexts, and levels of health literacy. Understanding the needs and preferences of diverse populations is essential for designing inclusive and equitable wearable health interventions. Some studies mention privacy concerns, but there is a limited in-depth exploration of ethical and privacy considerations associated with wearable health devices. Establishing trust and guaranteeing the moral use of wearable health technology are crucial issues to address. Numerous studies highlight the potential of wearable devices in managing chronic and long-term diseases and engaging patients, yet there remains a void in comprehending the effective integration of these devices into clinical practice. While there is growing interest in using wearable devices for health-related monitoring, there is a gap in evidence regarding their effectiveness and validity in this context.

3.5 METHODS

The research objectives of this study are twofold: first, to explore the influence of technology savviness on millennials' attitudes towards using smart healthcare wearable devices; and second, to investigate the mediating role of perceived purposefulness in this relationship. Specifically, the study aims to assess the level of technology savviness among millennials, using measures such as digital literacy, comfort with technology, and previous technology adoption behaviours. Additionally, the study seeks to measure millennials' attitudes towards using smart healthcare wearable devices, encompassing perceptions, acceptance, and intentions to use these devices. Furthermore, the research aims to examine how perceived purposefulness, which includes perceived benefits, relevance, and utility of smart healthcare wearables, mediates the relationship between technology savviness and attitudes. Through these objectives, the study aims to contribute to a deeper understanding of the factors influencing millennials' adoption of smart healthcare technology, with implications for healthcare providers, technology developers, and policymakers aiming to enhance the uptake and effectiveness of such devices among tech-savvy populations.

3.6 PARTICIPANTS

The participants in this study are selected from the millennial demographic, specifically focusing on individuals who are potential users of smart healthcare wearable devices. Participants were selected from diverse backgrounds to ensure a varied sample in terms of education, occupation, and socioeconomic status. The selection process involved purposive sampling, aiming to include millennials with varying levels of technology savviness. This will ensure a comprehensive exploration of attitudes towards smart healthcare wearables across different tech-savvy profiles.

As shown in Table 3.2, the demographic breakdown of participants, with 54.4% identified as male and 44.1% as female. A significant proportion of respondents were

TABLE 3.2
Demographic Profile of Respondents

	Frequency	Percentage	
Gender			
Male	74	54.4	1.57(.525) M(SD)
Female	60	44.1	2 Median
Prefer not to mention	2	1.5	.276 Var.
Age			
18-25	78	57.3	
26-33	28	21.3	27(7.31) M(SD)
34-41	21	15.3	25 Median 53.445 Var.
41 & above	9	6.5	
Education			
Bachelor	39	28.7	
Master	65	47.8	2.99 (1.35) M(SD)
Professional	25	18.4	4 Median 1.822 Var.
Sr. Secondary	7	5.1	
Occupation			
Professional	35	25.7	8.38(1.525) M(SD)
Students	91	66.9	9 Median
Others	10	7.1	2.32 Var.

N=136

students. The study included individuals aged 18 to 41 years and older. On average, participants were 41.27 years old, with a median age of 27, reflecting a cohort recognised for their adeptness and ease with technology.

3.7 PROCEDURE

The research design for this study employed a quantitative approach, utilising the simple mediation model proposed by Hayes (2013) to investigate the relationship between technology savviness, attitudes towards using smart healthcare wearable devices, and the mediating role of perceived purposefulness. This cross-sectional study targeted millennials, specifically potential users of smart healthcare wearable devices. The research design involves survey-based data collection, where participants were asked to complete measures assessing their technology savviness, attitudes towards smart healthcare wearables, and perceived purposefulness related to these devices. The collected data were analysed using correlation analysis to examine initial relationships, followed by mediation analysis using Hayes' simple mediation model to test the indirect effect of technology savviness on attitudes via perceived purposefulness.

3.8 MEASURES

Measures of technology savviness, attitudes towards smart healthcare wearables, and perceived purposefulness were assessed using validated scales to ensure the reliability and validity of the data. The reliability statistics are presented in Table 3.3.

The three constructs used in the model have Cronbach's alpha values of .8, .838, and .773 in that order. This suggests that the internal consistency of the scale items, which ranges from fair to good, is dependable for the study population under consideration (Zikmund et al., 2016).

3.9 ANALYSIS AND RESULTS

In this research paper, the simple mediation model is employed to analyse the relationship between the independent variable, technology savviness, and the dependent variable, attitudes towards smart healthcare wearable devices, with perceived purposefulness as the mediator.

TABLE 3.3
Descriptive & Reliability Statistics

Constructs	No. of Items	Cronbach's Alpha	Cronbach's Alpha Based on Standardised Items
Technology Savviness	5	.800	.805
Perceived Purposefulness	3	.838	.840
Consumer's attitude towards adoption	4	.773	.778

The simple mediation model examines how an independent variable (X) affects a dependent variable (Y) through a mediator variable (M). The model consists of three equations:

1. **The effect of X on M (Path a):** $M{=}i1{+}aX{+}e1$
2. **The effect of M on Y, controlling for X (Path b):** $Y{=}i2{+}c'X{+}bM{+}e2$
3. **The total effect of X on Y (Pathc):** $Y{=}i3{+}cX{+}e3$

In these equations:

- $i1$, $i2$, and $i3$ are the intercepts.
- a is the coefficient for the effect of X on M.
- b is the coefficient for the effect of M on Y.
- c' is the coefficient for the direct effect of X on Y, controlling for M.
- c is the coefficient for the total effect of X on Y.
- $e1$, $e2$, and $e3$ are the error terms.

The mediation effect (indirect effect) of X on Y through M is represented as the product of paths a and b (i.e., ab). The total effect (c) is the sum of the direct effect (c') and the indirect effect (ab): $c{=}c'{+}ab$

The study begins with data collection through surveys that measure participants' technology savviness, perceived purposefulness, and attitudes towards smart healthcare wearables using validated scales. Initial correlation analysis explores the relationships among these variables. The core analysis utilises Hayes' PROCESS macro for SPSS, which facilitates testing the direct and indirect effects within the mediation framework. The mediation model involves calculating the direct effect (c') of technology savviness on attitudes towards smart healthcare wearables, controlling for perceived purposefulness. The indirect effect (a*b) is examined by analysing two paths: the effect of technology savviness on perceived purposefulness (path a) and the effect of perceived purposefulness on attitudes towards smart healthcare wearables (path b). Bootstrapping, a non-parametric resampling method, is used to generate confidence intervals for the indirect effect, assessing its significance. The results interpretation focuses on the significance of the indirect effect, which indicates whether perceived purposefulness mediates the relationship between technology savviness and attitudes towards smart healthcare wearables. Additionally, the direct effect (c') is evaluated to determine if technology savviness still significantly impacts attitudes after accounting for perceived purposefulness.

3.9.1 Hypothesis for the Study

H1: Perceived purposefulness mediates the relationship between Tech Savviness and Attitude towards Smart Healthcare Wearable Devices of consumers.

The study adopted (Hayes, 2013) the recommended strategy to evaluate the hypothesis (H1). Model 4 was used, with 5000 bootstrapped samples, for the attitude towards smart healthcare wearable devices was the outcome variable, perceived purposefulness served as the mediator, and consumer's Tec Savviness was the independent variable in this model.

3.9.2 The Effect of X on M

The analysis results reported in Table 3.4 show that, people who scored high on Tech savviness perceive smart healthcare wearable devices as more useful ($\beta = 0.15, p < 0.05$).

3.9.3 The Effect of M on Y, Controlling for X

The perceived purposefulness of the consumers statistically influences the attitude towards smart healthcare wearable devices ($\beta = .5617, p < 0.05$) as shown in Table 3.5.

3.9.4 The Total Effect of X on Y

Afterwards, the analysis of the total effect also reported a statistically significant effect (indirect effect: .3362, p < .05, 95%-LLCI = .187 to 95%-ULCI = .4855) as shown in Table 3.6. For the constant, the 95% confidence interval's lower and upper bounds are 2.2107 and 3.3201, respectively. This indicates that there is a 95% confidence interval inside which the correct constant is located. Therefore, the total effect

TABLE 3.4
Model: Effect of X on M

	Coeff	SE	T	P	LLCI	ULCI
Constant	3.53	0.2757	12.8035	0.0000	2.9844	4.0749
Techsavy	0.1524	0.0742	2.0539	0.0419	0.0056	0.2991

TABLE 3.5
Model: Effect of M on Y

	coeff	se	t	p	LLCI	ULCI
constant	0.7828	0.35	2.2368	0.027	0.0906	1.4751
Tech Savvy	0.2507	0.0641	3.908	0.0001	0.1238	0.3775
PerPur	0.5617	0.0735	7.6369	0	0.4162	0.7072

TABLE 3.6
Total Effect Model

	coeff	se	t	p	LLCI	ULCI
constant	2.7654	0.2805	9.8603	0	2.2107	3.3201
Tech Savvy	0.3362	0.0755	4.4557	0	0.187	0.4855

TABLE 3.7
Indirect Effect Model

	Effect	BootSE	BootLLCI	BootULCI
PerPur	0.0856	0.0524	0.0094	0.1999

TABLE 3.8
Model Summary

The effect of X on M (Path a)	Tec Savvy ➔ Perceived purposefulness	Significant
The effect of M on Y, controlling for X (Path b):	Perceived purposefulness ➔ Attitude	Significant
The total effect of X on Y (Path c):	Tec Savvy➔ Attitude	Significant
Indirect Effect	Tec Savvy ➔ Perceived purposefulness ➔ Attitude	Significant

model indicates that technology savviness has a significant positive effect on attitudes towards smart healthcare wearable devices.

3.9.5 Indirect Effect Model

The Indirect effect as shown in Table 3.7 also reported a statistically significant effect (indirect effect: .0856, 95%-LLCI = .0094 to 95%-ULCI = .1999). Therefore, the total effect model indicates that technology savviness has a significant positive effect on attitudes towards smart healthcare wearable devices. This suggests that perceived purposefulness significantly mediates the relationship between technology savviness and attitudes towards smart healthcare wearable devices within the given sample and confidence level.

The analysis is summarised for all the models in Table 3.8.

3.10 DISCUSSION

Using a basic mediation model, the study's findings offer a thorough knowledge of the links between technology savviness (X), perceived purposefulness (M), and attitudes toward smart healthcare wearable devices (Y). The impact of technological savvy on the perception of purposefulness is investigated in the first pathway (Path a). The findings show a strong positive correlation between these factors, indicating that those who are more tech-savvy are more likely to believe wearable smart healthcare equipment has a purpose. This suggests that tech-savvy people are better at appreciating the benefits, applicability, and significance of these devices, which increases their perceived usefulness. This result is consistent with previous research indicating that comfort and familiarity with technology might improve opinions about its uses and advantages. After adjusting for technological savvy, the second pathway (Path b) examines the impact of perceived purposefulness on attitudes regarding wearable smart healthcare technologies. The findings demonstrate a strong positive correlation, suggesting that people are more inclined to see smart healthcare wearables favourably when they believe they serve a greater purpose. The significance of perceived purposefulness as a crucial factor influencing attitudes towards technology adoption is highlighted by this research. Users are more likely to have positive attitudes toward the usage of technology when they perceive its obvious advantages and applicability. The total effect (Path c') represents the association between attitudes towards smart healthcare wearables and technological savviness. This combined effect includes both the direct impact of technological savvy and the indirect impact of perceived purposefulness. Through perceived purposefulness, the mediation analysis demonstrates a strong indirect effect of tech-savviness on views towards wearable smart healthcare devices. This strong indirect effect implies that perceived purposefulness acts as a mediator in part of the relationship between consumer's attitudes and their technological savviness. Put another way, those who are tech-savvy tend to see smart healthcare wearables favourably in part because they believe they serve a greater purpose. This mediation emphasises how crucial perceived purposefulness is to increasing tech-savvy users' adoption and acceptance of healthcare innovations. Increased technology self-efficacy can assist people in cultivating more favourable attitudes toward smart wearables, which will increase their use of these gadgets (Chandrasekaran et al., 2020). One of the studies also supported that respondents who were aware of wearable fitness trackers had a stronger inclination to adopt them than those who were not (Lee & Lee, 2018).

There are several *limitations* to the study that should be acknowledged. First, the generalisability of the results may be impacted by the sample size not being large or diverse enough to represent the larger population adequately. Furthermore, because the research's cross-sectional methodology only records data at one particular moment in time, it is more difficult to determine causality or track changes in attitudes and behaviours over time. Because self-reported data is used, there is a risk of bias, including social desirability bias, where individuals give answers, they think are more socially acceptable than what they think. Potential confounding factors that could affect opinions towards such devices, such as socioeconomic status, education level, and cultural influences, were not taken into account in this study. Due to the swift progress of technological improvements in smart healthcare wearables, the findings may become obsolete rapidly. Therefore, future studies should take into account the continuous technological changes. Finally, although the study briefly acknowledges the impact of design and aesthetics, it does not extensively investigate these factors. This implies that further research is necessary to completely examine these elements. By recognising these constraints, future investigations can expand upon the discoveries of this study to provide a more all-encompassing comprehension of the aspects that impact the acceptance of intelligent healthcare wearables.

3.11 IMPLICATION

The results of this study have important consequences for the acceptance and approval of smart healthcare wearable devices. The presence of a highly positive relationship between technological proficiency and a perceived sense of purpose suggests that improving one's knowledge and skills in technology might greatly enhance how users view the usefulness of wearable health technologies. This implies that educational programmes focused on enhancing technological proficiency could promote a stronger recognition of and acceptance of these devices. Furthermore, the study highlights the significance of perceived purposefulness as a mediator in influencing favourable sentiments towards wearable health devices. Users' adoption and utilisation of these gadgets are more likely to increase when they comprehend and have confidence in the tangible advantages and suitability of these technologies. Developers and marketers should focus on highlighting the tangible benefits and significant uses of their products to increase user acceptance, as this has practical consequences. Furthermore, to meet the changing demands and preferences of users, it is crucial to do continuous research and development on wearable fitness trackers and the accompanying third-party applications. This will ensure that these devices remain up-to-date and generally accepted as the technology in this field advances.

3.12 CONCLUSION

Improving consumers' perceptions of the purposefulness of smart healthcare wearables is critical to changing attitudes toward these devices. Should wearable healthcare innovations yield numerous benefits for both patients and consumers, the public sector must provide consumers with more precise and comprehensive information about the gadgets. This can be accomplished by using focused communication techniques that draw attention to the advantages, applicability, and relevance of the gadgets. Developers and marketers of smart healthcare wearables should focus on conveying to potential customers the tangible and evident features of their products. Illustrating practical advantages and uses can improve perceived intent and, in turn, user attitudes. The quantity or quality of readily available applications might have a significant impact on a consumer's inclination to adopt them. Overall, this study emphasises the crucial significance of perceived purposefulness and offers insightful information on the mechanisms via which technological savvy influences attitudes regarding smart healthcare wearables. These results provide stakeholders with useful suggestions to improve healthcare technology adoption and reception.

REFERENCES

Abdo, N., & Almuraqab, S. (2021). Determinants that Influence Consumers' Intention to Purchase Smart Watches in the UAE: A Case of University Students. *Advances in Science, Technology and Engineering Systems Journal, 6*. https://doi.org/10.25046/aj0601142

Chandrasekaran, R., Katthula, V., & Moustakas, E. (2020). Patterns of Use and Key Predictors for the Use of Wearable Health Care Devices by US Adults: Insights from a National Survey. *Journal of Medical Internet Research, 22*(10), e22443. https://doi.org/10.2196/22443

Cheung, M. L., Chau, K. Y., Sum Lam, M. H., Tse, G., Ho, K. Y., Flint, S. W., Broom, D. R., Tso, E. K. H., & Lee, K. Y. (2019). Examining Consumers' Adoption of Wearable Healthcare Technology: The Role of Health Attributes. *International Journal of Environmental Research and Public Health, 16*(13). https://doi.org/10.3390/IJERPH16132257

Ferreira, J. J., Fernandes, C. I., Rammal, H. G., & Veiga, P. M. (2021). Wearable technology and consumer interaction: A systematic review and research agenda. *Computers in Human Behavior, 118*, 106710. https://doi.org/10.1016/J.CHB.2021.106710

Hayes, A. F. (2013). *From Guilford Introduction to Mediation, Moderation, and Conditional Process Analysis AF2E. 7006*, 9–10. https://www.guilford.com/books/Introduction-to-Mediation-Moderation-and-Conditional-Process-Analysis/Andrew-Hayes/9781462549030

Huarng, K. H., Yu, T. H. K., & Lee, C. Fang, C. (2022). Adoption model of healthcare wearable devices. *Technological Forecasting and Social Change*, *174*, 121286. https://doi.org/10.1016/J.TECHFORE.2021.121286

Keikhosrokiani, P., Mustaffa, N., & Zakaria, N. (2018). Success factors in developing iHeart as a patient-centric healthcare system: A multi-group analysis. *Telematics and Informatics*, *35*(4), 753–775. https://doi.org/10.1016/J.TELE.2017.11.006

Lee, S. Y., & Lee, K. (2018). Factors that influence an individual's intention to adopt a wearable healthcare device: The case of a wearable fitness tracker. *Technological Forecasting and Social Change*, *129*, 154–163. https://doi.org/10.1016/J.TECHFORE.2018.01.002

Manas, M., Sinha, A., Sharma, S., & Mahboob, M. R. (2018). A novel approach for IoT based wearable health monitoring and messaging system. *Journal of Ambient Intelligence and Humanized Computing*, *10*(7), 2817–2828. https://doi.org/10.1007/S12652-018-1101-Z

Misra, S., Adtani, R., Singh, Y., Singh, S., & Thakkar, D. (2023). Exploring the factors affecting behavioral intention to adopt wearable devices. *Clinical Epidemiology and Global Health*, *24*, 101428. https://doi.org/10.1016/J.CEGH.2023.101428

Park, E. (2020). User acceptance of smart wearable devices: An expectation-confirmation model approach. *Telematics and Informatics*, *47*, 101318. https://doi.org/10.1016/J.TELE.2019.101318

Perez, A. J., & Zeadally, S. (2018). Privacy Issues and Solutions for Consumer Wearables. *IT Professional*, *20*(4), 46–56. https://doi.org/10.1109/MITP.2017.265105905

Sivakumar, C. L. V., Mone, V., & Abdumukhtor, R. (2024). Addressing privacy concerns with wearable health monitoring technology. *Wiley Interdisciplinary Reviews: Data Mining and Knowledge Discovery*, *14*(3), e1535. https://doi.org/10.1002/WIDM.1535

Talukder, M. S., Sorwar, G., Bao, Y., Ahmed, J. U., & Palash, M. A. S. (2020). Predicting antecedents of wearable healthcare technology acceptance by elderly: A combined SEM-Neural Network approach. *Technological Forecasting and Social Change*, *150*. https://doi.org/10.1016/J.TECHFORE.2019.119793

Venn, R. A., Khurshid, S., Grayson, M., Ashburner, J. M., Al-Alusi, M. A., Chang, Y., Foulkes, A., Ellinor, P. T., McManus, D. D., Singer, D. E., Atlas, S. J., & Lubitz, S. A. (2024). Characteristics and Attitudes of Wearable Device Users and Nonusers in a Large Health Care System. *Journal of the American Heart Association*, *13*(1), 32126. https://doi.org/10.1161/JAHA.123.032126/SUPPL_FILE/JAH39113-SUP-0001-SUPINFO.PDF

Yoon, S. N., Lee, D. H., & Shin, Y. (2020). Innovative healthcare wearable device usage and service enhancement. *Global Business and Finance Review*, *25*(2), 1–10. https://doi.org/10.17549/GBFR.2020.25.2.1

Zhu, Y., Lu, Y., Gupta, S., Wang, J., & Hu, P. (2023). Promoting smart wearable devices in the health-AI market: the role of health consciousness and privacy protection. *Journal of Research in Interactive Marketing*, *17*(2), 257–272. https://doi.org/10.1108/JRIM-10-2021-0246/FULL/XML

Zikmund, W. G., Babin, B. J., Carr, J. C., Adhikari, A., & Griffin, M. (2016). *Business research methods: a South-Asian perspective*. Cengage Learning.

4 OralMedIE
Fine-tuning Biomedical Language Model for Clinical Information Extraction for Oral Medicine and Radiology

V. S. Anoop and R. Ardra

4.1 INTRODUCTION

Natural Language Processing (NLP) bridges human language and computers, facilitating effective interaction and communication. Recently, a significant surge of interest was visible in the field of NLP due to its ability to computationally understand and analyze human language (Khurana et al., 2023; Anoop and Asharaf, 2019; Anoop, 2023; Chandran et al., 2022). The fundamental aim of natural language processing is to reduce the burden of users on tasks with the advancements of NLP. As a result, industries such as health care, customer service, E-Commerce, and retail significantly benefited from the advancements of NLP (Anoop et al., 2024a, Anoop et al., 2024b). The massive digitization caused the accumulation of extensive amounts of data throughout all industries. By leveraging advanced NLP algorithms, a significant quantity of data can be turned into actionable insights. Cutting-edge techniques in NLP include advancements in discourse analysis, automatic summarization, machine translation, co-reference resolution, named entity recognition, morphological segmentation, part of speech tagging, and optical character recognition. These state-of-the-art methodologies contribute to the refinement of NLP by enabling tasks such as analyzing discourse structures, generating concise summaries, facilitating accurate translation between languages, resolving co-references, identifying named entities, segmenting morphological units, assigning grammatical tags to words, and recognizing characters from images (Khurana et al., 2023). By leveraging these cutting-edge techniques in NLP, industries, and researchers gain the ability to explore human language, extract valuable insights derived from extensive volumes of data, and enhance various applications and services (Tho et al., 2024). The continuous advancements in NLP techniques contribute to the evolution of the field, allowing for enhanced precision and sophistication in comprehending and processing language.

DOI: 10.1201/9781003503385-4

Recent years have witnessed exponential growth in data generation in the biomedical field, particularly in areas such as clinical reports, medical research publications, and electronic health records (Anoop et al., 2016). The enhanced accessibility of biomedical literature in repositories such as Medline caused an upsurge in interest to extract relevant key features from the biomedical domain (Fu et al., 2024). Extracting these relevant entities and information is highly beneficial in the areas of patient care, public health, data integration and analysis, and drug discovery and development. This can be achieved with advancements in Biomedical Natural Language Processing (BioNLP). BioNLP is a subdomain of NLP that specifically focuses on the processing and analysis of textual data related to the biomedical field. To address the challenges in this domain, BioNLP techniques automate the extraction of knowledge derived from biomedical literature, alleviating the burden.

In the past few years, there has been a significant drift in the NLP field with the introduction of pre-trained language models like Bidirectional Encoder Representation from Transformers (BERT) (Chang et al., 2021; Sharaf and Anoop, 2023). Transformer-based pre-trained language models (T-PTLMs) have achieved remarkable success across a wide range of NLP tasks. These models, pioneered by GPT and BERT, leverage the power of transfer learning, self-supervised learning, and transformers. Through the process of self-supervised learning, T-PTLMs can acquire universal language representations by analyzing extensive text data, and subsequently apply this acquired knowledge to various subsequent tasks. This eliminates the necessity of training downstream models starting from the beginning and provides valuable background knowledge (Kalyan et al., 2021). Large Language Models (LLMs) like GPT-3 and GPT-4, have garnered recognition due to their remarkable performance, but their influence on BioNLP tasks and the development of methods has not been thoroughly investigated. Pre-trained language models have significant relevance in NLP as they offer a powerful framework for leveraging pre-existing linguistic knowledge. They have widespread applications in tasks such as language understanding, sentiment analysis, text generation, machine translation, and information extraction. By pre-training models on large text corpora, they can effectively capture linguistic patterns, contextual information, and semantic relationships, enabling better performance on downstream NLP tasks. Pre-trained models have facilitated advancements in natural language understanding, allowing researchers and practitioners to build more accurate and efficient NLP systems (Kalyan et al., 2021). This language model could solve many challenges such as OOV (out of vocabulary) and became popular in many downstream tasks BERT is not a domain-specific language model, but there are several fine-tuned BERT variations available that are used for domain-specific purposes. This has resulted in the reporting of domain-specific BERT variations such as BioBERT, FinBERT (Huang et al., 2023), medBERT (Bressem et al., 2024), Climedbert (Fard et al., 2022), and TweetBERT (Chandran et al., 2022). This chapter discusses an approach powered by a domain-specific BERT model for biomedical information extraction from unstructured clinical documents on oral medicine and radiology, using machine learning techniques. The core contributions of this chapter can be outlined as follows:

a. Discusses the role of named entity recognition in NLP, with a focus on clinical information extraction.

b. Proposes machine learning approaches using different text encoding techniques for efficient retrieval of biomedical named entities from unstructured clinical documents.
c. Experimentally verifies the proposed approaches with state-of-the-art machine learning approaches to establish the usability of the proposed approach.

4.2 NAMED ENTITY RECOGNITION IN BIOMEDICAL DOMAIN

Named Entity Recognition (NER) is the fundamental and basic step in many NLP pipelines. It refers to the extraction of entities from the text. NER performs as the cornerstone for various NLP tasks such as machine translation, information extraction, sentiment analysis, and question answering, among others (Cao et al. 2024, Anoop 2021). Through the identification of named entities, NER facilitates a more comprehensive analysis, thereby enabling seamless information retrieval, efficient data mining, and effective knowledge extraction (Rajimol and Anoop, 2020, Chavan et al. 2022, Lee et al. 2020). The field of biomedical literature is growing rapidly, emphasizing the need to extract relevant information from this huge amount of data. Biomedical Named Entity Recognition (BioNER) refers to identifying named entities such as medical conditions, symptoms, and treatments from a biomedical context (Ardra et al., 2023). It plays an essential role in biomedical text mining as it facilitates the precise identification of named entities, subsequently contributing to other related tasks. To leverage the possibilities of automatic feature extraction, various deep learning techniques have been developed for BioNER (Devika et al., 2023). BioNER is a bit more challenging when compared to traditional NER since it demands extensive domain-specific knowledge. Apart from the general domain, the biomedical field contains complex terminologies that are challenging for individuals without specialized knowledge to comprehend. This indicates the relevance of domain-specific models and techniques. BioNER acts as a building block for constructing various NLP pipelines such as biomedical relation extraction (BioRE), healthcare text comprehension, healthcare information retrieval, health ontology creation, and health question answering.

4.3 RELATION EXTRACTION IN BIOMEDICAL DOMAIN

Knowledge is a formal way of understanding the world around us. It involves gathering information, facts, and insights about different things. When we have knowledge, it helps us think and make decisions, similar to how humans do. A reliable way to automatically acquire this knowledge called Relation Extraction (RE), plays a key role in NLP (Sarol et al., 2024). The objective of RE is to identify unknown relationships from plain text. The outputs of RE can be utilized to construct a knowledge base, enabling the accomplishment of various downstream tasks such as question answering, knowledge completion, summarization, and text generation (Guo et al., 2024).

With the rapid growth of textual data available, extracting relevant entities and relations from data is extremely important (Sreelakshmi and Anoop, 2023). Extracting relations between biomedical concepts is highly important in the field of biomedicine. BioRE emphasizes identifying and extracting biomedical entities and their relation in biomedical data. It enhances biomedical research, accelerates drug discovery, and improves healthcare outcomes (Li et al., 2024). Since the biomedical domain consists of abbreviations, specialized terminologies, and domain-specific context, it is challenging for RE. Furthermore, the lack of labeled training data, the presence of unambiguous sentence structures, and the need for domain-specific knowledge further complicate the process. The extracted relationship can be utilized to build knowledge bases, such as ontologies or biological networks, which serve as an essential tool for practitioners and biomedical researchers (Anoop and Asharaf, 2019).

4.4 STATE-OF-THE-ART IN BIOMEDICAL INFORMATION EXTRACTION

NER holds great importance in the field of NLP. Furthermore, it serves as a critical component within knowledge extraction pipelines. Methods for NER are highly influenced by the availability of labeled data. In earlier days, researchers were focused on handcrafted rules and small-scale corpora; recent advancements in machine learning and deep learning have resulted in better approaches. However, low-resource languages still depend on rules and conventional machine learning methods for performing NER tasks. The authors discussed four types of methods that are typically employed in the context of implementing NER systems. The author stated that deep learning techniques have replaced rule-based and traditional machine models in NER. A study has been carried out on clinical data, and classification is employed using ML framework and NLP techniques. Usually, doctors and nurses review the medical data and forward it to relevant authorities; the proposed model in this paper automates this process. The model makes use of a machine learning framework that integrates a bidirectional long short-term memory-conditional random field (LSTM-CRF) technique, which is initialized with pre-trained word embeddings. The proposed model integrates various machine learning algorithms such as naive Bayes, support vector machine (SVM), decision tree, logistic regression, random forest, and light GBM. Among all the models, light GBM outperformed with an accuracy of 99.58%. According to this study, the author asserts that traditional rule-based approaches and dictionary-based approaches face challenges due to the diverse writing styles of clinicians; machine learning-based approaches have demonstrated their effectiveness in tackling these issues (Ravikumar and Ramakanth, 2021).

Another approach proposed a model for disease-named entity recognition, which utilizes a bidirectional long short-term memory-conditional random field (LSTM-CRF) approach for sequence tagging, which is embedded with pre-trained word embeddings such as BERT (Jarashanth and Nawarathna, 2022). To generate sequence tags, they integrate BERT, a transformer-based neural network with a Conditional Random Fields (CRF) layer. Apart from traditional pre-trained word embeddings, BERT improves context-dependent representation by considering neighboring tokens. The BERT embeddings are obtained from tokenizing input text, and these embeddings are fed into the CRF layer to produce tags. In this study, the proposed BERT+CRF model achieved an F1-score of 85.30% and outperformed the CollaboNet model (SOTA model) on the BC5CDR dataset. Furthermore, it is worth noting that BERT+SVM accuracy was lower when compared to BERT+CRF, which indicates the relevance of the CRF layer in determining final outcomes (Jarashanth and Nawarathna, 2022). Another novel framework proposed for BioNER is DTranNER (Hong and Lee, 2020). The proposed model integrates deep learning to capture label-label transition relations, considering the contextual information present in input sequences. Unary-Network and Pairwise-Network are the two deep learning neural networks that comprise the proposed model. The Unary-Network is dedicated to individual labeling, while the Pairwise-Network evaluates the suitability of label transitions. To generate precise labels, these layers are embedded with CRF. The authors express their intention to extend DTranNER to unlabeled biomedical data. DTranNER outperformed all other models with an F1-score of 94.16% (Hong and Lee, 2020).

A study has been conducted on the impact of the latest transformer-based models, such as BERT, RoBERTa, and XLNet, on clinical RE (Yang et al., 2021). The authors' goal is to build an open-source package with clinical pre-trained transformer-based models for smooth RE in the clinical domain. The results indicate that the RoBERTa-clinical RE model outperforms on 2018 MADE1.0 dataset, while the XLNet-clinical model achieves good performance on the 2018 n2c2 dataset. The methods and models developed in this study are made publicly available, with the intention of improving existing approaches in clinical RE and other NLP tasks relevant to the biomedical field. The study exhibited the efficiency of transformer-based models for clinical RE and discovered significant details that can contribute to the design of transformer-based solutions (Yang et al., 2021). Recently a research investigation has been carried out on identifying causal relationships among events and entities within biomedical texts. To attain insights, the authors carried out a series of experiments using various techniques. They implemented and evaluated multiple models, including a Multiview CNN (MVC), attention-based BiLSTM models, and word embedding models such as ELMo and transformer architectures like BioBERT. In addition, they explored the use of a graph LSTM and a baseline rule-based system. Also, they employed oversampling techniques to address the problem of class imbalance in the annotated data. The results of the study demonstrated a significant improvement in the performance of state-of-the-art systems when using the random oversampling technique to reduce class imbalance (Akkasi and Moens, 2021). In another paper, the author proposes a novel approach for RE called the relation knowledge graph (RKG), which combines linguistic knowledge extracted from a large-scale corpus and classification knowledge obtained from labeled training data. The RKG is of two subgraphs; one is for mining linguistic knowledge, and the remaining one is for acquiring classification knowledge. In this study, they consider relation classification as a link prediction problem. The authors propose a Chunk Graph LSTM network that uses statistical and neural network reasoning to segment sentences into entity chunks and learn their representations (Huang et al., 2021). The proposed model outperforms recent approaches on multiple RE tasks according to experiments on standard datasets. The GloVe model, LLE algorithm, and the proposed node representation method are compared, with the results indicating the effectiveness of the proposed approach.

4.5 ORALMEDIE: INFORMATION EXTRACTION FRAMEWORK FOR ORAL MEDICINE AND RADIOLOGY

This section discusses the methodology proposed for developing a BioNER System for oral medicine. The flowchart outlining the proposed approach can be found in Figure 4.1.

The first step involves data collection from PubMed, where 800 PubMed abstracts on Oral Medicine and Radiology were obtained using the Python library Pymed. The collected data were then pre-processed and labeled using the BIOES tagging scheme using Label Studio, accessible at https://labelstud.io/. Figure 4.2 depicts an example of data labeling and provides an illustration of how the extracted labeled entities appear. To ensure accuracy, domain experts verified the labeled data before proceeding with the experiments. Various feature encoding techniques and embeddings, including TF-IDF, CountVectorizer, Word2Vec, GloVe, BioWordVec, BERT, and BioBERT, were employed in this approach. These techniques were used in conjunction with multiple machine learning and deep learning algorithms to train the classifiers.

The following algorithms were implemented in this study:

a. **Support Vector Machine:** The SVM algorithm is a supervised ML algorithm commonly used for classification and regression tasks. It represents each data point as a point in an n-dimensional space, where n corresponds to the number of features in the dataset. SVM aims to find a hyperplane that separates data points into corresponding classes. If the data is not linearly separable, the algorithm applies the kernel trick, which introduces an additional dimension to the data to make it separable.
b. **Logistic Regression:** The logistic regression algorithm is a supervised ML algorithm basically used for classification tasks. Its objective is to calculate the probability of input belonging to a particular class. The output of logistic regression is always a value between 0 and 1, representing the probability of the input being part of the class. The logistic regression model is trained by minimizing a cost function, aiming to reduce the error between predicted

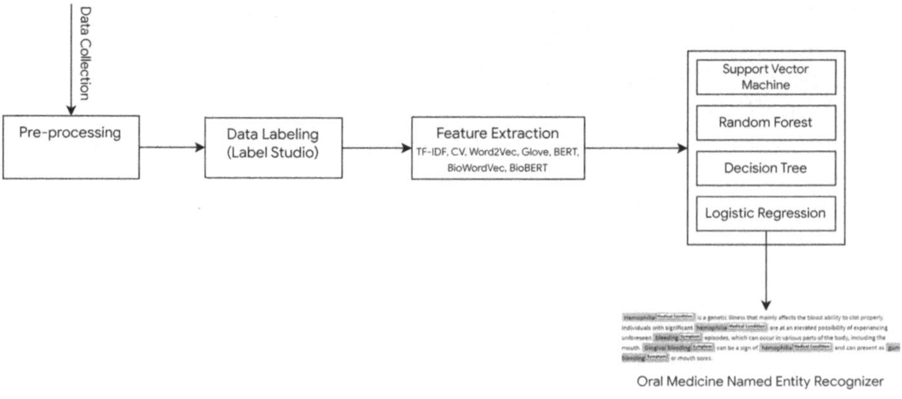

FIGURE 4.1 The overall workflow of the proposed approach.

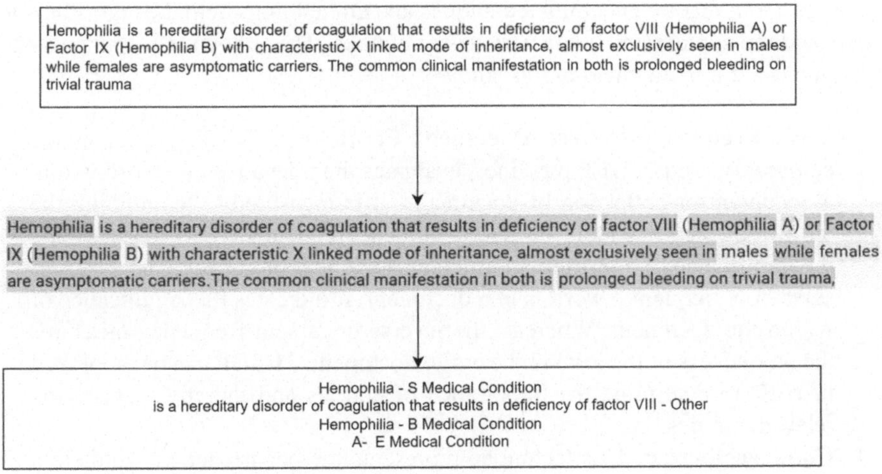

FIGURE 4.2 The input text and corresponding identified entities.

and actual values. This model is capable of handling both categorical and continuous input data.

c. **Random Forest:** The random forest algorithm is a supervised machine learning classification algorithm that utilizes an ensemble technique and operates in a similar manner to a decision tree. The RF algorithm employs the bootstrap aggregating technique, where it combines predictions from multiple individual decision trees. The final prediction is determined by aggregating the majority votes from each tree. To build the forest of decision trees, the algorithm randomly selects a subset of data. By utilizing multiple decision trees, the algorithm mitigates the risk of overfitting and improves accuracy.
d. **Decision Tree:** One commonly used machine learning algorithm, which is suitable for both regression and classification tasks, is extensively employed. It divides the input space into regions and independently classifies each region. The algorithm recursively partitions the input space and performs classification at the lowest level of the tree. Text classification is accomplished by the leaf nodes. The decision tree's splitting criterion, an essential characteristic, determines how the data should be divided to maximize performance.

Feature encoding techniques involve transforming textual input data into numerical representations that can be effectively processed using algorithms. These techniques capture the key characteristics of input text, such as linguistic features, word frequencies, or syntactic patterns, and transform them into numerical values. By doing so, these techniques facilitate the algorithms in learning and understanding comprehensively and contribute to making better predictions. On the other hand, embeddings are used to represent words or phrases in a vector space. These embeddings capture their semantic meaning or contextual relationships. There are numerous pre-trained word embeddings available, which effectively capture the semantic relationship between the words. Both feature encoding techniques and embeddings help the algorithms to understand the context and characteristics of entities. The following techniques and embeddings are implemented in this study:

a. **Term Frequency-Inverse Document Frequency:** TF-IDF, a technique commonly used in NLP pipelines, evaluates the relevance of a word within a document or collection of documents. It is measured by combining the term frequency (TF) and inverse document frequency (IDF) to determine the importance of a term to a particular document or corpus. The TF measures how frequent a word is in a document; it indicates the significance of within the document. Whereas, the inverse document frequency measures the uniqueness of the term in the entire document. TF-IDF can be employed in NER to determine the importance of entities and thereby identify the relevant entities.
b. **CountVectorizer:** This technique represents the occurrence of words in a document as a vector TF. In CountVectorizer, it splits each document into tokens and computes the occurrence of each token. This method builds a vocabulary of unique words and assigns a numerical value to each term based on their occurrence. It provides a simple and effective way of encoding text data into numerical values. This technique is much more useful in the NER system since it considers the occurrence of each term in the corpus, thereby identifying the relevant entities.
c. **Word2Vec:** This technique aims to represent words as dense vectors in a continuous vector space. It captures the semantic relationships and contextual information between words by learning word embeddings from large text corpora. In Word2Vec, similar words are located closer to each other; this facilitates capturing semantic similarities and relationships between words, even if they do not occur together frequently in the training data. Through the utilization of Word2Vec embeddings, NER systems can leverage the acquired semantic relationships to improve the performance of the system.
d. **Glove:** GloVe embeddings are a vector representation of words that are responsible for capturing semantic relationships and contextual information. These embeddings are trained on large corpora using a co-occurrence matrix, which measures the likelihood of words appearing together in a given context. GloVe embeddings offer a comprehensive understanding of word meanings and relationships, allowing NER systems to generalize from known examples to identify unseen entities. These embeddings boost the model's ability to distinguish synonyms, related terms, and contextual variations, leading to superior results.
e. **BioWordVec:** BioWordVec embeddings are specialized word embeddings specifically designed for biomedical text data. These embeddings are capable of understanding semantic relationships and domain-specific knowledge present in biomedical data. These domain-specific embeddings are trained on a large set of corpora, such as PubMed abstracts and articles, using techniques similar to Word2Vec and GloVe. BioWordVec embeddings offer

significant assistance and contribute to effectiveness in NER in biomedicine. By leveraging domain-specific knowledge encoded in these embeddings, NLP models can better understand and interpret biomedical text, leading to superior performance and accuracy in NLP applications.

f. **Bidirectional Encoder Representations from Transformers:** BERT is a state-of-the-art transformer-based model for NLP. It revolutionized various NLP tasks by introducing the concept of pre-training and fine-tuning specific downstream tasks. Unlike traditional models, BERT processes text in a bidirectional manner. To generate word representations of a word BERT model considers context from both the preceding and succeeding words. This bidirectional modeling facilitates BERT to capture rich contextual information and understand word dependencies in a sentence. NER using BERT can be implemented through two primary approaches: fine-tuning and contextual embeddings. The study conducted focused on generating contextual embeddings using BERT and subsequently integrating them into various models to enhance performance. These embeddings capture the contextual information of each word, considering its surrounding context.
g. **BioBERT:** BioBERT is a domain-specific variant of BERT that is specially trained and designed for biomedical text. BioBERT is built by pre-training BERT on a large corpus of biomedical literature and clinical texts and offers to capture the unique language and domain-specific knowledge present in these texts. BioBERT is capable of handling complex terminologies and abbreviations commonly found in biomedical literature. BioBERT brings the power of BERT's contextual understanding to the biomedical domain, enabling more accurate analysis and extraction of information from biomedical texts.

4.6 RESULTS AND DISCUSSIONS

The findings acquired from implementing the study are presented and discussed in this section.

In the case of the TF-IDF feature, the SVM classifier achieved 62.1%, 96%, 63%, and 76% for the A, P, R, and F values, while the Logistic Regression algorithm yielded 66.7%, 96%, 67%, and 79% for the same. Similarly, the Random Forest classifier attained 80.6%, 96%, 81%, and 88%, respectively, and the Decision Tree classifier obtained 77.4%, 96%, 77%, and 85% for the same metrics. The SVM classifier using Count Vectorizer achieved 62.9%, 96%, 63%, and 76%, respectively. The LR classifier obtained 66.8%, 96%, 67%, and 79% for the same metrics. The RF classifier obtained 80%, 96%, 80%, and 87% for A, P, R, and F, respectively, and the DT classifier achieved 76.9%, 96%, 77%, and 85%. For Word2Vec embedding, the A, P, R, and F values were 62.09%, 95%, 62%, and 74% for SVM; 62%, 95%, 62%, and 74% for LR; 75%, 97%, 76%, and 85% for RF; and 75%, 97%, 75% and 84% for DT classifier. For GloVe embedding with the SVM classifier, we have achieved 40.6%, 96%, 40%, and 56% as the A, P, R, and F values, and with LR, these values were 40.6%, 96%, 41%, and 56%; for RF classifier we have achieved 57.7%, 97%, 58%, and 73%; and for DT classifier these values were 57%, 96%, 57%, and 72%, respectively.

For BioWordVec embedding, the SVM has given 68.1% for A, 96% for P, 71% for R, and 82% for F-measure, and the LR algorithm has achieved 70.9% for A, 96% for P, 71% for R, and 82% for F. For the RF and DT classifiers, these values were 73%, 96%, 73%, and 83%, and 71.9%, 96%, 72%, and 82%, respectively. For all the feature types, the random forest algorithm outperformed all other models in accuracy, recall, and F-measure except for the recall and F-measure of Word2Vec. All models exhibit equivalent precision through all features. The graphs showing the accuracy, precision, recall, and F-measure values for the encoding techniques using TF-IDF, CountVectors, Word2Vec, and GloVe are shown in Figures 4.3–4.6 respectively.

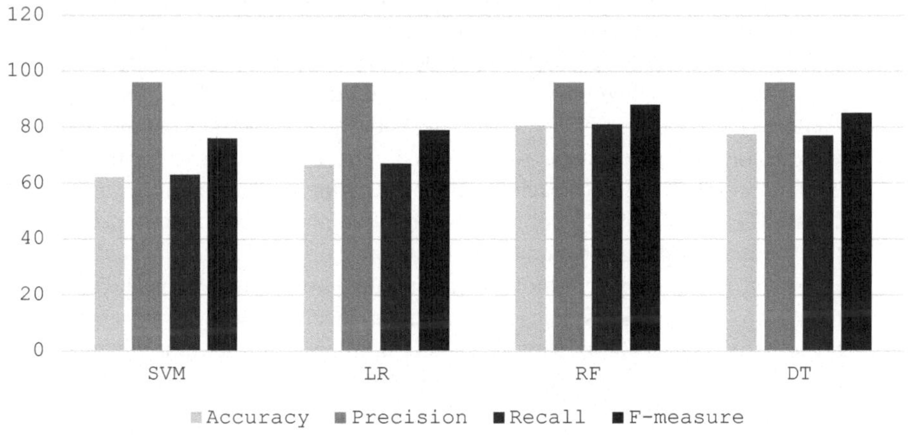

FIGURE 4.3 The precision, recall, accuracy, and F-measure comparison of different machine learning algorithms using TF-IDF approach.

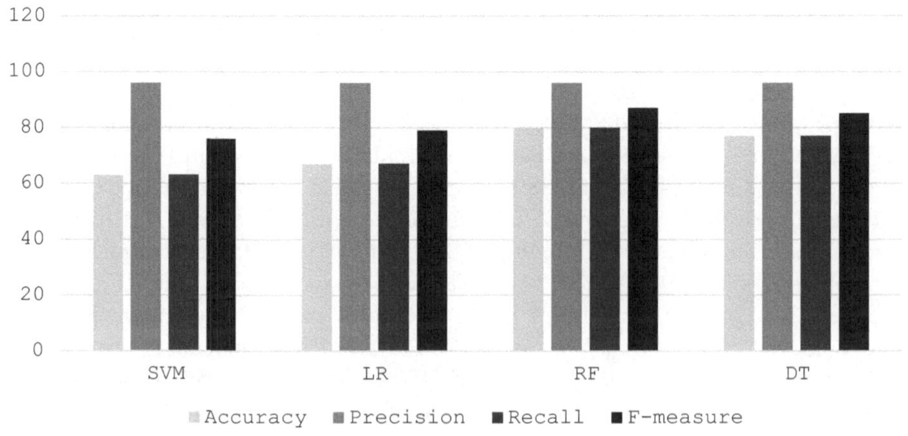

FIGURE 4.4 The precision, recall, accuracy, and F-measure comparison of different machine learning algorithms using the count vectorizer approach.

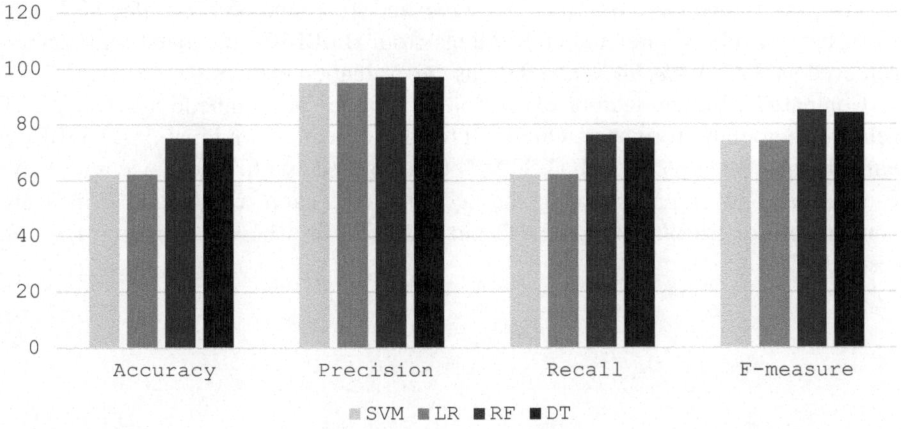

FIGURE 4.5 The precision, recall, accuracy, and F-measure comparison of different machine learning algorithms using Word2Vec approach.

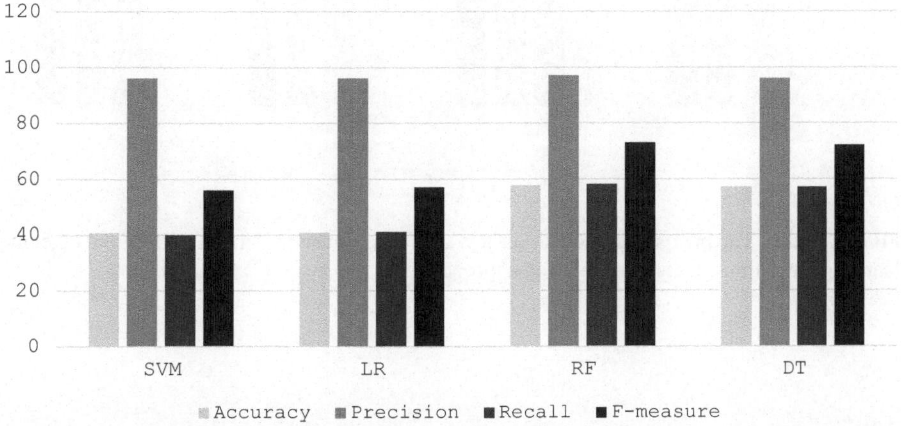

FIGURE 4.6 The precision, recall, accuracy, and F-measure comparison of different machine learning algorithms using GloVe approach.

In the experiment, BioBERT and BERT are also used as embeddings for models. For BERT embedding along with SVM, we achieved 72.1%, 95%, 73%, and 83% as A, P, R, and F values, respectively. For LR 74.8%, 96%, 75%, and 84%; for RF 87.1%, 96%, 87%, and 91%; and for DT 85.6%, 96%, 85%, and 90% are values for the same metric. In this instance, BERT embeddings and RF classifier outperformed all other BERT-classifier combinations. BioBERT is a fine-tuned pre-trained language model of BERT trained on a large biomedical corpus. The SVM classifier using BioBERT embedding obtained 84.4%, 97%, 84%, and 90%, respectively. The LR classifier achieved 72.2%, 96%, 72%, and 82% as A, P, R, and F values. For RF and DT, the values were 87.2%, 97%, 87%, and 92%, and 85.2%, 97%, 85%, and 91%, respectively. Contextual embeddings from BioBERT integrated with LSTM achieved 94.38%, 91%, 94%, and 93% as the evaluation metrics.

Compared to other feature extraction techniques and embeddings, BioBERT achieved a good performance. Out of all feature-classifier combinations, BioBERT embeddings integrated with LSTM outperformed with good accuracy and F-measure. The graphs showing the accuracy, precision, recall, and F-measure comparison for BioWordVec, BERT, and BioBERT are shown in Figures 4.7–4.9, respectively.

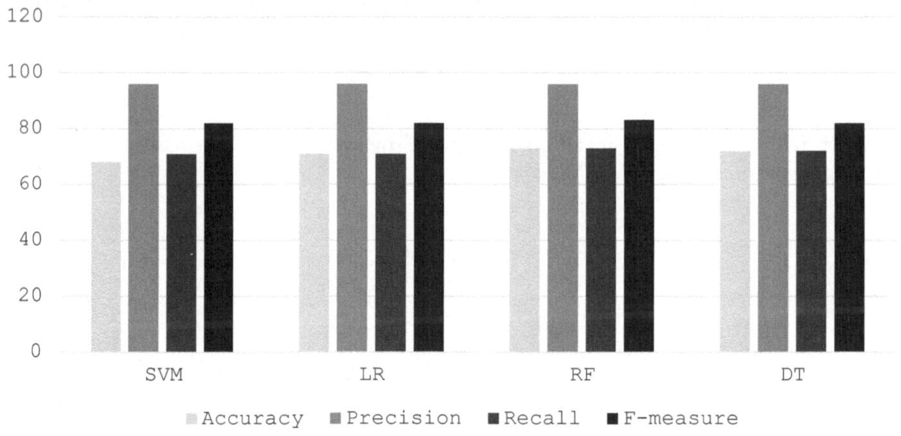

FIGURE 4.7 The precision, recall, accuracy, and F-measure comparison of different machine learning algorithms using BioWordVec approach.

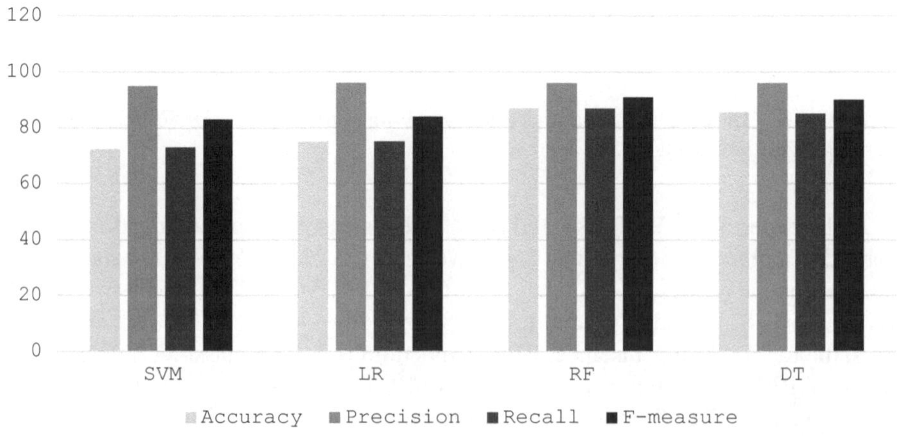

FIGURE 4.8 The precision, recall, accuracy, and F-measure comparison of different machine learning algorithms using BERT approach.

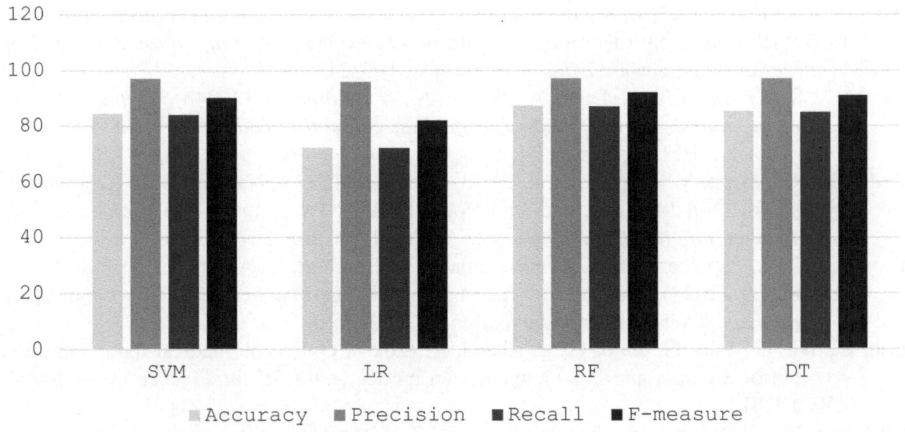

FIGURE 4.9 The precision, recall, accuracy, and F-measure comparison of different machine learning algorithms using BioBERT approach.

4.7 CONCLUSIONS AND FUTURE WORK

BioNER and Biomedical Relation Extraction (BioRE) serve as fundamental components of the BioNLP pipeline. It involves the identification and detection of relevant entities and the extraction of relations between them from biomedical texts. In this study, a novel methodology is proposed, leveraging the power of BioBERT, a state-of-the-art pre-trained language model specifically designed for the biomedical domain. In this study, multiple experiments have been conducted comparing BioBERT with other models and also combined with various features, and the results clearly demonstrate the superiority of BioBERT and LSTM in terms of performance. By leveraging the advanced language representation and understanding capabilities of BioBERT, along with LSTM's ability to capture long-term dependencies, this study paves the way for more accurate and efficient extraction of named entities in biomedical texts, thus contributing to advancements in the field of BioNLP.

REFERENCES

Akkasi, A., & Moens, M. F. (2021). Causal relationship extraction from biomedical text using deep neural models: A comprehensive survey. *Journal of Biomedical Informatics*, 119, 103820.

Anoop, V. S. (2021). Text mining and natural language processing for health informatics: recent trends and the way forward. In *Machine Learning and Data Analytics for Predicting, Managing, and Monitoring Disease* (pp. 111–121).

Anoop, V. S. (2023). Sentiment classification of diabetes-related tweets using transformer-based deep learning approach. In *International Conference on Advances in Computing and Data Sciences* (pp. 203–214). Cham: Springer Nature Switzerland.

Anoop, V. S., & Asharaf, S. (2019). Extracting conceptual relationships and inducing concept lattices from unstructured text. *Journal of Intelligent Systems*, 28(4), 669–681.

Anoop, V. S., Asharaf, S., & Deepak, P. (2016). Learning concept hierarchies through probabilistic topic modeling. arXiv preprint arXiv:1611.09573.

Anoop, V. S., Krishna, C. S., & Govindarajan, U. H. (2024a). Graph embedding approaches for social media sentiment analysis with model explanation. *International Journal of Information Management Data Insights*, 4(1), 100221.

Anoop, V. S., Krishnan, T. A., Daud, A., Banjar, A., & Bukhari, A. (2024b). *Climate Change Sentiment Analysis using Domain Specific Bidirectional Encoder Representations from Transformers*. IEEE Access.

Ardra, K. R., Anoop, V. S., & Panta, P. (2023). OralMedNER: A Named Entity Recognition System for Oral Medicine and Radiology. In *2023 9th International Conference on Smart Computing and Communications (ICSCC)* (pp. 262–267). IEEE

Bressem, K. K., Papaioannou, J. M., Grundmann, P., Borchert, F., Adams, L. C., Liu, L., ... & Löser, A. (2024). Medbert. de: A comprehensive german bert model for the medical domain. *Expert Systems with Applications*, 237, 121598.

Cao, L., Wu, C., Luo, G., Guo, C., & Zheng, A. (2024). Online biomedical named entities recognition by data and knowledge-driven model. *Artificial Intelligence in Medicine*, 150, 102813.

Chandran, N. V., Anoop, V. S., & Asharaf, S. (2022). A topic modeling-guided framework for aspect-oriented sentiment analysis on social media. In *Handbook of Research on Opinion Mining and Text Analytics on Literary Works and Social Media* (pp. 13–146). IGI Global.

Chang, Y., Kong, L., Jia, K., & Meng, Q. (2021). Chinese named entity recognition method based on BERT. In *2021 IEEE international conference on data science and computer application (ICDSCA)* (pp. 294–299). IEEE.

Chavan, T., Patankar, S., Kane, A., Gokhale, O., & Joshi, R. (2022). A twitter bert approach for offensive language detection in marathi. arXiv preprint arXiv:2212.10039.

Devika, N., Anoop, V. S., & Thekkiniath, J. (2023, August). Biomedical Named Entity Recognition from Malaria Literature using BioBERT. In *2023 9th International Conference on Smart Computing and Communications (ICSCC)* (pp. 239–244). IEEE.

Fard, B. J., Hasan, S. A., & Bell, J. E. (2022). Climedbert: A pre-trained language model for climate and health-related text. arXiv preprint arXiv:2212.00689.

Fu, L., Weng, Z., Zhang, J., Xie, H., & Cao, Y. (2024). MMBERT: a unified framework for biomedical named entity recognition. *Medical & Biological Engineering & Computing*, 62(1), 327–341.

Guo, B., Meng, J., Zhao, D., Jia, X., Chu, Y., & Lin, H. (2024). Integrating graph convolutional networks to enhance prompt learning for biomedical relation extraction. *Journal of Biomedical Informatics*, 157, 104717.

Hong, S. K., & Lee, J. G. (2020). DTranNER: biomedical named entity recognition with deep learning-based label-label transition model. *BMC Bioinformatics*, 21, 1–11.

Huang, A. H., Wang, H., & Yang, Y. (2023). FinBERT: A large language model for extracting information from financial text. *Contemporary Accounting Research*, 40(2), 806–841.

Huang, H., Lei, M., & Feng, C. (2021). Graph-based reasoning model for multiple relation extraction. *Neurocomputing*, 420, 162–170.

Jarashanth, S. T., & Nawarathna, R. D. (2022). Applying transformer models for disease named entity recognition. In *2022 2nd International Conference on Advanced Research in Computing (ICARC)* (pp. 272–277). IEEE.

Kalyan, K. S., Rajasekharan, A., & Sangeetha, S. (2021). Ammus: A survey of transformer-based pretrained models in natural language processing. arXiv preprint arXiv:2108.05542

Khurana, D., Koli, A., Khatter, K., & Singh, S. (2023). Natural language processing: state of the art, current trends and challenges. *Multimedia Tools and Applications*, 82(3), 3713–3744.

Lee, J., Yoon, W., Kim, S., Kim, D., Kim, S., So, C. H., & Kang, J. (2020). BioBERT: a pre-trained biomedical language representation model for biomedical text mining. *Bioinformatics*, 36(4), 1234–1240.

Li, Z., Tian, L., Jiang, Y., & Huang, Y. (2024). Relation extraction in biomedical texts: A cross-sentence approach. *IEEE/ACM Transactions on Computational Biology and Bioinformatics*. 21(6), 2156–2166.

Rajimol, R., & Anoop, V. S. (2020). A framework for named entity recognition for Malayalam—A Comparison of different deep learning architectures. *Natural Language Processing Research*, 1(1–2), 14–22.

Ravikumar, J., & Ramakanth, K. P. (2021). Machine learning model for clinical named entity recognition. *International Journal of Electrical and Computer Engineering*, 11(2), 1689.

Sarol, M. J., Hong, G., Guerra, E., & Kilicoglu, H. (2024). Integrating deep learning architectures for enhanced biomedical relation extraction: a pipeline approach. *Database*, 2024, baae079.

Sharaf, S., & Anoop, V. S. (2023). An analysis on large language models in healthcare: a case study of BioBERT. arXiv preprint arXiv:2310.07282.

Sreelakshmi, S., & Anoop, V. S. (2023). Cognitive computing and big data for digital health: Past, present, and the future. In *Era of Artificial Intelligence* (pp. 55–66). Chapman and Hall/CRC.

Tho, B. D., Nguyen, M. T., Le, D. T., Ying, L. L., Inoue, S., & Nguyen, T. T. (2024). Improving biomedical Named Entity Recognition with additional external contexts. *Journal of Biomedical Informatics*, 156: 104674.

Yang, X., Yu, Z., Guo, Y., Bian, J., & Wu, Y. (2021). Clinical relation extraction using transformer-based models. arXiv preprint arXiv:2107.08957

5 Generative AI for Healthcare Security

Addressing Privacy Challenges through Anomaly Detection in Healthcare Communications

Arul Kumar Natarajan, Kamal Upreti, Pravin R. Kshirsagar and Tan Kuan Tak

5.1 INTRODUCTION

The healthcare sector has become increasingly vulnerable to cyberattacks in recent years due to the rapid expansion of digital health records, telemedicine, and interconnected medical devices. The sensitive nature of healthcare data, which includes individuals' personal and medical information, makes it a prime target for malicious activities. Effective cybersecurity measures are crucial to safeguarding patient data, preserving the integrity of medical records, and ensuring the uninterrupted delivery of healthcare services. High-profile incidents, such as the 2020 attack on Universal Health Services, which disrupted services across 400 locations, highlight the pressing need for robust cybersecurity solutions tailored to the unique challenges of the healthcare industry (Falowo et al., 2024).

Generative AI has become a transformative force in cybersecurity, offering advanced methods for detecting and mitigating threats. Unlike traditional AI, which relies on predefined rules, generative AI uses sophisticated machine learning to create models that generate new data based on patterns. This approach is crucial for identifying novel and complex threats, with models like GANs and VAEs showing significant potential in improving threat detection and response.

Integrating AI into healthcare raises concerns about data privacy, ethical use, and regulatory compliance, necessitating adherence to HIPAA and GDPR to ensure secure patient information management (Said et al., 2023). Das (2024) explore the use of generative AI in analyzing phishing and cybersecurity metrics, offering a comprehensive examination of advanced methodologies for enhancing threat detection and response in cybersecurity. Agrawal et al. (2024) provide a comprehensive review

DOI: 10.1201/9781003503385-5

of generative models, specifically focusing on their application in generating synthetic attack data for cybersecurity, highlighting both the potential and challenges of using synthetic data to enhance deep learning models for cybersecurity.

Alwahedi et al. (2024) present a thorough review of machine learning techniques for enhancing IoT security, emphasizing current research trends, methodologies, and future directions with a focus on generative AI and large language models. Iturbe et al. (2023) introduce the AI4CYBER framework, which utilizes Artificial Intelligence to enhance cybersecurity by supporting incident response and recovery for critical systems. Ferrag et al. (2023) explore the use of generative AI for cyber threat-hunting in 6G-enabled IoT networks, highlighting its potential to enhance security measures in advanced network environments.

5.1.1 Major Contributions of the Chapter

- Provides an in-depth exploration of generative AI technologies and their application in cybersecurity, specifically within the healthcare sector.
- Demonstrates the practical application of BERT embeddings and Isolation Forest algorithms for anomaly detection in healthcare communications with a detailed case study.
- Highlights critical concerns about data privacy and ethical considerations in deploying AI technologies in healthcare, emphasizing regulatory compliance and responsible data management.

5.1.2 Generative AI for Cybersecurity

Recent AI models (GAI), such as Generative Adversarial Networks (GANs) and Variational Autoencoders (VAEs), have shown tremendous potential in various cybersecurity applications (Mohamed, 2023). These models learn to understand and replicate the underlying distributions of the training data, which can be leveraged to identify deviations indicative of cyber threats. In cybersecurity, generative AI can be used for the following purposes (Figure 5.1) (Sabuhi et al., 2021; Sarker, 2024).

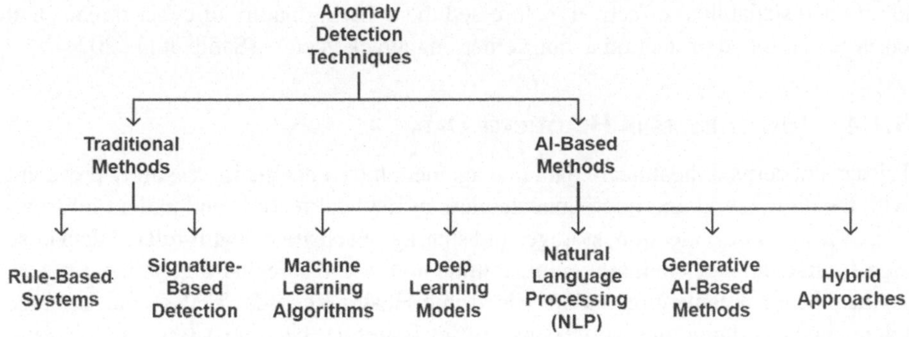

FIGURE 5.1 Generative AI for cybersecurity.

5.1.3 Mechanisms and Applications of Generative AI

Bidirectional Encoder Representations from Transformers (BERT) is a deep learning model designed to understand the context of words in a sentence, enabling it to generate high-quality textual representations (Bengesi et al., 2024). This ability to grasp context makes BERT particularly useful in cybersecurity applications, such as anomaly detection in email communications, where understanding the nuances of language is critical. This section delves into the key mechanisms through which generative AI models enhance cybersecurity measures, particularly in healthcare communications. By examining processes such as data preprocessing and feature extraction, model training, embedding generation, anomaly detection, and performance evaluation, we can understand how these advanced technologies contribute to robust and proactive security systems. Leveraging models like BERT, generative AI improves threat detection accuracy and protects sensitive information while adhering to stringent privacy and regulatory standards (Alwahedi et al., 2024; Thirunavukarasu et al., 2023; Sai et al., 2024).

The following are the various mechanisms of Generative AI in Cybersecurity.

- Data Preprocessing and Feature Extraction
- Model Training
- Embedding Generation
- Anomaly Detection
- Evaluation and Interpretation

Generative AI algorithms can autonomously generate data, which can be utilized to augment existing datasets for training robust cybersecurity models. This augmentation enables the development of more comprehensive and representative models, thereby enhancing their effectiveness in identifying and mitigating emerging threats (Yinka-Banjo & Ugot, 2020). Furthermore, generative AI algorithms excel in detecting subtle patterns and anomalies within vast datasets, thereby enabling early detection and proactive response to potential security breaches. By continuously analyzing data streams in real-time, these algorithms can provide organizations with actionable insights, allowing them to thwart attacks before they escalate into full-fledged breaches. Additionally, generative AI-powered cybersecurity solutions have demonstrated remarkable adaptability and scalability, effectively addressed the evolving nature of cyber threats, and ensured continued protection against emerging attack vectors (Saddi et al., 2024).

5.1.4 Privacy Issues in Healthcare Data

Privacy concerns in healthcare data management have become increasingly prevalent with the digitization and interconnectedness of medical records and patient information systems. The collection, storage, and sharing of sensitive health-related data pose significant challenges in maintaining confidentiality and safeguarding patient privacy. As healthcare organizations adopt Electronic Health Records (EHRs) and embrace telemedicine technologies, addressing privacy issues has become paramount to ensure compliance with regulatory requirements and uphold patient trust (Iyanna et al., 2022).

5.1.5 Sensitivity of Healthcare Data

Healthcare data is inherently sensitive, encompassing a wide range of personal and medical information that can uniquely identify individuals and reveal intimate details about their health status, medical history, and treatment plans. This includes Protected Health Information (PHI) such as patient demographics, medical diagnoses, laboratory test results, prescription medications, and medical procedures (Xiang & Cai, 2021). The sensitivity of healthcare data necessitates stringent privacy safeguards to prevent unauthorized access, disclosure, or misuse, thereby preserving patient confidentiality and mitigating the risk of harm or discrimination.

5.1.6 Examples of Privacy Breaches

Despite efforts to secure healthcare data, privacy breaches continue, resulting in significant repercussions for patients and healthcare providers. Examples of privacy breaches include unauthorized access to EHRs, data breaches resulting from cyberattacks or insider threats, accidental disclosures of sensitive information, and improper handling of PHI by healthcare personnel.

The 2015 Anthem data breach exposed the personal information of 78.8 million individuals, highlighting significant vulnerabilities in healthcare data security and underscoring the need for robust cybersecurity measures (Pool et al., 2024). Another example is the inadvertent disclosure of patient information through unsecured communication channels, such as emails or messaging platforms. In such cases, accidental disclosures of PHI can result in breaches of patient confidentiality and violations of regulatory requirements, leading to potential legal and regulatory repercussions for healthcare organizations. These examples underscore the importance of addressing privacy challenges in healthcare data management and implementing comprehensive safeguards to protect patient privacy and maintain trust in the healthcare system (Bada, 2023).

5.2 ANOMALY DETECTION

Effective anomaly detection in healthcare communications is essential for maintaining robust cybersecurity measures, protecting patient data, and ensuring the seamless delivery of healthcare services.

5.2.1 Types of Anomalies

In healthcare communications, anomalies can manifest in various forms, each posing distinct threats to data security and system integrity. Key types of anomalies include:

Phishing Attacks: Phishing attacks use deceptive emails to trick recipients into revealing sensitive information or downloading malicious software. In a healthcare context, phishing can target healthcare professionals or administrative staff, leading to compromised login credentials, unauthorized access to patient data, and potential disruptions in service delivery (Basit et al., 2021).

Unauthorized Access: Detecting unauthorized access attempts is crucial to prevent data breaches and protect sensitive patient information from exploitation or misuse (Adek & Ula, 2020).

Data Exfiltration: Data exfiltration involves unauthorized data transfer from healthcare systems to external locations. This can occur through various channels, including email, removable media, or network breaches. Detecting unusual data transfer patterns can help identify and prevent potential data exfiltration incidents, safeguard patient privacy, and maintain data integrity (Sabir et al., 2021).

Insider Threats: Anomalies in access patterns, data usage, or communication behaviors can signal insider threats, necessitating robust detection and response mechanisms to mitigate such risks (Le & Zincir-Heywood, 2021).

5.2.2 Impact on Healthcare Security

The impact of undetected anomalies in healthcare communications can be profound, leading to significant security breaches and operational disruptions (Šabić et al., 2021; Palakurti, 2024; Chatterjee & Ahmed, 2022). Key consequences include.

5.3 EXISTING ANOMALY DETECTION TECHNIQUES

Detecting anomalies in healthcare communications is crucial for identifying potential security threats and mitigating risks to patient data and system integrity. Various techniques have been developed to detect these anomalies, from traditional methods to advanced AI-based approaches (Figure 5.2).

5.3.1 Traditional Methods

Traditional anomaly detection methods rely on predefined rules and statistical models to identify deviations from normal behavior. These methods include:

Rule-Based Systems: Here, rules are manually crafted based on known threats and typical anomalous behavior. For instance, an email filter might flag messages containing specific keywords or originating from suspicious domains. This system encounters challenges in getting constant updates. (Sadikin & Kumar, 2020).

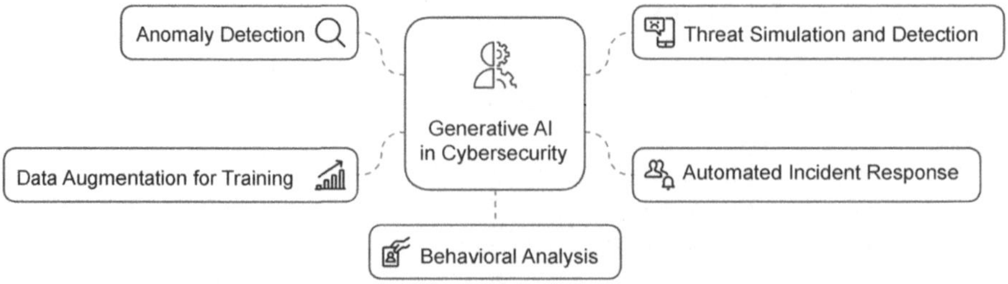

FIGURE 5.2 Existing anomaly detection techniques.

Statistical Analysis: Techniques such as mean, standard deviation, and clustering are commonly used for detection. For example, unusual spikes in data transmission volumes or access attempts could indicate a potential anomaly. However, statistical methods often require large datasets to establish accurate baselines and can be prone to false positives if normal behavior varies widely (Nassif et al., 2021).

Signature-Based Detection: It relies on a database of known threat signatures or patterns. Whenever an abnormal activity matches a signature in the database, it is flagged as anomalous. Antivirus software and intrusion detection systems often use signature-based methods. These methods are effective against known threats but are ineffective against novel or zero-day attacks that do not have existing signatures (Kwon et al., 2022).

5.3.2 AI-Based Methods

AI-based methods offer more advanced and adaptive solutions for anomaly detection. These methods include:

Machine Learning Algorithms: Machine learning algorithms can automatically adapt to new data, improving their detection capabilities (Nassif et al., 2021). For instance, an Isolation Forest algorithm, as used in the case study presented in this chapter, can effectively identify outliers in a dataset, flagging anomalous email communications.

Deep Learning Models: Deep-learning autoencoders can learn to reconstruct normal data patterns and identify anomalies based on reconstruction errors. RNNs are useful for detecting anomalies in time-series data (Choi et al., 2021).

Natural Language Processing (NLP): NLP techniques like BERT can generate embeddings that capture the semantic meaning of the text, allowing for more accurate anomaly detection. By leveraging NLP, AI-based methods can identify subtle linguistic patterns and deviations indicative of phishing attempts or other malicious communications (Das et al., 2020).

Generative AI-Based Methods: GANs and VAE methods can then compare real-time data against the synthetic models to identify anomalies. (Sabuhi et al., 2021).

Hybrid Approaches: Combining traditional methods with AI-based techniques can enhance the overall effectiveness of anomaly detection systems. Hybrid approaches leverage the strengths of both methods, using rule-based systems and statistical models for initial detection and AI-based methods for deeper analysis and adaptation to new threats.

5.4 ANOMALY DETECTION IN HEALTHCARE COMMUNICATIONS USING BERT

This section presents a case study that uses BERT embeddings and the Isolation Forest algorithm for anomaly detection in healthcare communications. The aim is to showcase how combining these methods effectively identifies unusual patterns and potential threats in healthcare emails, such as phishing attempts or unauthorized access.

The diagram of the proposed work for detecting anomalies is given in Figure 5.3. The following is the general algorithm developed for this case study:

1. *Initialization*:
   a. *Import necessary libraries: os, BeautifulSoup, BertTokenizer, BertModel, torch, IsolationForest, numpy.*
2. *Data Extraction*:
   b. *BeautifulSoup will parse the HTML content and extract plain text.*
3. *Load HTML Files*:
   a. *List all HTML files.*
   b. *Extract text from each HTML file.*
4. *Load BERT Model and Tokenizer*:
   a. *Load a pre-trained BERT model and tokenizer.*
5. *Generate BERT Embeddings*:
   a. *Define a function get_bert_embeddings(text) to generate BERT embeddings for the given text.*
   b. *Tokenize the text, obtain embeddings using the BERT model, and extract the [CLS] token's embedding.*
6. *Compute Embeddings for Emails*:
   a. *Generate embeddings for each extracted email text.*
   b. *Convert the list of embeddings into a numpy array.*
7. *Train Isolation Forest*:
   a. *Initialize and train an Isolation Forest algorithm with a specified contamination rate (e.g., 0.1).*
   b. *Fit the Isolation Forest model on the email embeddings.*
8. *Predict Anomalies*:
   a. *Use the trained Isolation Forest to compute anomaly scores for each email embedding.*
   b. *Classify each email as normal or anomalous based on the anomaly score.*
9. *Output Results*:
   a. *Print the classification and anomaly score for each email file.*
   b. *Highlight specific emails (e.g., email6.html) if required.*

5.5 RESULTS AND ANALYSIS

In this study, sample HTML files containing email communications were uploaded to the Google Colab environment for anomaly prediction using the developed model. The following results summarize the process of anomaly detection and the evaluation of the model's performance.

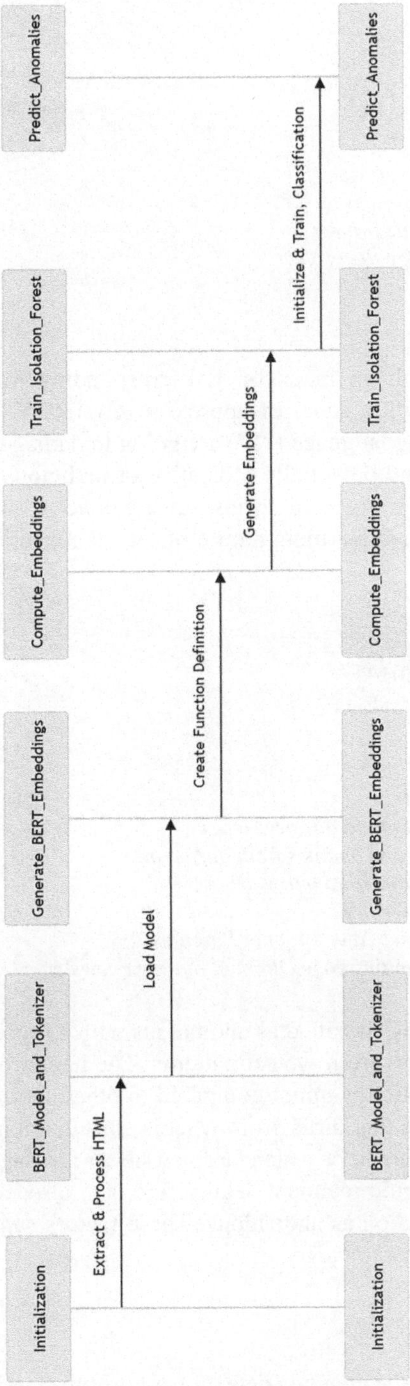

FIGURE 5.3 Sequence diagram of the proposed work.

5.5.1 Anomalous Emails

Email6.html

- Anomaly Score: 0.0257
- Classification: Anomalous
- Email Content

Greetings,
I am going to accept the project.
We are going to damage the project.
Best,
The Team

Analysis: The email with an index of 1, corresponding to "email6.html," was flagged as anomalous with a score of approximately 0.0257. The content of this email includes threatening language ("We are going to damage the project"), which is highly inappropriate and potentially indicative of malicious intent. Such content deviates significantly from expected norms, raising concerns about safety, security, or legality. The unusual and alarming nature of the language justifies its classification as anomalous.

Email2.html

- Anomaly Score: -0.0145
- Classification: Anomalous
- Email Content

Welcome to Our Newsletter
Thank you for subscribing to our newsletter.
Here's the latest news and updates from our team:
Exciting new features added to our website
Upcoming events and webinars
Customer success stories After Product Purchase
Stay tuned for more exciting New Offers in our next newsletter!

Analysis: Email2.html was classified as anomalous with a score of -0.0145, indicating that its content deviates from typical patterns. The negative anomaly score suggests that while the deviation is minor compared to other anomalous emails, it may still exhibit characteristics that differ from what is considered normal. Although the content of the email appears to be a standard newsletter message, its lack of personalization, absence of specific recipient details, and lack of sender information may contribute to its classification as anomalous. These factors suggest that it could be part of a phishing or spam campaign.

5.5.2 Normal Emails

For the remaining emails, the anomaly detection algorithm classified them as normal, as detailed in Table 5.1.

TABLE 5.1
Classification and Anomaly Scores of Normal Emails

File	Anomaly Score	Classification
Email3.html	0.0421	Normal
Email4.html	0.0145	Normal
Email5.html	0.0334	Normal
Email6.html	0.0228	Normal

Analysis: Emails 3, 4, 5, and 6 were classified as normal based on their anomaly scores, which indicate that their content closely aligns with the majority of emails in the dataset. The positive scores suggest that these emails are typical of normal communications, with higher scores reflecting a greater similarity to the norm. As a result, these emails do not show significant deviations and are therefore considered normal according to the anomaly detection algorithm.

5.6 ETHICAL CONSIDERATIONS

Deploying AI in healthcare requires adherence to ethical standards to ensure patient safety, fairness, and trust. Ethical considerations are critical in guiding the development and implementation of AI technologies.

Key ethical considerations include:

- Informed Consent: Patients must be fully informed about AI's role in their care, including its usage, potential risks, and benefits, and must provide their consent.
- Accountability: Clear frameworks should define responsibility for AI-driven decisions, address errors or adverse outcomes, and establish recourse mechanisms.
- Ethical Guidelines and Oversight: Develop and enforce ethical guidelines for AI in healthcare, supported by oversight bodies to ensure compliance and address ethical breaches.

Balancing innovation with privacy and ethical considerations is crucial in leveraging generative AI for healthcare security. By addressing privacy concerns and maintaining high ethical standards, integrating AI technologies can enhance healthcare cybersecurity while safeguarding patient trust and safety.

5.7 FUTURE WORK

In the book chapter, future endeavors focus on advancing anomaly prediction through the following strategies:

- Fine-tuning BERT on a relevant task: Explore the potential of refining the BERT model using labeled data specific to anomaly detection or similar

tasks. This process aims to tailor the model's parameters to the intricacies of the task, potentially amplifying its predictive capability.
- Optimizing hyperparameters: During the fine-tuning phase, experiment with various hyperparameters to fine-tune the model's performance.

5.8 CONCLUSION

The chapter concludes by emphasizing the pivotal role of generative AI in enhancing cybersecurity within the healthcare sector, particularly through applying BERT embeddings combined with the Isolation Forest algorithm for anomaly detection in healthcare communications. It highlights the efficacy of this approach in identifying potential security breaches and privacy violations, thereby safeguarding sensitive patient data and ensuring the integrity of healthcare systems. The case study elucidates the practical implementation of these advanced AI techniques, showcasing their ability to detect anomalies in real-time and mitigate emerging threats effectively. Furthermore, the findings underscore the importance of continual refinement and adaptation of cybersecurity measures to address evolving threats, ultimately contributing to the ongoing efforts to secure healthcare systems against cyberattacks while upholding patient confidentiality and regulatory compliance.

REFERENCES

Adek, R. T., & Ula, M. (2020, July). A survey on the accuracy of machine learning techniques for intrusion and anomaly detection on public data sets. In *2020 International Conference on Data Science, Artificial Intelligence, and Business Analytics (DATABIA)* (pp. 19–27). IEEE.

Agrawal, G., Kaur, A., & Myneni, S. (2024). A review of generative models in generating synthetic attack data for cybersecurity. *Electronics*, 13(2), 322.

Alwahedi, F., Aldhaheri, A., Ferrag, M. A., Battah, A., & Tihanyi, N. (2024). Machine learning techniques for IoT security: Current research and future vision with generative AI and large language models. *Internet of Things and Cyber-Physical Systems*.

Bada, M. (2023). A clinician's guide to cybersecurity and data protection: How to ensure client confidentiality? In *A Practitioner's Guide to Cybersecurity and Data Protection* (pp. 25–37). Routledge.

Basit, A., Zafar, M., Liu, X., Javed, A. R., Jalil, Z., & Kifayat, K. (2021). A comprehensive survey of AI-enabled phishing attacks detection techniques. *Telecommunication Systems*, 76, 139–154.

Bengesi, S., El-Sayed, H., Sarker, M. K., Houkpati, Y., Irungu, J., & Oladunni, T. (2024). Advancements in Generative AI: A Comprehensive Review of GANs, GPT, Autoencoders, Diffusion Model, and Transformers. *IEEE Access*, 12, 69812–69837.

Chatterjee, A., & Ahmed, B. S. (2022). IoT anomaly detection methods and applications: A survey. *Internet of Things*, 19, 100568.

Choi, K., Yi, J., Park, C., & Yoon, S. (2021). Deep learning for anomaly detection in time-series data: Review, analysis, and guidelines. *IEEE Access*, 9, 120043–120065.

Das, R. (2024). *Generative AI: Phishing And Cybersecurity Metrics*. CRC Press.

Das, S., Ashrafuzzaman, M., Sheldon, F. T., & Shiva, S. (2020, December). Network intrusion detection using natural language processing and ensemble machine learning. In *2020 IEEE Symposium Series on Computational Intelligence (SSCI)* (pp. 829–835). IEEE.

Falowo, O. I., Ozer, M., Li, C., & Abdo, J. B. (2024). Evolving Malware & DDoS Attacks: Decadal Longitudinal Study. *IEEE Access*, 12, 39221–39237.

Ferrag, M. A., Debbah, M., & Al-Hawawreh, M. (2023, May). Generative ai for cyber threat-hunting in 6g-enabled iot networks. In *2023 IEEE/ACM 23rd International Symposium on Cluster, Cloud and Internet Computing Workshops (CCGridW)* (pp. 16–25). IEEE.

Iturbe, E., Rios, E., Rego, A., & Toledo, N. (2023, August). Artificial Intelligence for next generation cybersecurity: The AI4CYBER framework. In *Proceedings of the 18th International Conference on Availability, Reliability and Security* (pp. 1–8).

Iyanna, S., Kaur, P., Ractham, P., Talwar, S., & Islam, A. N. (2022). Digital transformation of healthcare sector. What is impeding adoption and continued usage of technology-driven innovations by end-users?. *Journal of Business Research*, 153, 150–161.

Kwon, H. Y., Kim, T., & Lee, M. K. (2022). Advanced intrusion detection combining signature-based and behavior-based detection methods. *Electronics*, 11(6), 867.

Le, D. C., & Zincir-Heywood, N. (2021). Anomaly detection for insider threats using unsupervised ensembles. *IEEE Transactions on Network and Service Management*, 18(2), 1152–1164.

Mohamed, M. (2023). Comparative Evaluation of VAEs, VAE-GANs, and AAEs for Anomaly Detection in Network Intrusion Data. *EMITTER International Journal of Engineering Technology*, 11(2), 160–173.

Nassif, A. B., Talib, M. A., Nasir, Q., & Dakalbab, F. M. (2021). Machine learning for anomaly detection: A systematic review. *IEEE Access*, 9, 78658–78700.

Palakurti, N. R. (2024). Challenges and Future Directions in Anomaly Detection. In *Practical Applications of Data Processing, Algorithms, and Modeling* (pp. 269–284). IGI Global.

Pool, J., Akhlaghpour, S., Fatehi, F., & Burton-Jones, A. (2024). A systematic analysis of failures in protecting personal health data: a scoping review. *International Journal of Information Management*, 74, 102719.

Šabić, E., Keeley, D., Henderson, B., & Nannemann, S. (2021). Healthcare and anomaly detection: using machine learning to predict anomalies in heart rate data. *AI & Society*, 36(1), 149–158.

Sabir, B., Ullah, F., Babar, M. A., & Gaire, R. (2021). Machine learning for detecting data exfiltration: A review. *ACM Computing Surveys (CSUR)*, 54(3), 1–47.

Sabuhi, M., Zhou, M., Bezemer, C. P., & Musilek, P. (2021). Applications of generative adversarial networks in anomaly detection: a systematic literature review. *IEEE Access*, 9, 161003–161029.

Saddi, V. R., Gopal, S. K., Mohammed, A. S., Dhanasekaran, S., & Naruka, M. S. (2024, March). Examine the role of generative AI in enhancing threat intelligence and cyber security measures. In *2024 2nd International Conference on Disruptive Technologies (ICDT)* (pp. 537–542). IEEE.

Sadikin, F., & Kumar, S. (2020, May). ZigBee IoT Intrusion Detection System: A Hybrid Approach with Rule-based and Machine Learning Anomaly Detection. In *IoTBDS* (pp. 57–68).

Sai, S., Gaur, A., Sai, R., Chamola, V., Guizani, M., & Rodrigues, J. J. (2024). Generative AI for Transformative Healthcare: A Comprehensive Study of Emerging Models, Applications, Case Studies and Limitations. IEEE Access.

Said, A., Yahyaoui, A., & Abdellatif, T. (2023, November). HIPAA and GDPR Compliance in IoT Healthcare Systems. In *International Conference on Model and Data Engineering* (pp. 198–209). Cham: Springer Nature Switzerland.

Sarker, I. H. (2024). Generative AI and Large Language Modeling in Cybersecurity. In *AI-Driven Cybersecurity and Threat Intelligence: Cyber Automation, Intelligent Decision-Making and Explainability* (pp. 79–99). Cham: Springer Nature Switzerland.

Thirunavukarasu, A. J., Ting, D. S. J., Elangovan, K., Gutierrez, L., Tan, T. F., & Ting, D. S. W. (2023). Large language models in medicine. *Nature Medicine*, 29(8), 1930–1940.

Xiang, D., & Cai, W. (2021). Privacy protection and secondary use of health data: strategies and methods. *BioMed Research International*, 2021.

Yinka-Banjo, C., & Ugot, O. A. (2020). A review of generative adversarial networks and its application in cybersecurity. *Artificial Intelligence Review*, 53, 1721–1736.

6 Navigating the Ethereal
Ethical Frameworks in AI for Healthcare

Bodhibrata Nag, Mahesh Devnani and Ranjan Pal

6.1 INTRODUCTION

Artificial intelligence (AI) has been used in healthcare since the 1970s, reaching the market size shown in Figure 6.1, with more than 300 AI/ML technologies approved by the FDA. Prominent market players include Koninklijke Philips, Intel, Microsoft, IBM, Siemens Healthineers, Nvidia, Google, General Electric, Amazon Web Services, Medtronic, Micron Technology, Johnson & Johnson, General Vision, and CloudmedX. AI-driven technologies include virtual health assistants, personalized therapies, diagnostics, clinical decision-making, smart digital medications, and remote robotic procedures (Pasricha, 2023; Guan, 2019). In 2018, the FDA approved Idx-DR for detecting retinopathy, showing the impact of AI in diagnosing eye conditions. Healthcare platforms use AI to monitor user interactions for mental health issues, but may face privacy and consent issues. Other applications include (Pham, 2021; Xing, Giger, & Min, 2021; Najarian, 2022; Lidstromer & Ashrafian, 2022):

- Machine learning methods are being used to generate sophisticated disease models that replicate sickness development using advanced computing and computer vision techniques. Clinicians may use these models to forecast cancer and cardiovascular disease outcomes and establish proactive treatment plans.
- Predictive models in healthcare harness data from electronic health records, genomics, wearable devices, and clinical trials to forecast patient health outcomes. These algorithms identify disease-risk people for earlier interventions and individualized treatment. AI may, however, misdiagnose patient deterioration using predictive analytics.
- AI systems are transforming diagnostics by utilizing machine learning algorithms for early detection and prediction of medical issues. These algorithms scan medical imaging, genetic profiles, and electronic health records for illness trends. Predictive models provide genetic markers of illness susceptibility, enabling timely interventions and targeted treatments.
- AI and data science offer personalized treatment plans by analyzing health profiles, including genetics, lifestyle, and clinical history. Wearable technology provides real-time physiological data for early prevention and

DOI: 10.1201/9781003503385-6

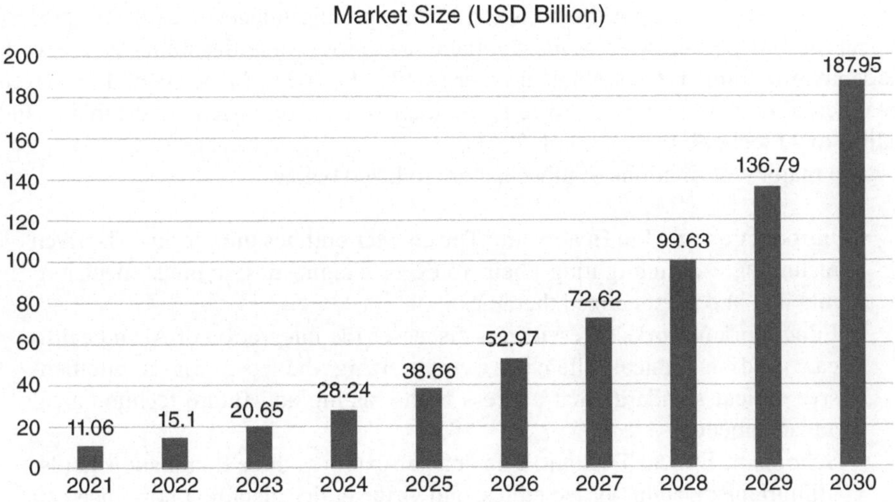

FIGURE 6.1 Size of AI in Healthcare Market.

Source: Chart generated using data from Precedence Research Report (Precedence Research, 2023).

intervention. Smart gadgets using AI can detect minute changes in patients' bodies that may indicate illness or disease progression, making it easier to monitor them outside of hospitals.

- Electronic health records centralize a patient's information, making it easier for doctors and nurses to access and lowering the number of tests needed.
- IBM's Watson personalized cancer treatments using patient data, but hazardous and inaccurate therapies cast doubt on AI's accuracy. Issues included unsupervised machine use and speculative training data.
- Google's DeepMind has been used to improve the NHS's ability to identify specific health conditions in patients by studying medical photos. However, using patient data without permission was criticized. This showed the necessity of AI transparency and patient acceptability.

Healthcare practitioners have historically prioritized high-quality care, patient autonomy, and fairness to build trust with patients. Early embryo screening and sex selection avoid genetic problems but raise eugenics concerns (Schneiderman, 1990). The application of AI in otolaryngology raises ethical concerns related to the notion of autonomy, as patients may need detailed information regarding the potential hazards and advantages connected with AI technology (Arambula & Bur, 2020). These issues demonstrate the importance of ethics in healthcare.

However, AI in the healthcare sector has raised ethical questions that challenge long-held ideas about patient care and decision-making (Kasula, 2024; Chukwuka, 2023). AI-powered healthcare is a major shift in how we conceptualize, provide, and manage healthcare. AI and robotics have changed healthcare practitioners' roles, as they now oversee AI algorithms instead of interpreting images. Healthcare professionals and AI/robotic systems must collaborate to foster interdisciplinary teamwork and maximize human-technological synergy (Elendu, 2023). In the era of data-driven healthcare, doctors may need to redefine their roles as knowledge custodians and adjust to AI technologies (Arnold, 2021).

The major contributions of this chapter are listed below:

- Introduction of AI in Healthcare: The chapter outlines the various AI-driven technologies, highlighting their roles in diagnostics, clinical decision-making, and personalized therapies.
- Ethical Frameworks Overview: It discusses the integration of AI in healthcare and its ethical dilemmas, emphasizing the need for comprehensive ethical standards that address both existing and future technological advancements.
- Schools of Ethical Thought: The chapter explores three dominant schools: utilitarianism, rights-based ethics, and virtue ethics, detailing how each can govern AI ethics effectively.
- Principles-Based Ethical Frameworks: Various frameworks like the Ken Blanchard and Norman Vincent Peale framework, and the Markkula Center Framework are described, offering structured methods for high-level decision-making in AI ethics.
- Key Ethical Principles in Healthcare: The core principles such as autonomy, confidentiality, beneficence, non-maleficence, justice, and transparency are elaborated, explaining their importance in the ethical application of AI in healthcare.
- Practical Applications and Issues: The chapter highlights practical applications of AI in healthcare like personalized treatment plans and predictive diagnostics, while also addressing the potential issues such as data privacy, patient autonomy, and AI transparency.
- Future Directions and Challenges: It discusses the evolving nature of ethical frameworks necessary to handle new challenges posed by AI in a technologically advanced world, emphasizing the importance of continuous updates and stakeholder involvement in ethical governance.

6.2 ETHICAL FRAMEWORKS

Ethics is a systematic study of right and wrong, with morality being the common term for good and bad (Kazim & Koshiyama, 2021). Computer ethics analyzes the social impact of computer technology and the formulation of ethical policies (Moor, 2006). Machine ethics focuses on providing ethical principles for machines to resolve ethical dilemmas and make ethical decisions (Anderson, 2011). Law and ethics are closely intertwined for accountability and enforcement. As we enter this historic moment, it is crucial to create comprehensive ethical standards and principles that address existing issues and adapt to future technological advancements in AI. These frameworks must be efficient and adaptable to address existing challenges and ensure accountability and enforcement in the healthcare industry.

6.2.1 Schools of Ethical Thought

AI ethics can be governed ethically through three dominant schools of normative ethics: utilitarianism, rights-based ethics, and virtue ethics. Utilitarianism (also known as teleology is associated with Jeremy Bentham and John Stuart Mill) focuses on the consequences of actions and decisions made by AI systems, aiming for the maximization of overall happiness and reduction of suffering (Candee & Puka, 1984). It requires frameworks to weigh benefits against potential harms, such as ensuring automated decisions don't exacerbate existing healthcare disparities (Portmore, 2020). Rights-based ethics (also known as deontology and is often associated with Immanuel Kant) emphasizes respecting and protecting the rights of individuals, ensuring that actions align with established moral norms (Candee & Puka, 1984). This approach enforces data privacy and security regulations, ensuring that patients' sensitive health data are handled ethically. Virtue ethics, also known as axiology, focuses on the character and moral virtues that individuals and AI systems should exhibit. It encourages AI systems to foster virtues like honesty, justice, and empathy, supporting human flourishing by promoting ethical behavior and decision-making that aligns with human values. Virtue-based frameworks also emphasize the continuous cultivation of trustworthiness in AI, ensuring that systems remain reliable and aligned with the fundamental goals of improving patient care (Orsi, 2015).

These ethical theories contribute to frameworks that guide the responsible development, implementation, and use of AI in healthcare. Ethical frameworks provide a comprehensive set of principles, values, and processes to govern high-level decision-making, providing flexibility for interpretation and implementation in various situations and scenarios. Two well-known frameworks include the Ken Blanchard and Norman Vincent Peale framework, which focuses on legality, fairness, and emotional impact, and the Markkula Center Framework, which identifies five approaches (including the utilitarianism approach, rights approach, fairness or justice approach, common good approach, and virtue approach).

6.2.2 Key Components of Ethical Frameworks

The Hippocratic Oath embodies a historical ethical framework that still influences modern medical practice. Other principles include the World Medical Association's 1964 resolution (also known as the Helsinki Declaration) and the 1979 Belmont Report on ethical principles governing medical research using human subjects. The core principles of healthcare ethical frameworks include autonomy, confidentiality, beneficence, nonmaleficence, justice and equity, and transparency (Pasricha, 2023). Autonomy respects patients' rights to make informed decisions, while confidentiality ensures personal information is shared only with authorized individuals (Vuori, 1977). Beneficence promotes patient well-being and enhances care quality. Non-maleficence avoids harm to the patient, preventing physical harm and guarding against psychological impacts. Justice and equity ensure the fair distribution of healthcare resources and treating all patients equitably. Transparency entails the practice of openly communicating the functions, judgments, and data of AI systems, which helps to cultivate confidence among users.

An example of a principles-based approach is the Google's AI Principles (Google, 2023). The objective is to ensure that AI is useful to society, eliminates unfair bias, prioritizes safety in development and testing, remains accountable to individuals, incorporates privacy design principles, maintains high scientific standards, and is accessible for uses that align with these principles.

The Asilomar AI Principles (Future of Life Institute, 2017), published by Future of Life Institute in 2017, is a second example of principles-based approach. It emphasizes the utmost need for ensuring the safety and security of AI systems during their entire lifespan. They also emphasize failure transparency, judicial transparency, responsibility, value alignment, human values, personal privacy, liberty and privacy, shared benefit, shared prosperity, human control, non-subversion, risks, and recursive self-improvement.

The Montreal Declaration for Responsible AI (Morandín-Ahuerma, 2023) is a third example of principles-based approach. It strives to meet accessibility, justifiability, and intelligibility standards; promote justice and equality; protect social and cultural variety; be cautious in AI development; and ensure environmental sustainability. It also promotes the well-being of all sentient beings, respects autonomy, protects privacy and intimacy against intrusion, and data acquisition and archiving systems (DAAS).

The Ethics Guidelines for Trustworthy AI (European Commission High-Level Expert Group on AI, 2019), published in 2019, by the High-Level Expert Group on Artificial Intelligence of the European Commission is a fourth example of principles-based approach. It introduced "trustworthy AI" and listed seven requirements: privacy, accountability, human agency and oversight, and human agency and oversight. The IEEE Global Initiative on Ethics of Autonomous and Intelligent Systems (IEEE, 2019) introduced the Ethically Aligned Design document, which recommends values-based design and provides a framework for ethical discussions.

Rules or guidelines are explicit instructions that restrict behavior or decision-making under certain conditions. They aim to limit harmful consequences while advising governments and AI practitioners on establishing socially beneficial AI systems. They give precise instructions, usually in the form of standards. International guidelines include the GDPR (European Union, 2016), the AMA's Policy on Augmented Intelligence in Medicine (American Medical Association, 2018), and the WHO's Guidelines on Ethics and Governance for AI in Health (World Health Organisation, 2021; Katirai, 2023).

The comprehensive Responsible Research and Innovation (RI) framework addresses risks and uncertainties associated with developing technologies like AI. (Guan, 2019). Establishing stakeholder trust and resolving AI technology risks and uncertainties promotes ethical governance. The European Commission's Ethics Guidelines for Trustworthy AI describe "trustworthy AI" and prescribe ethical AI development, implementation, and use. The framework's principles include autonomy, damage prevention, justice, and explicability.

An ethical framework commonly includes protocols for resolving ethical difficulties. This process involves participating in talks with relevant parties, assessing the prospective results of different options, and reaching a balanced compromise between conflicting principles. This dynamic structure must adapt to new challenges, especially in a connected and technologically advanced world.

AI integration in healthcare requires regular evaluations and audits to ensure protocol compliance and ethical purity (Hisan & Amri, Artificial Intelligence for Human Life: A Critical Opinion from Medical Bioethics Perspective—Part II, 2022b). To keep rules relevant and address new ethical issues as AI technology advances, regulatory frameworks must be adaptive.

AI healthcare must follow non-discrimination rules to maintain legal accountability and individual rights. Legal systems must be integrated and standardized to handle legal issues and ensure ethical AI use in healthcare (Dokter & Kedokteran, 2023).

Cultural diversity, dynamic contexts, clashing values, balancing innovation and ethical compliance, and changing regulatory landscapes are all challenges for AI ethics. Cultural diversity can lead to different ethical concepts, making it difficult to create universal standards (Coeckelbergh, 2020). AI regulation debates center on international and national government roles. Some advocate strong international AI restrictions, while others prefer customized ones. Global AI ethical norms are necessary for trust and collaboration between states for equitable AI technology development and use. The geographic concentration of AI ethics guidelines, predominantly from economically developed countries, may contribute to bias (Gupta & Heath, 2020) and promote inequalities in the Global South (Astobiza, 2022). Addressing data poverty is essential for inclusive and representative health data (Amini, 2023).

Some researchers advocate for a human rights approach (HRA) as a guiding framework for those involved in AI development, transcending national boundaries and offering a common normative language. (Wong, 2019) elucidates that the use of human rights in HRA serves a dual purpose: first, it establishes a normative benchmark to identify, anticipate, and assess the adverse (or beneficial) effects of AI technologies; and second, it provides a set of legal and institutional measures to prevent, mitigate, and address the harm caused by these technologies within existing legal and institutional frameworks (Yeung, Howes, & Pogrebna, 2019) proposed a comprehensive rationale for a governance framework centered on human rights principles in design, deliberation, and oversight. This framework is built on human rights norms and principles, uses a cohesive and integrated set of technical, organizational, and evaluative tools and methods, is accountable to legally mandated external oversight by an independent regulatory body with appropriate investigative and enforcement authority, and facilitates meaningful engagement and consultation with stakeholders and the public (Wong, 2019; Yeung, Howes, & Pogrebna, 2019).

6.3 CORE PRINCIPLES

The core principles of AI in healthcare are confidentiality, data protection, beneficence, non-maleficence, justice and equity, transparency, and patient autonomy, as shown in Figure 6.2. These principles enable trust building as well as regulatory compliance.

6.3.1 Patient Autonomy and AI

Healthcare relies on patient autonomy to let patients make informed decisions about their care. AI in healthcare presents new challenges and opportunities for this principle. AI can improve decision-making by analyzing massive amounts of data and

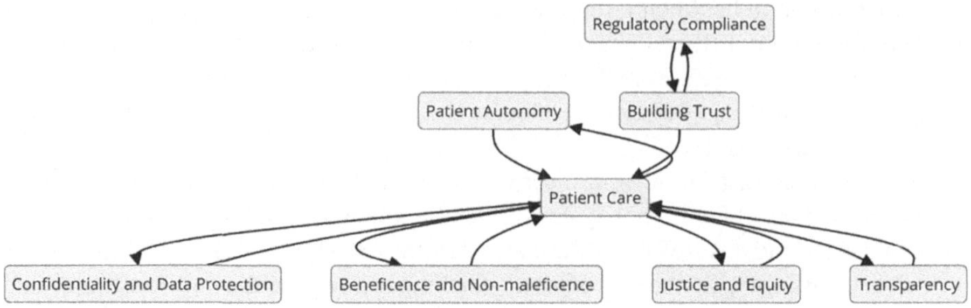

FIGURE 6.2 Core Principles of AI in Healthcare.

Source: Generated by authors.

providing insights, but it also hinders patient autonomy. AI technology must be balanced with patient agency to preserve patient autonomy (Pasricha, 2023).

6.3.2 Confidentiality and Data Protection

Another ethical issue in healthcare AI is how patient data is used to train AI systems. Maintaining patient trust and following data protection laws requires strong data protection and privacy (Pasricha, 2023).

The healthcare industry's use of AI has raised concerns about data security and confidentiality (Jeyaraman, 2023a, 2023b; Anyanwu, 2024). Given the large amounts of personal health information (PHI) AI systems handle, they must be designed to protect sensitive data. Internationally, HIPAA and GDPR govern healthcare data privacy and security. These regulations require healthcare providers and organizations that handle PHI to implement sufficient security measures to protect data integrity and confidentiality. AI systems should use encryption, access controls, and audit trails to protect PHI and restrict data access to authorized personnel. Another relevant concept is data owner rights in healthcare AI applications. Understanding and communicating these rights to data owners is essential for ethical data practices (Amini, 2023).

Advanced technical safeguards are employed to counter the risks associated with digital data management, including state-of-the-art encryption techniques, rigorous access controls, and regular security audits. AI algorithms must be designed to inherently protect data using techniques like differential privacy, homomorphic encryption, secure multiparty computation, and convolutional neural networks (Jeyaraman, 2023a, 2023b). To safeguard data and ensure data privacy, legislation defining the purposes of data collection, organizational measures governing data handling practices, administrative measures, and technical measures focusing on the physical security of premises, encryption, access controls, and other technical safeguards are essential (Vuori, 1977).

6.3.3 Beneficence and Non-maleficence

AI technologies can analyze medical data and find patterns that humans may miss, improving patient outcomes. Beneficence involves prioritizing patient well-being.

Non-maleficence requires healthcare professionals to prevent harm, which is difficult with AI. AI system accuracy is a major concern because misdiagnoses can lead to ineffective treatments that endanger patients. For instance, the patient may receive needless and possibly hazardous treatments if an AI system misclassifies a benign ailment as malignant (Kelly, 2019). To uphold the principle of non-maleficence, rigorous testing and validation are crucial. Robust cybersecurity measures are essential to protect patient data and prevent AI systems from becoming sources of harm (Naik, 2022).

6.3.4 Justice and Equity in AI

Justice and equity in healthcare AI deployments are ethical issues. It aims to give all patients fair access to AI technologies and services. This principle is essential for healthcare equity (Pasricha, 2023) and social welfare. AI applications should undergo careful examination to assess their technical effectiveness and evaluate their effects on various demographic groups. This includes training diagnostic algorithms using diverse datasets and subjecting them to rigorous testing in real-world environments.

However, the "digital divide," which can result in differences in the accessibility of AI-enhanced services, makes it difficult to achieve this level of fairness. Making AI tools accessible and usable across all healthcare infrastructures—especially in underserved areas—is necessary to address this. Furthermore, AI systems have the ability to reinforce or duplicate preexisting biases in historical health data, which can result in unequal treatment outcomes (Pasricha, 2023; Hisan & Amri, 2022a, 2022b). To adapt to new data and patient needs, healthcare organizations should use transparent data collection and algorithm training and monitor and update AI systems. Multidisciplinary oversight boards can ensure ethical AI deployment.

6.3.5 Transparency and Interpretability

AI systems' operations, decisions, and data must be disclosed for ethical healthcare AI deployment. Maintaining accountability and building trust with patients, healthcare professionals, and stakeholders requires transparency. Health AI transparency includes system functionality, decisions, and data use. Without transparency, it becomes challenging to ensure accountability and understand the reasoning behind AI-generated recommendations (Upadhyay, 2023). Transparency also requires clearly communicating the limitations of AI systems. Healthcare stakeholders should be informed about the scenarios where AI might not perform well, reducing the risk of overreliance or misuse.

Understanding the system's operational capabilities is key to understanding AI tool decision-making. Healthcare professionals must possess a comprehensive understanding of the reasoning process employed by an AI tool in order to verify its efficacy and incorporate it into clinical decision-making. For instance, a radiologist using an AI tool to detect abnormalities in imaging must comprehend why the system flagged certain anomalies. However, AI-based healthcare devices often operate as black boxes due to the proprietary nature of the algorithms.

Interpretability in AI refers to the ability to understand and explain how machine learning algorithms make decisions or predictions. Interpretability focuses on understanding the inner workings of the models, while explainability focuses on explaining the decisions made. Consequently, interpretability requires a greater level of detail than explainability (Amini, 2023). Tools for evaluating interpretability can help stakeholders comprehend AI processes, leading to more informed decision-making and improved patient outcomes (Morgan & Mates, 2023).

Privacy and security are also essential aspects of transparency. AI developers and healthcare organizations must provide clear information on data privacy practices and measures taken to secure sensitive health information. Patients should be granted the privilege to provide informed consent regarding the utilization of their data, with a comprehensive understanding of the individuals or entities that will have access to it and the specific intentions for which it will be used.

6.4 IMPLICATIONS ON SOCIETY

6.4.1 Role and Impact of Explainable AI (XAI) Frameworks in Society

Explainable AI (XAI) helps healthcare providers and patients understand and track AI decision-making processes, ensuring AI operations comply with ethical standards of transparency and accountability. People trust AI systems more with XAI. Knowing how AI systems handle and protect PHI makes stakeholders more likely to trust them with sensitive data. XAI also simplifies compliance with laws that require precise data handling and use of records.

Explainable AI (XAI) frameworks aim to make AI systems more transparent, understandable, and accountable, which is crucial in maintaining public trust and ethical integrity in AI applications across various sectors, including healthcare, finance, and law enforcement (Saranya & Subhashini, 2023; Hassija, 2024; Ali, 2023; Chamola, 2023).

XAI also enhances regulatory compliance by providing tools and methodologies that clarify how decisions are made, aiding in adherence to laws such as the GDPR, which requires explainability as part of its right to explanation provision. This leads to better outcomes in AI governance, ensuring that AI acts in the public's interest and respects human rights. The approaches used to achieve explainability are given in Table 6.1.

TABLE 6.1
Approaches to Meet Explainability Requirements

AI Explainability Requirement	Approach to Address the Requirement
Explainability for model developers	Visualization of model internals and testing that verifies operation at the model boundary and beyond
Grounds for automated decision	Computation of relative importance of factors, often portrayed through vertical charts or highlighting of factors in the source stream
Impact of modifying input factors	Combination of sensitivity analysis and forward model operation
Confidence associated with decisions	Computation of uncertainty associated with a given decision
Fairness and impartiality	Analysis and modification of the dataset used for model training using tools for bias evaluation

Source: Bhattacharya and Ramesh (2020).

6.4.2 The Role and Impact of XAI Frameworks in Healthcare

XAI contributes to upholding the ethical principle of autonomy in healthcare. By providing clear explanations of AI-driven decisions, XAI enables patients to make more informed decisions about their treatments, thereby enhancing their autonomy (Jeyaraman, 2023a, 2023b).

XAI requires the implementation of robust mechanisms to ensure data security and patient confidentiality. This leads to strengthened protections against data breaches and unauthorized access to sensitive health information (Anyanwu, 2024).

6.4.3 Challenges of XAI

- Complexity in Implementation: Creating models that are both highly accurate and inherently explainable can be challenging. The trade-off between performance and explainability remains a significant hurdle (Upadhyay, 2023; Amini, 2023).
- Subjectivity in Explanations: What is considered a satisfactory explanation can vary widely among different stakeholders, making standardized approaches difficult.
- Risk of Misinterpretation: Explanations provided by XAI systems could be misinterpreted by users, leading to incorrect conclusions about the AI's decision-making process (Hulsen, 2023).
- Data Privacy Concerns: Generating explanations often requires access to sensitive data, raising concerns about privacy and data protection.
- Scalability Issues: Applying XAI effectively in large-scale systems can be resource-intensive and technically demanding.
- Limited Scope of Explanations: Current XAI methods may not provide the depth of explanation necessary to fully understand complex AI models, particularly in deep learning.
- Bias in Explanations: If not carefully designed, the explanations themselves can be biased, which might mislead users or obscure the presence of biases in AI decisions (Longo, 2024).
- Overreliance on AI: Effective explanations might lead to overreliance on AI systems, assuming that explainability equates to infallibility (Pasricha, 2023).
- Regulatory and Standardization Challenges: Developing regulations that adequately cover the broad spectrum of XAI applications is challenging and requires international cooperation.
- Cost of Development and Maintenance: Developing and maintaining explainable AI systems can be significantly more expensive than traditional AI systems.

6.5 CONCLUSION

AI is revolutionizing the healthcare sector, but it presents contrasting approaches and challenges (Pasricha, 2023). Traditional medical ethics emphasize transparency, accountability, and patient autonomy, while AI ethics struggle to explain complex algorithms and determine accountability. While AI risks algorithmic bias and patient autonomy, traditional medical ethics emphasize equity.

Evolving ethical standards, global regulatory harmonization, and continuous monitoring and compliance are necessary. By addressing these differences and aligning ethical frameworks with technological advances, stakeholders can promote ethical AI integration while protecting patient welfare and healthcare ecosystem trust.

All stakeholders—patients, healthcare providers, AI technologists, ethicists, and policymakers—must collaborate to integrate AI into healthcare (Solanki, 2022). The digital divide and bias can prevent equitable access to AI-enhanced healthcare. Transparency about AI systems' pros and cons build public trust in AI.

To increase awareness of ethical issues among developers, healthcare professionals, and students, ethical education in AI development and healthcare curricula is essential (Pasricha, 2023). In the end, ethical principles and fair healthcare outcomes for all stakeholders can be maintained while medical training advances by implementing responsible AI design techniques (Sqalli, 2023). The inclusion of ethicists in the development process can facilitate the early identification and resolution of ethical considerations (Pasricha, 2023). Finding and resolving ethical issues with AI-based healthcare technologies requires conducting ethical analyses at every stage of the product lifecycle.

AI should serve as a supplementary tool, rather than a substitute for clinical expertise (Petersson, 2023). The purpose of AI is to enhance care and offer supplementary assistance to clinicians, rather than supersede or substitute their expertise.

Due to the ethical and legal implications of using AI in medicine, the lack of regulations is concerning. Without clear guidelines and standards, data breaches, decision-making biases, and patient privacy and safety issues are possible. The lack of regulatory frameworks can make AI-driven healthcare interventions' accountability and responsibility unclear (Naik, 2022; Elendu, 2023; Goirand, 2021).

In conclusion, diverse stakeholders must be involved in AI integration to ensure ethical, patient-centric, and ethical solutions. AI in healthcare requires an adaptable ethical framework, diverse stakeholders, and practical solutions. Patients, healthcare providers, AI technologists, and ethicists participate in healthcare AI development to ensure multiple perspectives shape AI solutions. Explainable artificial intelligence (XAI) is essential for stakeholder trust and understanding. Healthcare AI must be approached ethically. Our ethical and regulatory frameworks must evolve with technology. AI has great potential in healthcare, but it also carries a responsibility. To strengthen medical ethics with AI, we must prioritize morality.

REFERENCES

Ali, S. (2023). Explainable Artificial Intelligence (XAI): What we know and what is left to attain Trustworthy Artificial Intelligence. *Information Fusion*.

American Medical Association. (2018). *Augmented intelligence in health care*. Retrieved from AMA: https://www.ama-assn.org/system/files/2019-01/augmented-intelligence-policy-report.pdf

Amini, M. (2023). Artificial Intelligence Ethics and Challenges in Healthcare Applications: A Comprehensive Review in the Context of the European GDPR Mandate. *Machine Learning & Knowledge Extraction*, *5*(3), 1023–1035.

Anderson, M. &. (2011). *Machine ethics*. Cambridge: Cambridge University Press.
Anyanwu, E. (2024). Artificial Intelligence in healthcare: a review of ethical dilemmas and practical applications. *International Medical Science Research Journal*, *4*(2), 126–140.
Arambula, A. M., & Bur, A. M. (2020). Ethical Considerations in the Advent of Artificial Intelligence in Otolaryngology. *Otolaryngology–Head and Neck Surgery*, *162*(1), 38–39.
Arnold, M. H. (2021). Teasing out Artificial Intelligence in Medicine: An Ethical Critique of Artificial Intelligence and Machine Learning in Medicine. *Bioethical Inquiry*, 121–139.
Astobiza, A. M. (2022). Ethical Governance of AI in the Global South: A Human Rights Approach to Responsible Use of AI. *MDPI Proceedings*, 1–5.
Bhattacharya, P., & Ramesh, N. (2020). *Explainable AI: A practical perspective*. Retrieved from Infosys Knowledge Institute: https://www.infosys.com/about/knowledge-institute/insights/documents/explainable-ai-practical-perspective.pdf
Candee, D., & Puka, B. (1984). An analytic approach to resolving problems in medical ethics. *Journal of Medical Ethics*, 30, 61–70.
Chamola, V. (2023). A Review of Trustworthy and Explainable Artificial Intelligence (XAI). *IEEE Access*, 11, 2169–3536.
Chukwuka, E. (2023). Ethical implications of AI and robotics in healthcare: A review. *Medicine*.
Coeckelbergh, M. (2020). *AI Ethics*. Cambridge: The MIT Press.
Dokter, P., & Kedokteran, F. (2023). Legal Consideration in Implementing Artificial Intelligence when Dealing with Patients in Healthcare Services. *Jurnal Sapientia et Virtus*, 210–224.
Elendu, C. (2023). Ethical implications of AI and robotics in healthcare. *Medicine*, 102, 1–7.
European Commission High-Level Expert Group on AI. (2019, April 8). *Ethics guidelines for trustworthy AI*. Retrieved from European Commission: https://digital-strategy.ec.europa.eu/en/library/ethics-guidelines-trustworthy-ai
European Union. (2016, April 27). *General Data Protection Regulation*. Retrieved from Intersoft Consulting: https://gdpr-info.eu/
Future of Life Institute. (2017, August 11). *Asilomar AI Principles*. Retrieved from Future of Life Institute: https://futureoflife.org/open-letter/ai-principles/
Goirand, M. (2021). Implementing Ethics in Healthcare AI-Based Applications: A Scoping Review. *Science and Engineering Ethics*, 27(5), 61.
Google. (2023). *RESPONSIBILITY: Our Principles*. Retrieved from Google AI: https://ai.google/responsibility/principles/
Guan, J. (2019). Artificial Intelligence in Healthcare and Medicine Promises, Ethical Challenges and Governance. *Chinese Medical Sciences Journal*, 76–83.
Gupta, A., & Heath, V. (2020, September 14). AI ethics groups are repeating one of society's classic mistakes. *MIT Technology Review*. Retrieved from.
Hassija, V. (2024). Interpreting Black-Box Models: A Review on Explainable Artificial Intelligence. *Cognitive Computation*, 45–74.
Hisan, U., & Amri, M. (2022a). Artificial Intelligence for Human Life: A Critical Opinion from Medical Bioethics Perspective – Part I. *Journal of Public Health Sciences*, 1(2), 100–111.
Hisan, U., & Amri, M. (2022b). Artificial Intelligence for Human Life: A Critical Opinion from Medical Bioethics Perspective – Part II. *Journal of Public Health Sciences*, 112–130.
Hulsen, T. (2023). Explainable Artificial Intelligence (XAI): Concepts and Challenges in Healthcare. *AI*, 1(2), 652–666.
IEEE. (2019). *The IEEE Global Initiative on Ethics of Autonomous and Intelligent Systems*. Retrieved from IEEE: https://sagroups.ieee.org/global-initiative/wp-content/uploads/sites/542/2023/01/ead1e.pdf
Jeyaraman, M. (2023a, August 10). *Unraveling the Ethical Enigma: Artificial Intelligence in Healthcare*. Retrieved from PubMed Central: https://www.ncbi.nlm.nih.gov/pmc/articles/PMC10492220/

Jeyaraman, M. (2023b). Unraveling the Ethical Enigma: Artificial Intelligence in Healthcare. *Cureus*, 2–6.

Kasula, B. (2024). Ethical Implications and Future Prospects of Artificial Intelligence in Healthcare: A Research Synthesis. *International Meridian Journal*, 1–7.

Katirai, A. (2023). The ethics of advancing artificial intelligence in healthcare: analyzing ethical considerations for Japan's innovative AI hospital system. *Frontiers of Public Health.*

Kazim, E., & Koshiyama, A. S. (2021). A high-level overview of AI ethics. *Patterns*, 2, 1–12.

Kelly, C. (2019). Key challenges for delivering clinical impact with artificial intelligence. *BMC Medicine*, 17, 1–9.

Lidstromer, N., & Ashrafian, H. (2022). *Artificial Intelligence in Medicine*. Cham, Switzerland: Springer Nature.

Longo, L. (2024). Explainable Artificial Intelligence (XAI) 2.0: A manifesto of open challenges and interdisciplinary research directions. *Information Fusion.*

Moor, J. (2006). The Nature, Importance, and Difficulty of Machine Ethics. *IEEE Intelligent Systems*, 18–21.

Morandín-Ahuerma, F. (2023, September 20). *Montreal Declaration for Responsible AI: 10 Principles and 59 Recommendations*. Retrieved from OSF Preprints: https://osf.io/preprints/osf/sj2z5

Morgan, M., & Mates, J. (2023). Ethics of Artificial Intelligence in Breast Imaging. *Journal of Breast Imaging*, 5(2), 195–200.

Naik, N. (2022). Legal and Ethical Consideration in Artificial Intelligence in Healthcare: Who Takes Responsibility? *Frontiers in Surgery*, 9, 862322.

Najarian, K. (2022). *Artificial Intelligence in Healthcare and Medicine*. Boca Raton, Florida: CRC Press.

Orsi, F. (2015). *Value Theory*. London: Bloomsbury.

Pasricha, S. (2023). AI Ethics in Smart Healthcare. *IEEE Consumer Electronics Magazine*, 12(4), 12–20.

Petersson, L. (2023). Ethical considerations in implementing AI for mortality prediction in the emergency department. *Digital Health*, 9, 20552076231206588.

Pham, T. D. (2021). *Advances in Artificial Intelligence, Computation, and Data Science For Medicine and Life Science*. Cham, Switzerland: Springer.

Portmore, D. W. (2020). *The Oxford Book of Consequentialism*. New York: Oxford University Press.

Precedence Research. (2023, February). *Artificial Intelligence in Healthcare Market Size, Share, and Trends 2024 to 2034*. Retrieved from Precedence Research: https://www.precedenceresearch.com/artificial-intelligence-in-healthcare-market

Saranya, A., & Subhashini, R. (2023). A systematic review of Explainable Artificial Intelligence models and applications: Recent developments and future trends. *Decision Analytics Journal*, 7(2023), 100230.

Schneiderman, L. J. (1990). Still Saving the Life of Ethics. *The Hastings Center Report*, 22–24.

Solanki, P. (2022). Operationalising ethics in artificial intelligence for healthcare: a framework for AI developers. *AI and Ethics*, 3(1), 223–240.

Sqalli, M. (2023). Humanizing AI in medical training ethical framework for responsible design. *Frontiers in Artificial Intelligence*, 6, 1189914.

Upadhyay, U. (2023). Call for the responsible artificial intelligence in the healthcare. *BMJ Health & Care Informatics*, 30(1), 1–4.

Vuori, H. (1977). Privacy, confidentiality and automated health information systems. *Journal of Medical Ethics*, 174–178.

Wong, P. (2019). Cultural differences as excuses? Human rights and cultural values in global ethics and governance of AI. *Philosophy & Technology*, 33(4), 705–715.

World Health Organisation. (2021, June 28). *Ethics and governance of artificial intelligence for health-WHO Guidance*. Retrieved from World Health Organisation: https://www.who.int/publications/i/item/9789240029200

Xing, L., Giger, M., & Min, J. (2021). *Atificial Intelligence in Medicine-Technical Basis and Clinical Applications*. London: Elsevier Academic Press.

Yeung, K., Howes, A., & Pogrebna, G. (2019). AI governance by human rights-centred design, deliberation and oversight: An end to ethics washing. In M. Dubber, & F. Pasquale, *The Oxford Handbook of AI Ethics*. Oxford: Oxford University Press.

7 Case Study on Explainable Artificial Intelligence in Healthcare Diagnostics

Muskan Jalan, Malhar Desai, Sunik Malik and Gurpreet Kaur Grewal

7.1 INTRODUCTION

"Health" is defined by the World Health Organisation (WHO) as a condition of whole mental, bodily, and social well-being rather than just the absence of illness or disability. A variety of diagnostic tests are available on the market to detect diseases and aid in health investigations. New research has emerged on artificial intelligence (AI) in healthcare, which plays a key part in disease diagnostics, patient profiles, and precision medicine (Loh et al., 2022). AI is defined as a computer's ability to fulfill tasks which usually need human intelligence, like image processing, decision-making, and speech recognition (Joiner, 2018). Machine learning (ML) is a part of AI, while Deep Learning (DL) is a component of ML, and the backbone of DL consists of neural networking. AI has numerous applications in different fields, including education, finance, marketing, E-commerce, social media, chatbots, agriculture, and healthcare. AI has been used in the detection of Alzheimer's, skin disease, liver disease, chronic diseases, cancer, and tuberculosis so far (Y. Kumar et al., 2022). Conventional Neural Networking (CNN) and Artificial Neural Networking (ANN) are the two types of neural networks used in clinical diagnosis by analysis and interpretation of medical images (Shahid et al., 2019; Sarvamangala & Kulkarni, 2021).

Because the internal algorithms are opaque and only the input and output programs can be seen, AI has been rendered as a "black box" (Durán & Jongsma, 2021). Patients and physicians have no idea how it works, making it difficult for them to trust the results of AI-generated diagnoses (Xu & Shuttleworth, 2024). DL models are extremely complex to understand, making it challenging to catch and rectify any errors in the event of an incorrect diagnosis, which may lead to the death of the patient in extreme cases. This makes it one of the primary reasons behind the complications of using AI models in healthcare, owing to the increased liability and safety issues due to its "black box" nature, as per the European General Data Protection Regulation (GDPR) (May, 2018), which deals with a patient's life and

 DOI: 10.1201/9781003503385-7

data privacy (Holzinger et al., 2022). One of the major limitations of black box AI is that it compromises personal values such as patient data privacy when it comes to diagnosis, which is an issue not only for the patients but also for the physicians treating them (Chan, 2023). To address the lack of transparency, privacy concerns, explanation, and predictability of AI, (Xu & Shuttleworth, 2024) a new model known as Explainable Artificial Intelligence (XAI) has been developed to transform black box AI into a transparent glass box, attempting to explain the algorithms to humans (Allen, 2024; Holzinger et al., 2022).

In this chapter, we have described XAIs and its principles as well as the detailed classifications of XAI. We have also elaborated on XAI models put in use for healthcare.

- **Section 7.2** discusses the features and models of explainable artificial intelligences
- **Section 7.3** covers various case studies of XAI models used in diagnoses of various diseases
- **Section 7.4** focuses on limitations of XAI
- **Section 7.5** describes conclusion and future directions

7.2 EXPLAINABLE ARTIFICIAL INTELLIGENCE (XAI)

In recent years, many studies have been put forward to explain the complex models of DL, ML, and neural networking, but XAI has been widely considered to resolve the black box of AI. XAI is a promising AI discipline which brings transparency to the opaque AI algorithm, which is complex for the laypeople to understand (Samek, 2023). The term Explainable Artificial intelligence was coined by DARPA (Defence Advanced Research Projects Agency), USA, in May 2017 (Holzinger et al., 2022). According to DARPA, *XAI is a new generation machine learning technique that can explain its logic and can define its weaknesses and strengths.* XAI is also called the "third wave of AI" of the DARPA program, where ML and their explanatory models allow them to understand the real world and environment (Sholapur, 2022). The core aim of XAI is explaining the reason behind AI outcomes for both humans and computers (Sudar et al., 2022). To date, XAI has been used in various fields such as demand forecasting, finance, agriculture, computer vision, remote sensing and signal processing, and the healthcare domain. The application of XAI in various fields is based on three features, viz. interpretability, transparency, and explainability (Chaddad et al., 2023). XAI is classified into multiple types based on its scope (Kamakshi & Krishnan, 2023), stages (Hulsen, 2023), and specificity (Kamakshi & Krishnan, 2023), with different types of XAI models existing under each category (Figure 7.1).

7.2.1 Types of XAI Model

7.2.1.1 Surrogate-based XAI

The Local Interpretable Model-agnostic Explanation (LIME) seeks to elucidate classifier predictions based on locally located instances (ElShawi et al., 2020). It acts as a surrogate model that tries to fit a new model around the local instances of the AI

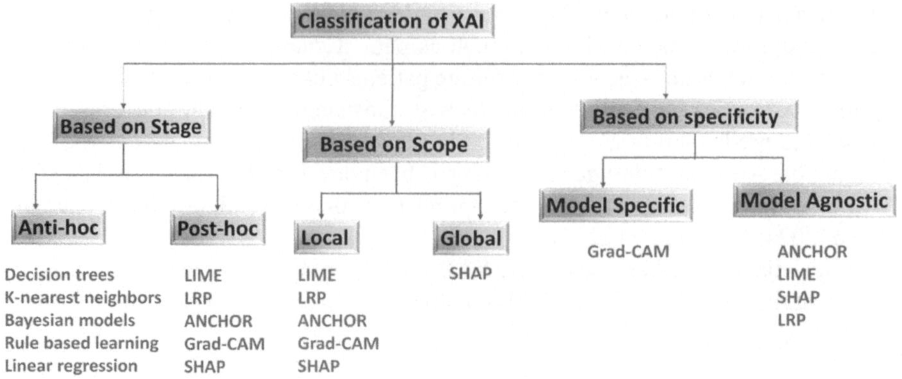

FIGURE 7.1 Classification of Explainable Artificial Intelligence (XAI) into different categories based on stage, scope, and specificity with their distinct subtypes.

* **SHAP: Shapley Additive Explanation, LRP: Layer Wise Relevance Propagation, LIME: Local Interpretability Model-agnostics Explanation, Grad-CAM: Gradient weighted Class Activation Mapping.**

decision boundary. LIME functions on the set of steps (Palatnik de Sousa et al., 2019). The image generated by the black box is nonlinear and consists of various groups of instances; LIME selects the local instance present near the classifier's decision boundary and constructs a surrogate linear model. LIME process involves creating a super pixel image, filling it with solid black, and using the kernel function to weight it appropriately. The next step in LIME is fitting a simple interpretable model, such as a Decision Tree Regressor, for predicting perturbed images and generate weights. The final step in LIME is to plot the super pixels of the perturbed image. This allows us to analyze the outcome based on the number of instances that contribute to the prediction. Different disease predictions, such as Parkinson's (Magesh et al., 2020), cardiovascular disease (Paudel et al., 2023), and COVID-19 (Chadaga et al., 2023) have been done using LIME.

7.2.1.2 Pixel-based XAI

Layer wise relevance propagation (LRP) is an XAI method used for explaining neural networks, with inputs such as MRI scans in the case of Alzheimer's. As for the methodology behind LRP, it operates by examining an image through backward propagation of the output. It works on each input feature, calculating a relevant score at each level, which is then combined to produce the expected output (Montavon et al., 2019). LPR is also known as pixel-wise explanation, in which a positive relevant score indicates that the pixels were relevant for prediction and a negative score indicates the opposite. This results in the generation of a heatmap, making it easier for people to identify the problem (Bach et al., 2015). In one recent study (Sudar et al., 2022), LRP was used to diagnose Alzheimer's disease using VGG 16.

7.2.1.3 Local and Global-based Model

Shapley Additive explanation (SHAP) is an agnostic model XAI tool used to assign the desired Shapley value (as introduced in 1951 by Lloyd Shapley (Hart, 2008)) to each feature based on the contribution of each feature to the desired outcome. Shapley value represents the weighted average contribution of a particular feature. It is centered on coalitional game theory, where the values are fairly distributed among the players, where the contributions of players are unequal. Diseases such as chronic kidney disease (Raihan et al., 2023), COVID-19 (Chadaga et al., 2023), and uterine fibroids (Mahmoud et al., 2014) have been predicted using SHAP.

7.2.1.4 Visualization-based Model

Class Activation Mapping (CAM) is an XAI approach which uses the last layer of conventional neural networks consisting of the most distinctive spatial features of our predictive class, which helps in creating the heatmap. In CAM, global averaging pooling is applied to each feature map of the last CNN layer. These pooled feature maps then act as the input layer for the fully connected layers (FC layers), which are used to connect two distinct layers and are made up of neurons and weights, and by assigning the weights to the previous CNN layer, the areas with greater characterization of CNN decision are highlighted as a heatmap.

The CAM model cannot be used for pre-trained networks or networks that do not follow the specified fully convolutional neural networking architecture, so to overcome this problem, Gradient-weighted Class Activation Mapping (Grad-CAM) is used (Angelov et al., 2021). Grad-CAM is mostly employed for the visualization of images, as it uses both forward and backward propagation for the localization of the objects in the CNN. Grad-CAM calculates the gradients for the class with respect to each feature map generated from the last CNN layer, then it averages all the gradients through Global Average Pooling (GAP) to assign a weight to a feature map, and the summation of each weighted map corresponds to the class. Also, as an activation function, it uses ReLU (Rectified linear unit) to get only the features influencing positive results of the class of interest and generating the desired heatmap (Selvaraju et al., 2019). Grad CAM++ is another version of Grad-CAM, which can be used for multi-classification of the data, where the variable weight assigned to each pixel allows the gradient feature map to detect the significance of each pixel distinctly. For high-resolution and class-discriminative visualization, an upgraded version of Grad-CAM have been designed, known as Guided Grad-CAM (Saranya & Subhashini, 2023). Studies have been performed where Grad-CAM has been used as a visualization tool to predict COVID-19 (Rajpal et al., 2021) and colon cancer (Sholapur & Indiramma, 2022).

7.2.1.5 Anchor

One of the drawbacks of LIME is that it is sometimes difficult to say that the explanation given by LIME for a specific attribute is applied to the area where the attribute is present. Anchor, a model-agnostic local explainer model, overcomes this limitation of LIME. Anchor works by finding the attributes that are sufficient for the specific prediction such that altering the other attributes does not affect the final prediction. It uses different approaches for the explanation, such as bottom-up approach, beam-search approach, and greedy approach. The beam-search approach is the most reliable approach because it upholds a set of candidate rules and guides the search in order to choose the anchor with the greatest coverage, from multiple potential anchors. Anchors ensure that predictions for instances in the same anchor are almost the same (ElShawi et al., 2020). The anchor model has been used for diagnosing COVID-19 using hematological markers (Chadaga et al., 2023).

7.3 CASE STUDIES

XAI models have been extensively applied in the field of healthcare when studying cardiac, pulmonary, and neurological diseases, among others, a few examples of which have been elaborated on in this section.

7.3.1 XAI for Brain

7.3.1.1 Alzheimer's Disease

Alzheimer's disease (AD) is one of the most typical kinds of dementia, where the patient suffers from mild memory loss at first, that gradually interferes with daily activities and causes irregular impairment in a person's personality, such as language, judgment, memory, reasoning, and identification. The major causes of AD are aging, autonomic nervous system degeneration (cholinergic and cortical pathways), genetic factors such as Beta-amyloid precursor protein aggression, and environmental factors (A. Armstrong, 2013). Diagnosis of AD can be done through magnetic resonance imaging (MRI), positron emission tomography (PET), and biomarkers by identifying them in the cerebrospinal fluid (Bomasang-Layno & Bronsther, 2021).

Case study: In a recent study (Sudar et al., 2022), LRP was used to diagnose AD and predict the most relevant region for AD using the generated heatmap. This work also included the combination of LRP with conventional neural networks, with Visual Geometry Group (VGG-16) being used as a CNN to classify MRI-scan images. They divided the dataset into four classes: non-demented, moderately demented, very mild demented, and mildly demented, and using VGG-16, researchers selected the Alzheimer-specific features that were present in a large amount. After applying VGG-16, the researchers used the XAI-based LRP to re-examine the image generated by VGG-16 through backward propagation of each input level. At each input level, the LRP accurately plotted the pixels of selected features and generated four different heatmaps for all four classes. Finally, the researchers were able to diagnose and explain Alzheimer's using a heatmap that depicted brain shrinkage in demented images.

7.3.2 XAI for Heart

Cardiovascular disorders (CVD): Disorders such as coronary artery disease (CAD), peripheral artery disease, aortic atherosclerosis, etc., are some of the major reasons for mortality globally. CAD is the most common heart disease affecting the blood vessels passing through the heart and may lead to acute myocardial infarction (heart attack) (Sjögren et al., 2015). Diabetes, hypertension, obesity, lack of exercise, and smoking are some of the causes of CVD (Flora & Nayak, 2019). There are various types of tests available for the prediction of heart diseases, such Electrocardiogram, echocardiogram, Chest-X-ray, Coronary CT angiography, MRI, and Chest CT etc. (Counseller & Aboelkassem, 2023).

Case study: An application of LIME was used for the prediction of an early Heart Attack with the aid of 4 ML models in one study from 2023 (Paudel et al., 2023). They extracted publicly available heart disease datasets from Kaggle with eight specific attributes (age, impulse, gender, pressure low, pressure height, creatine kinase-myocardial band (CK-MB), troponin, glucose). After pre-processing, out of 1319 samples, the data was split into an 80:20 train-test ratio in which 1055 samples were used for training and 264 samples for testing. All eight parameters were analyzed each by 4 ML models – Ada Boast Classifier (ABC), Random Forest (RF), Gradient Boasting (GB), and Light Gradient-Boasting Machine (LGBM) to classify the samples as normal and attack. Evaluation of each model was done based on Precision, Recall, F1 score, confusion matrix, and PR curve (AUC value), and the outcomes are displayed in Table 7.1. Out of four models, LGBM was seen with a maximum accuracy level of 99.33%. Along with the prediction of the models, explanation of each model's outcome was also performed using LIME. Table 7.2 highlights the analysis of LIME for each model based on instances responsible for heart attacks. With the help of LIME, researchers could identify CK-MB and Troponin as the two major indicators for heart disease.

7.3.3 XAI FOR LUNGS

COVID-19: COVID-19 is a communicable disease brought on by severe acute respiratory syndrome coronavirus 2 (SARS-Cov-2). It became a global health crisis as it led to more than 6 million deaths globally (Cascella et al., 2023). The symptoms of COVID-19 include fever, cough, sore throat, exhaustion, and difficulty breathing. In certain cases, these symptoms can escalate to pneumonia, acute respiratory distress syndrome (ADRS), and multidrug

TABLE 7.1
Prediction Percentages Based on the AUC Value as Predicted by Various Models

Category/Models	ABC	RF	GB	LGBM
Normal class	18%	0%	0%	0%
Attack class	82%	100%	100%	100%
AUC Values	99%	99%	99%	100%

Ada Boast Classifier (ABC), Random Forest (RF), Gradient Boasting (GB) and Light Gradient-Boasting Machine (LGBM) models were used to classify the samples as normal and attack.

TABLE 7.2
LIME Analysis of Various Models Based on Instances Contributing to Heart Attack

Instances/Models	ABC	RF	GB	LGBM
CK-MB	24%	43%	48%	48%
Troponin	13%	42%	48%	42%
Age	1%	2%	1%	
Pressure height	1%		2%	
Impulse	1%			
Gender				1%
Glucose				1%

creatine kinase-myocardial band (CK-MB), Models-Ada Boast Classifier (ABC), Random Forest (RF), Gradient Boasting (GB) and Light Gradient-Boasting Machine (LGBM).

dysfunction (Singhal, 2020). As of now, the two most common methods for detecting COVID-19 are Chest Computed Tomography (CT) scans and Real-Time Reverse Transcription Polymerase Chain Reaction (RT-PCR), with RT-PCR being the most widely utilized method (Zahan et al., 2022).

Case study: In one study (Rajpal et al., 2021), researchers attempted to analyze the Chest-X-rays (CXRs) of patients with pneumonia and COVID-19 distinctly, since both share similar symptoms and affect the lungs, leading many people to incorrectly diagnosing COVID-19 as pneumonia and vice versa. Differentiating CXR images obtained from COVID-19 and pneumonia patients is an arduous task. For better differentiation, Grad-CAM was used in this case study. For the dataset, 1560 images of CXRs were taken from various sources and divided into three classes: COVID-19, viral and bacterial pneumonia, and normal class.

Three modules were prepared to analyze the three classes to reduce the complexity of the features and increase the reliability of the result. First module consisted of the Conventional neural network tool ResNet50, which uses pre-processed CXR images and improves the overall model capacity which contained 2048 features. The second module was based on the handpicked features, which collected 252 pictures, and the 3rd module was the combination of both, reducing the features to 1000 using a dense layer. Employing the ReLU model, these 1000 features acted as an input that helped in assigning the sample to either one of the three classes. As a result, 97.9% accuracy was observed for COVID-19 prediction. For explaining the model, researchers used Grad-CAM as an XAI. It is a visualization explanation tool which uses a heatmap for the prediction of the disease, highlighting the area of interest with red color responsible for stimulating the last conventional layer of the network, while the blue area serves as verification for class identification. Researchers also confirmed their work with a radiologist who stated that the region of the lung highlighted by the heatmap in red color was indeed primarily affected in COVID-19. A basic overview has been illustrated in Figure 7.2.

7.3.4 XAI for Intestinal Disorders

Colon cancer: The gastrointestinal tract's colon and the rectum of the large intestine, can both be affected by colon cancer (also known as colorectal cancer). Polyp formation leads to colon cancer, where polyps are the small masses formed in the lumen of the colon. Abdominal pain, rectal bleeding, and change in bowel habits are the most common symptoms of this cancer, with change in bowel habits being the most prominent (Ballinger & Anggiansah, 2007) (Prc 2020). The diagnosing and treatment of colon cancer involve surgery, endoscopy, chemotherapy, pathological evaluation, radiotherapy, imaging evaluation, etc.

Case study: In a recently presented study (Sholapur & Indiramma, 2022), histopathological images of colon cancer taken from the Kaggle database were used as a dataset. For this study, the datasets were segregated into two classes: benign colon tissue and colon adenocarcinoma.

10000 images of colon cancer from a sample of 500 HIPPA (Health Insurance Portability and Accountability Act) compliant pictures of colon tissue (250 images of benign colon and colon adenocarcinoma each) were created. Furthermore, two kinds of AI models were employed for the prediction of colon cancer -Inception-ResNet-v2 and Inception V3 layer with validation accuracy of 99.6% and 99.8% respectively.

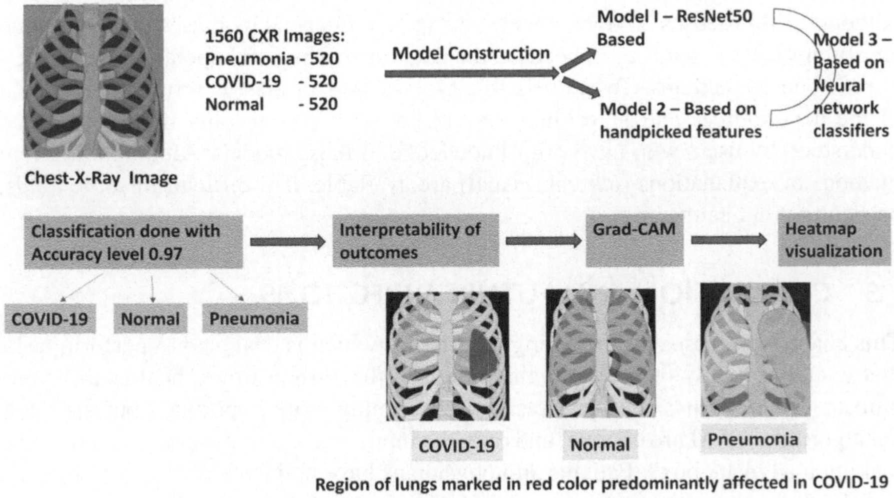

FIGURE 7.2 Workflow for classification of Chest X-ray Images (Rajpal et al., 2021). Three models were used to classify chest X-ray (CXR) lung image data into COVID-19, pneumonia, and normal. The XAI – Grad-CAM was used to generate the heatmap for visualization.

For the explanation of the models' results, researchers used Grad-CAM as an XAI. As mentioned previously, Grad-CAM works by considering the CNN's last layer, whose function in this specific case is an identification of polyp area in cancer. The heatmap was generated for the last conventional layer of the model. Through forward propagation, features were extracted from 768*768 pixels images to the final CNN layer (consisting of polyp region of cancer) and accordingly, feature maps were saved. Further, using the final CNN layer, backpropagation was performed, and weighted gradients were elected for each CNN layer, followed by GAP. For an explanation, heatmaps were generated for the images, highlighting the region of interest of cancer. The middle (near corner) area of heatmaps showed the maximum number of gradients in most of the images, demonstrating the presence of colon cancer.

7.4 LIMITATIONS

Though XAI has the potential to diagnose diseases, there are some limitations as well. There are few models that can interpret other AI models. Also, no explanation user interface (XUI) is available for XAI models. Explaining the model can be difficult at times because it requires the model to be opened up, which may include sensitive and personal information about the patient. It is simple for XAI to interpret CNN models, but it is difficult to develop tools and specific algorithms for DL methods due to their hierarchical architectures and abstract representations. As a result, signal data and biomedical text mining are less explored areas in healthcare. Following the laws and ethics of GPDR, HIPPA, and PIPL, which state that AI algorithms working with healthcare data should be transparent, it becomes more difficult to explain the complex AI algorithm, which is why as of now the explanation is only provided to researchers and not to doctors or patients. Life and Death are the top priorities in healthcare, so clinicians rely more on accuracy than explainability (Hulsen, 2023). Although XAI focuses on transparency, it can be influenced by biases in the data and algorithms used to analyze it, because the data for training and operating the models is provided by humans. To address this type of human bias, careful consideration of the data sources and algorithms should be used. AI can only be operated and understood by users who have prior knowledge of these models. Although different methods of explanations (textual, visual) are available, it is difficult in some fields, particularly in healthcare.

7.5 CONCLUSION AND FUTURE DIRECTIONS

This chapter discusses the emerging field of AI, which is designed to perform tasks that would normally require a human mind. In the current times, healthcare is one industry where AI has been progressively becoming more important., but the internal algorithms of AI are opaque, and only the input and output programs can be seen, making it a "black box". Patients and physicians have no idea how it works, making it difficult for them to trust the results of AI-generated diagnoses. To overcome the problem, DARPA launched Explainable AI, a new AI program that converts the black box to transparent, which is named Explainable AI. XAI is based on Interpretability, Explainability and Transparency, which helps the users to understand the outcome of AI models. From the case studies discussed in this chapter, we can say that XAI can be used in hospitals for the prediction of diseases, but due to certain ethics and laws, if we are working with AI algorithms in healthcare, they should be transparent, which becomes difficult for XAI when it comes to dealing with complex AI algorithms.

Future research projects should work on including healthcare professionals' feedback directed into AI to give accurate output, which can assist in improving clinical outcomes. Ethical concerns and regulatory frameworks need to be set up to protect the privacy rights of patients. Additionally, there is no rating system for different models used in XAI for diagnosis, which should be done to identify which model works best. With the ongoing efforts to resolve the problems with XAI, it will soon be possible to use it as an ideal tool in the field of healthcare. Thus, disease diagnosis in the healthcare sector with the use of XAI will reach a new milestone.

ABBREVIATIONS

AI	Artificial Intelligence
ML	Machine Learning
DL	Deep Learning
NN	Neural networking
CNN	Conventional neural networking
ANN	Artificial neural networking
XAI	Explainable artificial intelligence
LIME	Local Interpretable Model-agnostic Explanation
LRP	Layer wise relevance propagation
SHAP	Shapley Additive explanation
CAM	Class Activation Mapping
Grad-CAM	Gradient-weighted Class Activation Mapping
AD	Alzheimer disease
MRI	Magnetic Resonance imaging
CVD	Cardiovascular Disorder
CXR	Chest-X-ray
ABC	Ada Boast Classifier
RF	Random Forest
LGBM	Light Gradient-Boasting Machine
GB	Gradient Boasting

REFERENCES

Allen, B. (2024). The promise of explainable AI in digital health for precision medicine: a systematic review. *Journal of Personalized Medicine*, *14*(3). https://doi.org/10.3390/JPM14030277

Angelov, P. P., Soares, E. A., Jiang, R., Arnold, N. I., & Atkinson, P. M. (2021). Explainable artificial intelligence: an analytical review. *Wiley Interdisciplinary Reviews Data Mining and Knowledge Discovery*, *11*(5). https://doi.org/10.1002/widm.1424

Armstrong, R. A. (2013). Review article what causes alzheimer's disease? *Folia Neuropathologica*, *3*, 169–188. https://doi.org/10.5114/fn.2013.37702

Bach, S., Binder, A., Montavon, G., Klauschen, F., Müller, K., & Samek, W. (2015). On Pixel-Wise explanations for non-linear classifier decisions by layer-wise relevance propagation. *Plos One*, *10*(7), e0130140. https://doi.org/10.1371/journal.pone.0130140

Ballinger, A. B., & Anggiansah, C. (2007). Colorectal cancer. *BMJ*, *335*(7622), 715–718. https://doi.org/10.1136/bmj.39321.527384.be

Bomasang-Layno, E., & Bronsther, R. (2021). Diagnosis and treatment of Alzheimer's disease. *Delaware Journal of Public Health*, *7*(4), 74–85. https://doi.org/10.32481/djph.2021.09.009

Cascella, M., Rajnik, M., Cuomo, A., Dulebohn, S. C., & Di Napoli, R. (2023). Features, evaluation, and treatment of coronavirus (COVID-19). *StatPearls*. https://www.ncbi.nlm.nih.gov/books/NBK554776/

Chadaga, K., Prabhu, S., Bhat, V., Sampathila, N., Umakanth, S., & Chadaga, R. (2023). Artificial intelligence for diagnosis of mild–moderate COVID-19 using haematological markers. *Annals of Medicine*, *55*(1). https://doi.org/10.1080/07853890.2023.2233541

Chaddad, A., Peng, J., Xu, J., & Bouridane, A. (2023). Survey of explainable AI techniques in healthcare. *Sensors*, *23*(2), 634. https://doi.org/10.3390/s23020634

Chan, B. (2023). Black-box assisted medical decisions: AI power vs. ethical physician care. *Medicine Health Care and Philosophy*, *26*(3), 285–292. https://doi.org/10.1007/s11019-023-10153-z

Counseller, Q., & Aboelkassem, Y. (2023). Recent technologies in cardiac imaging. *Frontiers in Medical Technology*, *4*. https://doi.org/10.3389/fmedt.2022.984492

De Sousa, I. P., Vellasco, M. M. B. R., & Da Silva, E. C. (2019). Local Interpretable Model-Agnostic explanations for classification of lymph node metastases. *Sensors*, *19*(13), 2969. https://doi.org/10.3390/s19132969

Durán, J. M., & Jongsma, K. R. (2021). Who is afraid of black box algorithms? On the epistemological and ethical basis of trust in medical AI. *Journal of Medical Ethics*, medethics-106820. https://doi.org/10.1136/medethics-2020-106820

ElShawi, R., Sherif, Y., Al-Mallah, M., & Sakr, S. (2020). Interpretability in healthcare: a comparative study of local machine learning interpretability techniques. *Computational Intelligence*, *37*(4), 1633–1650. https://doi.org/10.1111/coin.12410

Flora, G. D., & Nayak, M. K. (2019). A brief review of cardiovascular diseases, associated risk factors and current treatment regimes. *Current Pharmaceutical Design*, *25*(38), 4063–4084. https://doi.org/10.2174/1381612825666190925163827

Hart, S. (2008). Shapley value. In *Palgrave Macmillan UK eBooks* (pp. 1–5). https://doi.org/10.1057/978-1-349-95121-5_1369-2

Holzinger, A., Saranti, A., Molnar, C., Biecek, P., & Samek, W. (2022). Explainable AI Methods - a brief overview. In *Lecture notes in computer science* (pp. 13–38). https://doi.org/10.1007/978-3-031-04083-2_2

Hulsen, T. (2023). Explainable Artificial Intelligence (XAI): Concepts and challenges in healthcare. *AI*, *4*(3), 652–666. https://doi.org/10.3390/ai4030034

Joiner, I. A. (2018). Chapter 1 – Artificial Intelligence: AI is Nearby. *Chandos Information Professional Series*, 1–22. https://www.sciencedirect.com/science/article/pii/B9780081022535000022

Kamakshi, V., & Krishnan, N. C. (2023). Explainable image classification: the journey so far and the road ahead. *AI*, *4*(3), 620–651. https://doi.org/10.3390/ai4030033

Kumar, Y., Koul, A., Singla, R., & Ijaz, M. F. (2022). Artificial intelligence in disease diagnosis: a systematic literature review, synthesizing framework and future research agenda. *Journal of Ambient Intelligence and Humanized Computing*, *14*(7), 8459–8486. https://doi.org/10.1007/s12652-021-03612-z

Loh, H. W., Ooi, C. P., Seoni, S., Barua, P. D., Molinari, F., & Acharya, U. R. (2022). Application of explainable artificial intelligence for healthcare: a systematic review of the last decade (2011–2022). *Computer Methods and Programs in Biomedicine*, *226*, 107161. https://doi.org/10.1016/j.cmpb.2022.107161

Magesh, P. R., Myloth, R. D., & Tom, R. J. (2020). An explainable machine learning model for early detection of Parkinson's disease using LIME on DaTSCAN imagery. *Computers in Biology and Medicine*, *126*, 104041. https://doi.org/10.1016/j.compbiomed.2020.104041

Mahmoud, M. Z., Alkhorayef, M., Alzimami, K. S., Aljuhani, M. S., & Sulieman, A. (2014). High-Intensity Focused Ultrasound (HIFU) in uterine fibroid treatment: review study. *Polish Journal of Radiology*, *79*(1), 384. https://doi.org/10.12659/PJR.891110

Montavon, G., Binder, A., Lapuschkin, S., Samek, W., & Müller, K. (2019). Layer-wise relevance propagation: an overview. In *Lecture notes in computer science* (pp. 193–209). https://doi.org/10.1007/978-3-030-28954-6_10

Paudel, P., Karna, S. K., Saud, R., Regmi, L., Thapa, T. B., & Bhandari, M. (2023). Unveiling key predictors for early heart attack detection using machine learning and explainable AI technique with LIME. *NSysS '23: Proceedings of the 10th International Conference on Networking, Systems and Security*. https://doi.org/10.1145/3629188.3629193

Prc, N. H. C. O. (2020). National guidelines for diagnosis and treatment of colorectal cancer 2020 in China (English version). *Chinese Journal of Cancer Research*, *32*(4), 415–445. https://doi.org/10.21147/j.issn.1000-9604.2020.04.01

Raihan, M. J., Khan, M. A., Kee, S., & Nahid, A. (2023). Detection of the chronic kidney disease using XGBoost classifier and explaining the influence of the attributes on the model using SHAP. *Scientific Reports*, *13*(1). https://doi.org/10.1038/s41598-023-33525-0

Rajpal, S., Lakhyani, N., Singh, A. K., Kohli, R., & Kumar, N. (2021). Using handpicked features in conjunction with ResNet-50 for improved detection of COVID-19 from chest X-ray images. *Chaos Solitons & Fractals*, *145*, 110749. https://doi.org/10.1016/j.chaos.2021.110749

Samek, W. (2023). Explainable deep learning: concepts, methods, and new developments. In *Elsevier eBooks* (pp. 7–33). https://doi.org/10.1016/b978-0-32-396098-4.00008-9

Saranya A, & Subhashini R. (2023). A systematic review of Explainable Artificial Intelligence models and applications: recent developments and future trends. *Decision Analytics Journal*, *7*, 100230–100230. https://doi.org/10.1016/j.dajour.2023.100230

Sarvamangala, D. R., & Kulkarni, R. V. (2021). Convolutional neural networks in medical image understanding: a survey. *Evolutionary Intelligence*, *15*(1), 1–22. https://doi.org/10.1007/s12065-020-00540-3

Selvaraju, R. R., Cogswell, M., Das, A., Vedantam, R., Parikh, D., & Batra, D. (2019). Grad-CAM: visual explanations from deep networks via gradient-based localization. *International Journal of Computer Vision*, *128*(2), 336–359. https://doi.org/10.1007/s11263-019-01228-7

Shahid, N., Rappon, T., & Berta, W. (2019). Applications of artificial neural networks in health care organizational decision-making: a scoping review. *PLoS ONE*, *14*(2), e0212356. https://doi.org/10.1371/journal.pone.0212356

Sholapur, P. N. (2022). Explainable AI and Deep Learning techniques for Colon Cancer Detection. *2022 4th International Conference on Advances in Computing, Communication Control and Networking (ICAC3N)*. https://doi.org/10.1109/icac3n56670.2022.10074383

Sholapur, P. N., & Indiramma, M. (2022). Explainable AI and Deep Learning techniques for Colon Cancer Detection. In *2022 4th International Conference on Advances in Computing, Communication Control and Networking (ICAC3N)* (pp. 1096–1105). IEEE.

Singhal, T. (2020). A review of coronavirus disease-2019 (COVID-19). *The Indian Journal of Pediatrics*, *87*(4), 281–286. https://doi.org/10.1007/s12098-020-03263-6

Sjögren, B., Bigert, C., & Gustavsson, P. (2015). Cardiovascular disease. In *Elsevier eBooks* (pp. 313–331). https://doi.org/10.1016/b978-0-444-59453-2.00016-0

Sudar, K. M., Nagaraj, P., Nithisaa, S., Aishwarya, R., Aakash, M., & Lakshmi, S. I. (2022). Alzheimer's Disease Analysis using Explainable Artificial Intelligence (XAI). *2022 International Conference on Sustainable Computing and Data Communication Systems (ICSCDS)*. https://doi.org/10.1109/icscds53736.2022.9760858

Xu, H., & Shuttleworth, K. M. J. (2024). Medical artificial intelligence and the black box problem: a view based on the ethical principle of "do no harm." *Intelligent Medicine*. https://doi.org/10.1016/j.imed.2023.08.001

Zahan, M., Habibi, H., Pencil, A., Abdul-Ghafar, J., Ahmadi, S., Juyena, N., Rahman, M., & Parvej. (2022). Diagnosis of COVID-19 in symptomatic patients: An updated review. *Vacunas (English Edition)*, *23*(1), 55–61. https://doi.org/10.1016/j.vacune.2022.04.002

8 Robust CNN based on LIME for Glaucoma Classification

Sonali Dash and V. Keerthi Kiran

8.1 INTRODUCTION

The damage to the blood vessels in the back of the eye (retina) caused by long-term diabetes is known as Diabetic Retinopathy (DR). The retina creates new, aberrant blood vessels if the person is affected with diabetes. If new blood vessels develop on the iris, the eye's fluid channels will close off, leading to increased intraocular pressure and the condition known as neovascular glaucoma disease. The absence of symptoms or pains, as well as normal vision in the early stages, makes glaucoma detection very difficult. When a patient loses 70% of their eyesight, it is clear that they are in the advanced stage. World Health Organization (WHO) projections indicate that the number of glaucoma patients will reach 111.8 million in 2040 [1], accounting for around 3–5% of all cases in adults aged 40–80. Manual screening of glaucoma is laborious and time-consuming, yet early discovery and ongoing screening have the potential to reduce the blindness rate by 50%.

Two main forms of glaucoma, such as open-angle and angle-closure, are distinguished by the presence or absence of elevated Intra-Ocular Pressure (IOP). In both forms of glaucoma, the accumulation of fluid known as Aqueous Humour (AH) causes an increase in IOP and impacts the Optic Nerve Head (ONH). Current research on glaucoma diagnosis has mostly relied on three main tools: IOP measurement, visual field testing, and ONH diagnosis. Skilled ophthalmologists often do glaucoma screenings by visually analysing retinal fundus images, measuring IOP, and determining the angle of drainage or outflow channel. The problem is that the hand-operated procedures and perceivable analyses of biomedical images are laborious, subjective, and can take anywhere from twenty to forty-five minutes. Therefore, ophthalmologists want a glaucoma-specific Computer-Aided Diagnostic (CAD) system that can quickly and thoroughly analyse medical pictures.

In order to diagnose glaucoma, the CAD system processes medical pictures by segmenting them and then classifying them. Before applying any filters or morphological procedures, etc., to an input picture, pre-processing is performed to eliminate any unwanted noise or outliers that can compromise the results of the subsequent analysis. In addition, segmentation involves splitting the input picture

DOI: 10.1201/9781003503385-8

into several sections in order to extract the Region of Interest (ROI), which is more relevant than other sections and allows for easier abnormality analysis. The last step is classification, which is a decision-making method for labelling photos as "normal" or "abnormal".

The categorization of glaucoma using a convolutional multi-layer neural network based on perceptrons was developed by Romany F. Mansour et al. [2]. By utilizing entropy-based estimate, the region between the optic disc and optic cup is able to be identified. Following the segmentation of the disc of the optic and border of the cup, the disc ratio and atomistic local characteristics are recovered using weighted least square fit. Various databases, together with Drishti-GS and Rim-ONE are used in perceptron-based convolutional multilayer neural network to improve the recognition rate of glaucoma in retinal pictures. The pre-trained models for glaucoma diagnosis are created by Jahanzaib Latif et al. [3] and are based on transfer learning. To evaluate the efficacy of transfer learning-based models that contain saliency maps in distinguishing between normal and glaucomatous pictures, various databases such as ORIGA, HRF, DRIONS-DB, etc. are utilized. Using classifier fusion and pre-trained convolutional neural network (CNN) techniques. Vijaya Kumar Velpula et al. [4] have presented an automated approach for glaucoma stage categorization. Different CNN models, such as ResNet50, AlexNet, VGG19, etc., are used in the suggested model. To evaluate the efficiency of the model, various databases like Drishti, ACRIMA, RIM-ONE, etc., are used. The goal of developing classifier fusion is to achieve maximal voting-based decision merging across all CNN models.

In a groundbreaking move, Shubham Joshi et al. [5] have put out the first-ever ensemble-based deep learning technique to detect the glaucoma disease. In order to classify glaucoma, three pre-trained CNNs are chosen. Among these networks, ResNet, VGGNet, and GoogLeNet are considered for visual geometry group network. A new technique presented by Álvaro S. Hervella et al., [6] enables the categorization of glaucomatic conditions with segmentation of optic disc and optic cup in retinal pictures. Niharika Thakur et al. [7] have introduced a novel set of reduced hybrid characteristics generated from structural and nonstructural data for classifying retinal fundus images. Recoverable properties of the model include cup-to-disc ratio and disc damage index.

Filip Tarcoveanu et al., [8] have utilized the following algorithms as classification tools: C4.5, Non-Nested Generalized Exemplars, Multilayer Perceptron, Random Forest, Random Tree, and k-Nearest Neighbours. The ORIGA database is utilized to evaluate the glaucoma pictures with the deep learning technique developed by M.B. Sudhan et al. [9] for the purpose of optic cup segmentation, a pre-trained transfer learning model and a U-Net architecture based on a deep learning algorithm are employed.

To diagnose and anticipate glaucoma in its early stages, Ramgopal Kashyap et al. [10] have put forth a deep learning-based solution. This suggested deep learning technique uses the glaucoma dataset to analyse glaucoma images. Transfer learning approaches with pre-trained are incorporated by the U-Net technique for segmentation of the optic cup using deep learning, while DenseNet-201 extracts feature and classify. Shyamalee et al. [11] have suggested a computer methodology for segmentation and categorize retina images for glaucoma identification. The attention U-Net that utilizes the ResNet50 model as its encoder backbone has achieved the highest accuracy of 97.53% in optic disc segmentation using the RIM-ONE dataset.

Ajitha S. et al. [12] have suggested an approach for identification of glaucomatic eyes more quickly by using R-CNN that is a subsection of AI-powered deep learning system. One part of Faster R-CNN is the Region Proposal Network (RPN), which is responsible to identify an object's region on an image, and the other part is a network that can identify items inside the suggested region. The best results were achieved by using a transfer learning technique using ResNet50 and VGG16. Kamesh Sonti et al. [13] have fine-tuned the hyperparameters of CNN to classify the glaucoma images. Law Kumar Singh et al. [14] have developed a hybrid optimization technique combined with random forest to achieve the higher accuracy in classification of fundus images. Table 8.1 represents the comparison of the various existing models.

According to the study of various methods discussed above few challenges are discussed below.

- Each research employs a different set of features for the purpose of categorization.
- There have been a very limited number of research that have utilized the combined feature set for categorization.
- The datasets that are utilized for analysing is different from one study to the next.

TABLE 8.1
Comparison of Few Models

Authors	Architecture	Strengths	Dataset	Accuracy (%)
Romany F. Mansour et al. [2]	Perceptron's CNN	Multi-Layer Neural network classification with Weighted Least Square Fit holistic feature extraction	Drishti-GS and Rim-ONE dataset	99% and 88% for Drishti-GS and Rim-ONE Dataset respectively
Jahanzaib Latif et al. [3]	ODGNet	Transfer learning-based models were used	ORIGA	95.75%
Kamesh Sonti et al. [13]	CNN	Implemented the model on a combination of balanced and unbalanced datasets	Private dataset, and Refuge dataset.	88.89% for the private dataset, and 89.17% for Refuge dataset
Law Kumar Singh et al. [14]	Random forest	Feature selection based on emperor penguin optimization	Customized dataset	95.41%

Therefore, in the suggested work following points are to be taken care.

- Four different existing CNNs are utilized to extract the features classified with the original dataset.
- In the second step, the low-light image enhancement technique is combined with individual CNN models and enhanced features are extracted. Afterwards the enhanced features are classified.
- In the third step all the original features are concatenated and classified.
- In the last step all the enhanced features are concatenated and classified.
- Various classifiers are utilized for the task of classification.
- To stay away from biases the experimentation is conducted for the same database.

The remainder of this article is organized as mentioned. Section 8.2 represents methods and materials; in Section 8.3 experimentation and the outputs are discussed. Section 8.4 concludes the work.

8.2 MATERIALS AND METHODS

Materials, methodology and dataset utilized are highlighted in this section.

8.2.1 Dataset

A total of 101 retinal fundus camera pictures labelled as "glaucoma" or "non-glaucoma" make up the DRISHTI-GS [15] dataset. The research scholars at IIIT Hyderabad in collaboration with Aravind Eye Hospital in Madurai have developed the soft segmented disc and cup maps, which serve as the basis for comparing the applied methods. As an important diagnostic criterion for glaucoma, it also comes with a .txt file including CDR values for every retinal picture. In addition, the experimental dataset includes photographs captured under different lighting conditions, and the subjects include individuals of diverse ages that visit the hospital. Some of the images of the dataset are given in Figure 8.1.

8.2.2 GoogLeNet

Google unveiled its GoogLeNet [16] model, which is based on the inception structure, during the 2014 ImageNet Large-Scale Visual Recognition Challenge (ILSVRC14).

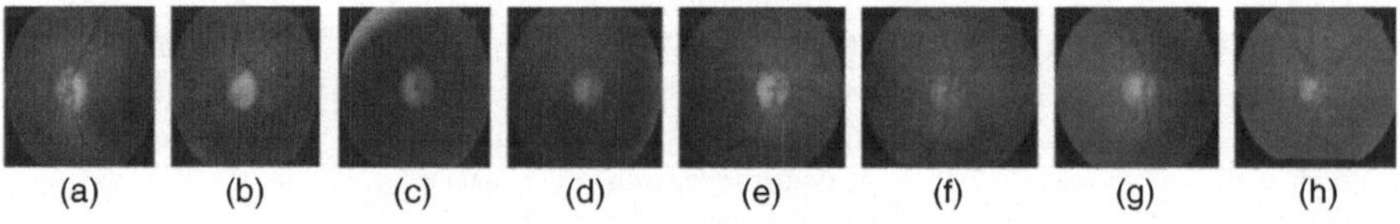

FIGURE 8.1 Samples of DRISHTI-GS dataset: (a–d) glaucoma images; (e–h) normal images.

The central component of this setup is an extended inner layer of the neural network that can produce different correlation distributions. This is based on the theory that each layer of the network can perform at its best when it can produce different probability distributions that are highly correlated with the input data. The outputs from four separate layers—1×1, 3×3, 5×5 convolution layers and a 3×3 max-pooling layer—are integrated into one data set in the fundamental GoogLeNet (inception v1) module.

8.2.3 Inception ResNet v2

Inception ResNet v2 [17, 18] is built on the framework of inception and the Residual connection. It utilizes residual connections to combine convolutional filters of different sizes. Residual connections prevent deterioration in deep structures and decrease training time. Figure 8.3 displays the fundamental network structure of Inception ResNet v2. While Inception v3 and v4 are pure convolutional networks, Inception ResNet v1 and Inception ResNet v2 are Inception-style networks that use residual connections instead of filter concatenation.

8.2.4 Xception

A continuation of the Inception framework, Francois Chollet presented the Xception architecture [19, 20]. These architectures are a linear group of deeply separated convolution layers with residual connections. Less computing cost and memory consumption are the goals of the depthwise separable convolution.

8.2.5 Methodology

The main focus of this work is to improve the existing CNN models based on enhancement techniques for glaucoma detection. Various original CNN models, such as GoogLeNet, Darknet53, Inception-ResNet-v2, and Xception, are combined with low-light image enhancement technique for the glaucoma detection. Four different computations are carried out for the suggested model. Initially, the original CNN model is considered for glaucoma detection. In the second step, the enhanced CNN models are used for glaucoma detection. In the third step, all the features extracted from the original CNN models are concatenated and classified for identification of glaucoma. Finally, all the features extracted from the enhanced CNN models are concatenated and classified for identification of glaucoma. For classification purposes, various classifiers like Binary tree, SVM, K-NN, NAÏVE BAYES, and Neural Network are utilized. For the verification of the suggested model DRISHTI-GS dataset is used.

Several classifiers have been employed in this study to classify images captured at the microscopic level. The suggested architecture takes advantage of four cutting-edge Convolutional Neural Networks (CNNs) (i.e., GoogLeNet, Darknet53, Inception-ResNet-v2, and Xception) to combine the features they acquired in respective feature extraction layers. Binary tree, SVM, K-NN, NAÏVE BAYES, and Neural Network are the five machine learning techniques that are used to provide classification outputs from the combined features. The block diagram of the proposed model is illustrated in Figure 8.2.

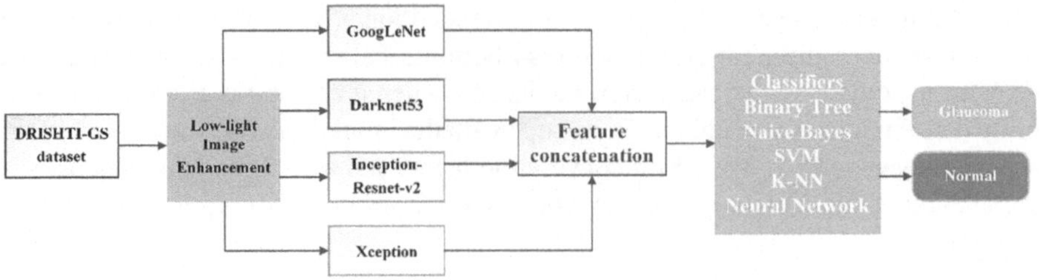

FIGURE 8.2 The schematic diagram of suggested concatenated model.

8.2.6 Preprocessing

The original DRISHTI-GS dataset has images of resolution ranging from 2045 × 1752 to 2466 × 1763. As the sizes of the raw images differ greatly, to make them fit into the pre-trained model, all the photographs are resized to 256 × 256 during the image pre-processing. The images are enhanced using Low-light Image Enhancement technique [14]. It describes about the low-light image generation:

$$m = i^{\circ} p \tag{8.1}$$

where m is the image taken and i is the desirable improvement. Additionally, p denotes the map of illumination. The above equation is the observation of image that is decomposed into the product of the desirable scene and the illumination of the image. It can be noticed that the estimated value of p is significant to the retrieval of i. Some of the enhanced images of DRISHTI-GS dataset are shown in Figure 8.3.

8.2.7 Feature Extraction

Here, we describe how the suggested approach for microscopical image categorization uses four deep CNN architectures specifically, GoogLeNet, Darknet53, Inception-ResNet-v2, and Xception—as feature extractors. Based on transfer learning theory, these CNNs may be used to extract discriminative features from biological pictures after being pre-trained on ImageNet, a collection of natural images, for unique generic image descriptors. Afterwards, the features are classified using various classifiers. Figure 8.4 illustrates the design flow of the suggested approach.

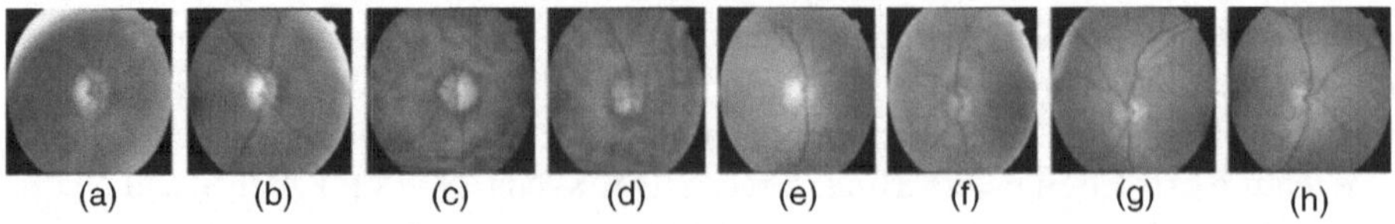

FIGURE 8.3 Samples of enhanced DRISHTI-GS dataset: (a-d) glaucoma images; (e-h) normal images.

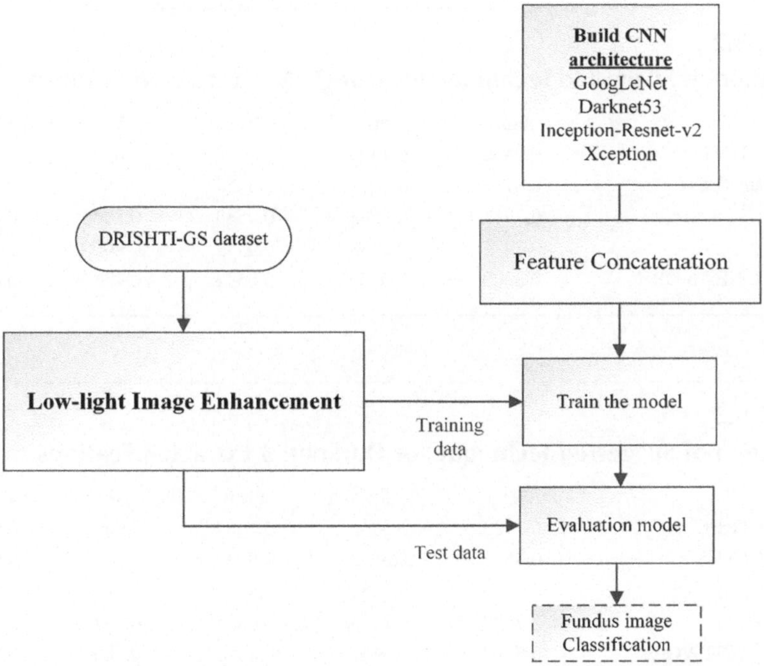

FIGURE 8.4 Design flow of proposed method.

8.3 EXPERIMENTAL RESULTS

The experiments were carried out on MATLAB 2023a on a Windows 10 operating system with 64 bits, an Intel Core i7-6500U CPU running at 2.50GHz, and an Intel HD 520 Graphics. As part of each experiment, we have selected 30% of the dataset at random to serve as the testing set. We refer to the remaining 70% of the dataset as the "training plus validation set", and then we arbitrarily split it up into five similar bunch in order to carry out the five-fold cross-validation. Afterwards, the network is trained on the training set, and evaluation is carried out on the validating set, and the outputs are recorded. The features are extracted using pre-trained networks GoogLeNet, Darknet53, Inception-ResNet-v2, and Xception and classified using prominent classifiers, i.e., Binary Tree, Naïve Bayes, SVM, k-NN, and Neural Network. Finally, the detection rate is considered as the baseline for selecting the finest model in classification of DRISHTI-GS dataset. The experiments are also performed by concatenation of features obtained by the three pre-trained networks mentioned above and compared with the accuracy obtained by individual networks. The performance of the suggested techniques for both original and enhanced are shown in Tables 8.2–8.13. Figures 8.5–8.14 demonstrate about the confusion matrices of every classifier for the different features extracted networks and concatenated features.

The comparison of the proposed model in terms of accuracy for original dataset and enhanced dataset for the concatenated features is shown in Table 8.12 and 8.13

TABLE 8.2
Evaluation of Suggested Technique for GoogLeNet Extracted Features

Classifier	Sen	Sp	Prec	Acc	F1 Score
BINARY TREE	0.7400	0.4500	0.7708	0.6571	0.7551
NAÏVE BAYES	0.8113	0.7059	0.8958	0.7857	0.8515
SVM	0.7931	0.8333	0.9583	0.8000	0.8679
K-NN	0.7931	0.8333	0.9583	0.8000	0.8679
NEURAL NETWORK	0.8200	0.6500	0.8542	0.7714	0.8367

TABLE 8.3
Evaluation of Suggested Technique for Darknet53 Extracted Features

Classifier	Sen	Sp	Prec	Acc	F1 Score
BINARY TREE	0.7273	0.3846	0.6667	0.6	0.6957
NAÏVE BAYES	0.8511	0.6522	0.8333	0.7857	0.8421
SVM	0.8036	0.7857	0.9375	**0.8000**	0.8654
K-NN	0.7627	0.7273	0.9375	0.7571	0.8411
NEURAL NETWORK	0.8367	0.6667	0.8542	0.7857	0.8454

TABLE 8.4
Evaluation of Suggested Technique for Inception-ResNet-v2 Extracted Features

Classifier	Sen	Sp	Prec	Acc	F1 Score
BINARY TREE	0.7143	0.3333	0.7143	0.6000	0.7143
NAÏVE BAYES	0.8491	0.7647	0.9184	0.8286	0.8824
SVM	0.8276	0.9167	0.9796	**0.8429**	0.8429
K-NN	0.8103	0.8333	0.9592	0.8143	0.8785
NEURAL NETWORK	0.8542	0.6364	0.8367	0.7857	0.8454

TABLE 8.5
Evaluation of Suggested Technique for Xception Extracted Features

Classifier	Sen	Sp	Prec	Acc	F1 Score
BINARY TREE	0.7778	0.4800	0.7292	0.6714	0.7527
NAÏVE BAYES	0.8367	0.6667	0.8542	0.7857	0.8454
SVM	0.7895	0.7692	0.9375	0.7857	0.8571
K-NN	0.8000	1.0000	1.0000	**0.8286**	0.8889
NEURAL NETWORK	0.9250	0.6333	0.7708	0.8000	0.8409

TABLE 8.6
Evaluation of Suggested Technique for Concatenated Features

Classifier	Sen	Sp	Prec	Acc	F1 Score
BINARY TREE	0.8000	0.5500	0.8163	0.7286	0.8081
NAÏVE BAYES	0.8302	0.7059	0.8980	**0.8000**	0.8627
SVM	0.7966	0.8182	0.9592	**0.8000**	0.8704
K-NN	0.7719	0.6154	0.8980	0.7429	0.8302
NEURAL NETWORK	0.8704	0.5714	0.8163	0.7429	0.8163

TABLE 8.7
Evaluation of Suggested Technique for GoogLeNet Features

Classifier	Sen	Sp	Prec	Acc	F1 Score
BINARY TREE	0.7222	0.3750	0.7959	0.6429	0.7573
NAÏVE BAYES	0.8261	0.5417	0.7755	**0.7286**	0.8000
SVM	0.7143	0.4286	0.9184	0.6857	0.8036
K-NN	0.7213	0.4444	0.8980	0.6857	0.8000
NEURAL NETWORK	0.7609	0.4167	0.7143	0.6429	0.7368

TABLE 8.8
Evaluation of suggested technique for Darknet-53 Features

Classifier	Sen	Sp	Prec	Acc	F1 Score
BINARY TREE	0.8222	0.5600	0.7708	0.7286	0.7957
NAÏVE BAYES	0.8163	0.6190	0.8333	0.7571	0.8247
SVM	0.8000	0.7333	0.9167	**0.7857**	0.8544
K-NN	0.7627	0.7273	0.9375	0.7571	0.8411
NEURAL NETWORK	0.7778	0.4800	0.7292	0.6714	0.7527

TABLE 8.9
Evaluation of Suggested Technique for Improved Inception-ResNet-v2 Features

Classifier	Sens	Sp	Prec	Acc	F1 Score
BINARY TREE	0.8302	0.7647	0.9167	0.8143	0.8713
NAÏVE BAYES	0.8148	0.7500	0.9167	0.8000	0.8627
SVM	0.8393	0.9286	0.9792	**0.8571**	0.9038
K-NN	0.7797	0.8182	0.9583	0.7857	0.8598
NEURAL NETWORK	0.8800	0.8000	0.9167	**0.8571**	0.8980

TABLE 8.10
Evaluation of Suggested Technique for Improved Xception Features

Classifier	Sen	Sp	Prec	Acc	F1 Score
BINARY TREE	0.7174	0.3750	0.6875	0.6000	0.7021
NAÏVE BAYES	0.7547	0.5294	0.8333	0.7000	0.7921
SVM	0.7377	0.6667	0.9375	0.7286	0.8257
K-NN	0.7500	1.0000	1.0000	**0.7714**	0.8571
NEURAL NETWORK	0.8039	0.6316	0.8542	0.7571	0.8283

TABLE 8.11
Evaluation of Suggested Technique for Concatenated Features of Enhanced Dataset

Classifier	Sen	Sp	Prec	Acc	F1 Score
BINARY TREE	0.8627	0.7368	0.8980	0.8286	0.8800
NAÏVE BAYES	0.8519	0.8125	0.9388	0.8429	0.8932
SVM	0.8033	1.0000	1.0000	0.8286	0.8909
K-NN	0.8305	1.0000	1.0000	**0.8571**	0.9074
NEURAL NETWORK	0.8600	0.7000	0.8776	0.8143	0.8687

TABLE 8.12
Comparison of Suggested Techniques for Original Dataset

	Accuracy (%)				
Classifier	GoogLeNet	Darknet53	Inception-ResNet-v2	Xception	Concatenated
BINARY TREE	65.7	60	60	67.1	72.9
NAÏVE BAYES	78.6	78.6	82.9	78.6	80
SVM	80	80	84.3	78.6	80
K-NN	80	75.7	81.4	82.9	74.3
NEURAL NETWORK	77.1	78.6	78.6	80	74.3

TABLE 8.13
Comparison of Suggested Techniques for Enhanced Dataset

	Accuracy (%)				
Classifier	GoogLeNet	Darknet53	Inception-ResNet-v2	Xception	Concatenated
BINARY TREE	64.3	72.9	81.4	60	82.86
NAÏVE BAYES	72.9	75.7	80	70	84.29
SVM	68.6	78.6	85.7	72.9	82.86
K-NN	68.6	75.7	78.6	77.1	**85.71**
NEURAL NETWORK	64.3	67.1	85.7	75.7	81.43

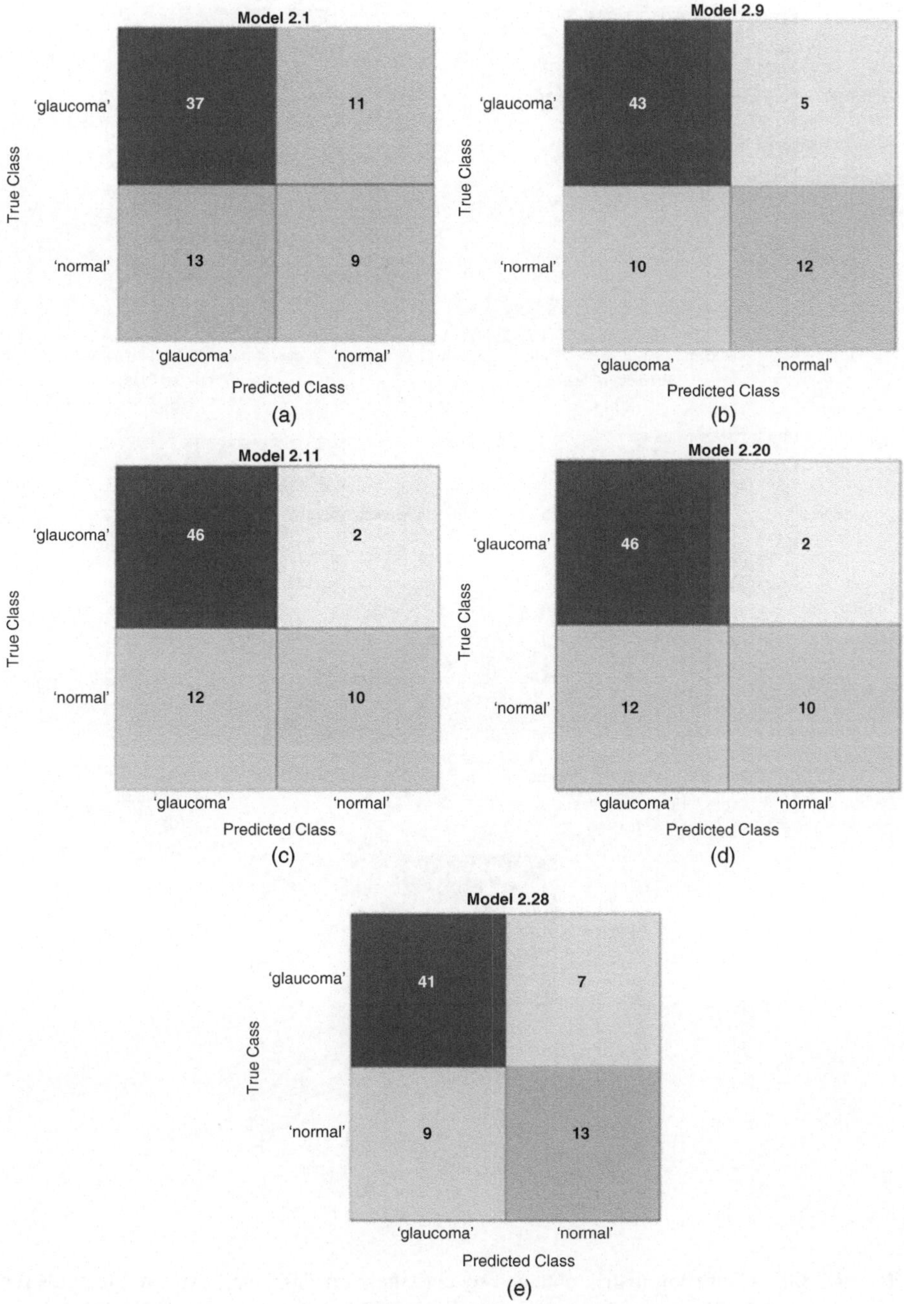

FIGURE 8.5 Confusion matrix obtained by classifiers for GoogLeNet extracted features for original dataset a) Binary tree b) NAÏVE BAYES c) SVM d) K-NN e) Neural Network.

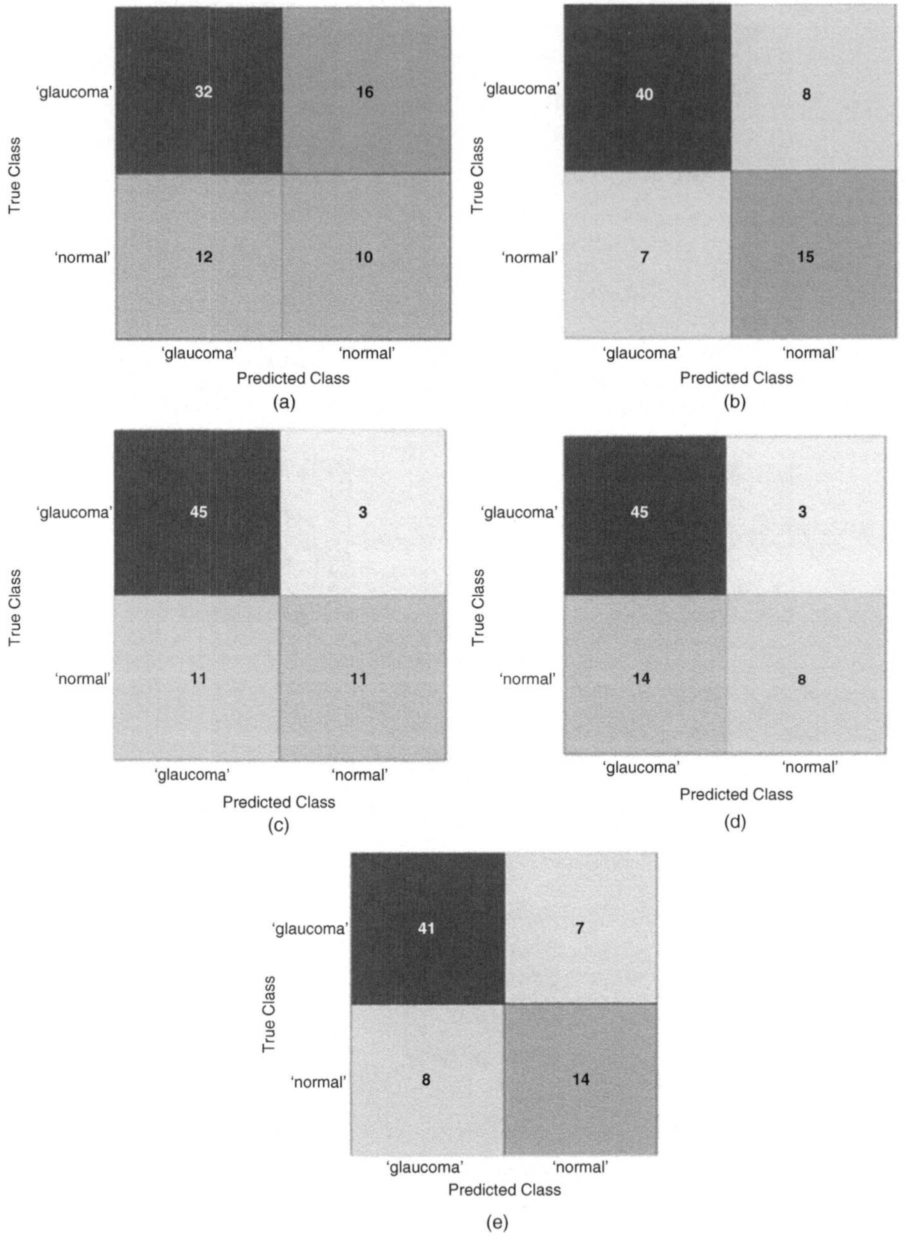

FIGURE 8.6 Confusion matrix obtained by classifiers for darknet53 extracted features for original dataset a) Binary tree b) NAÏVE BAYES c) SVM d) K-NN e) Neural Network.

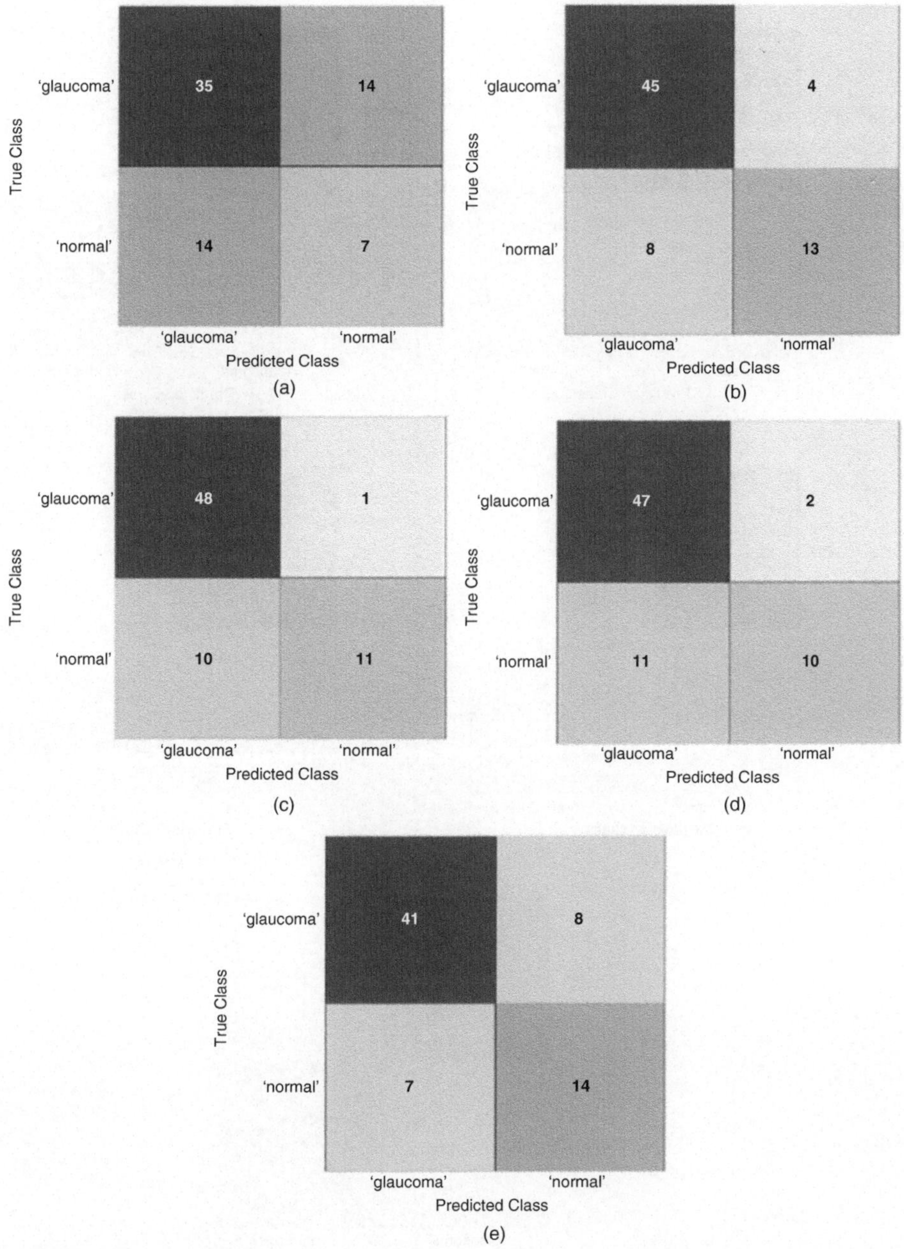

FIGURE 8.7 Confusion matrix obtained by classifiers for Inception-ResNet-v2 extracted features for original dataset a) Binary tree b) NAÏVE BAYES c) SVM d) K-NN e) Neural Network.

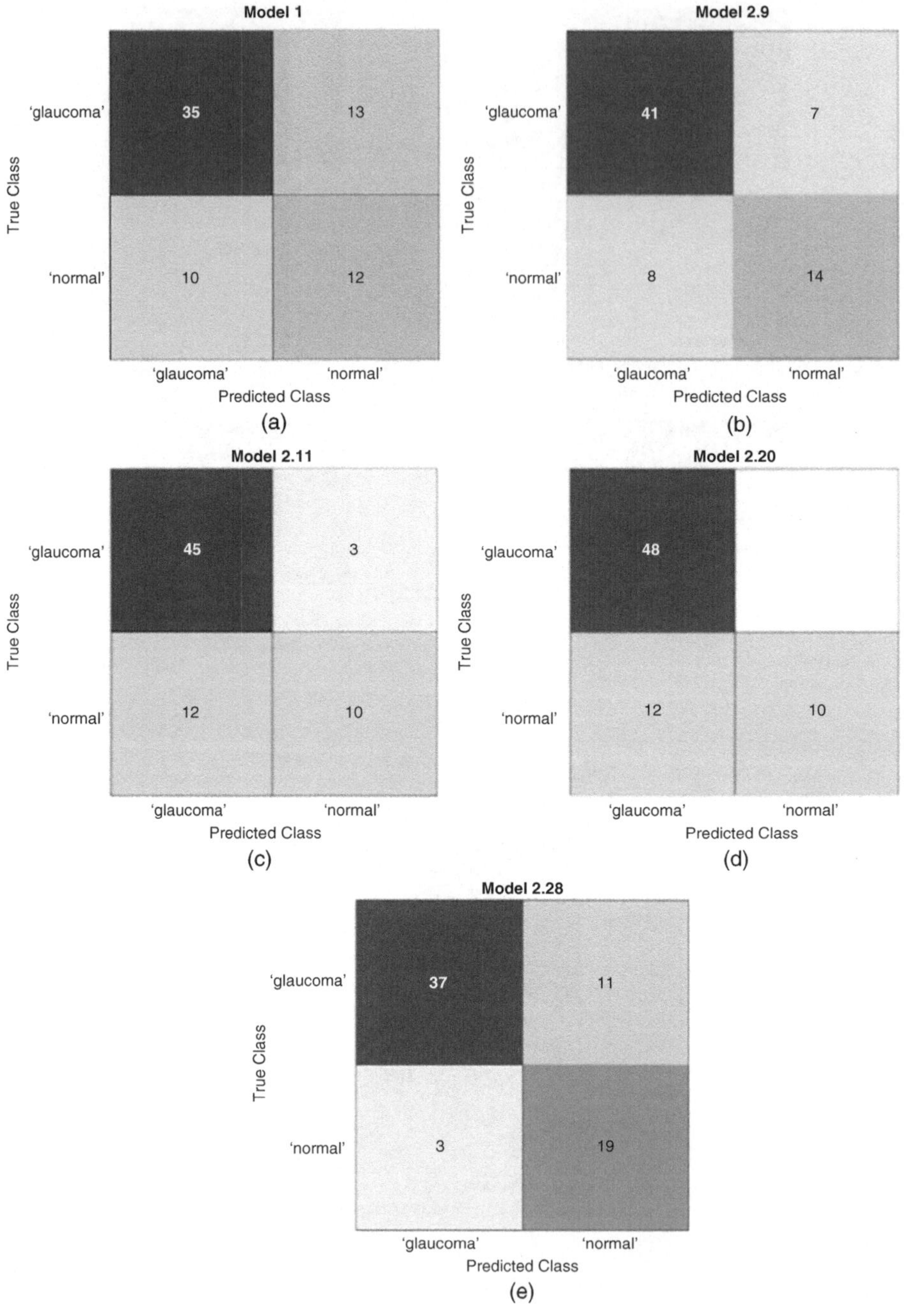

FIGURE 8.8 Confusion matrix obtained by classifiers for Xception extracted features for original dataset a) Binary tree b) NAÏVE BAYES c) SVM d) K-NN e) Neural Network.

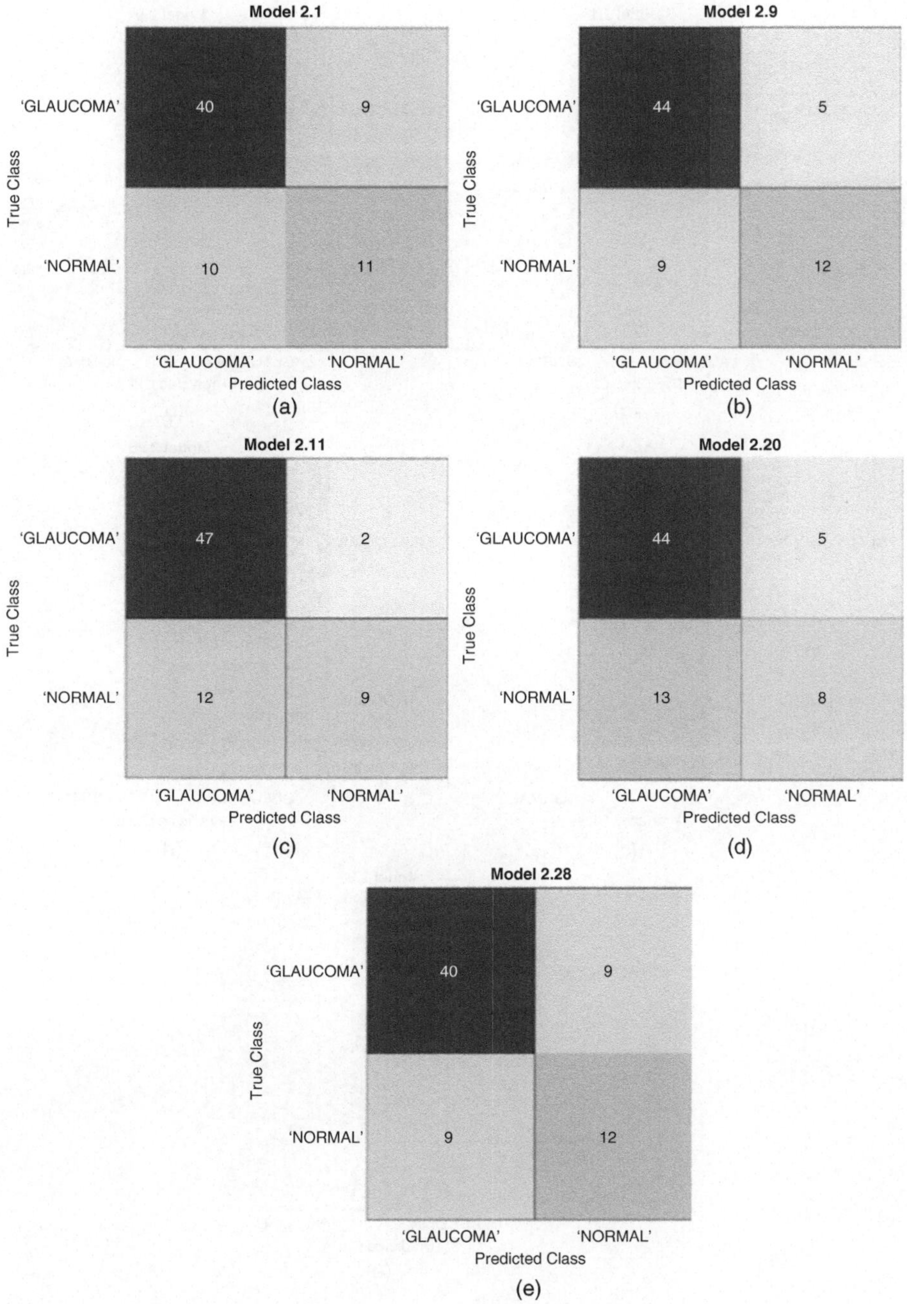

FIGURE 8.9 Confusion matrix obtained for concatenated features of original dataset by classifiers: a) Binary tree b) NAÏVE BAYES c) SVM d) K-NN e) Neural Network.

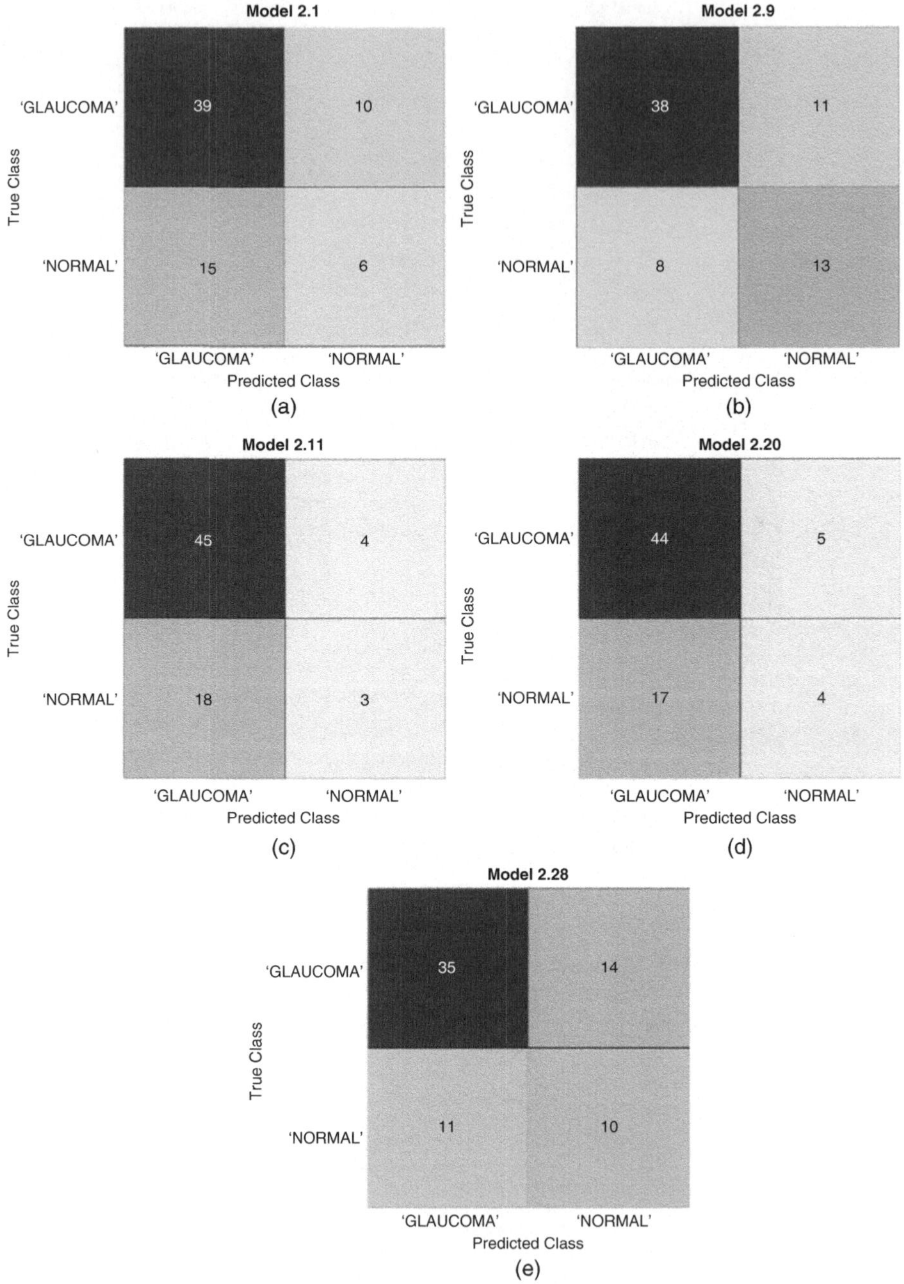

FIGURE 8.10 Confusion matrix obtained for GoogLeNet extracted features of enhanced dataset by classifiers: a) Binary tree b) NAÏVE BAYES c) SVM d) K-NN e) Neural Network.

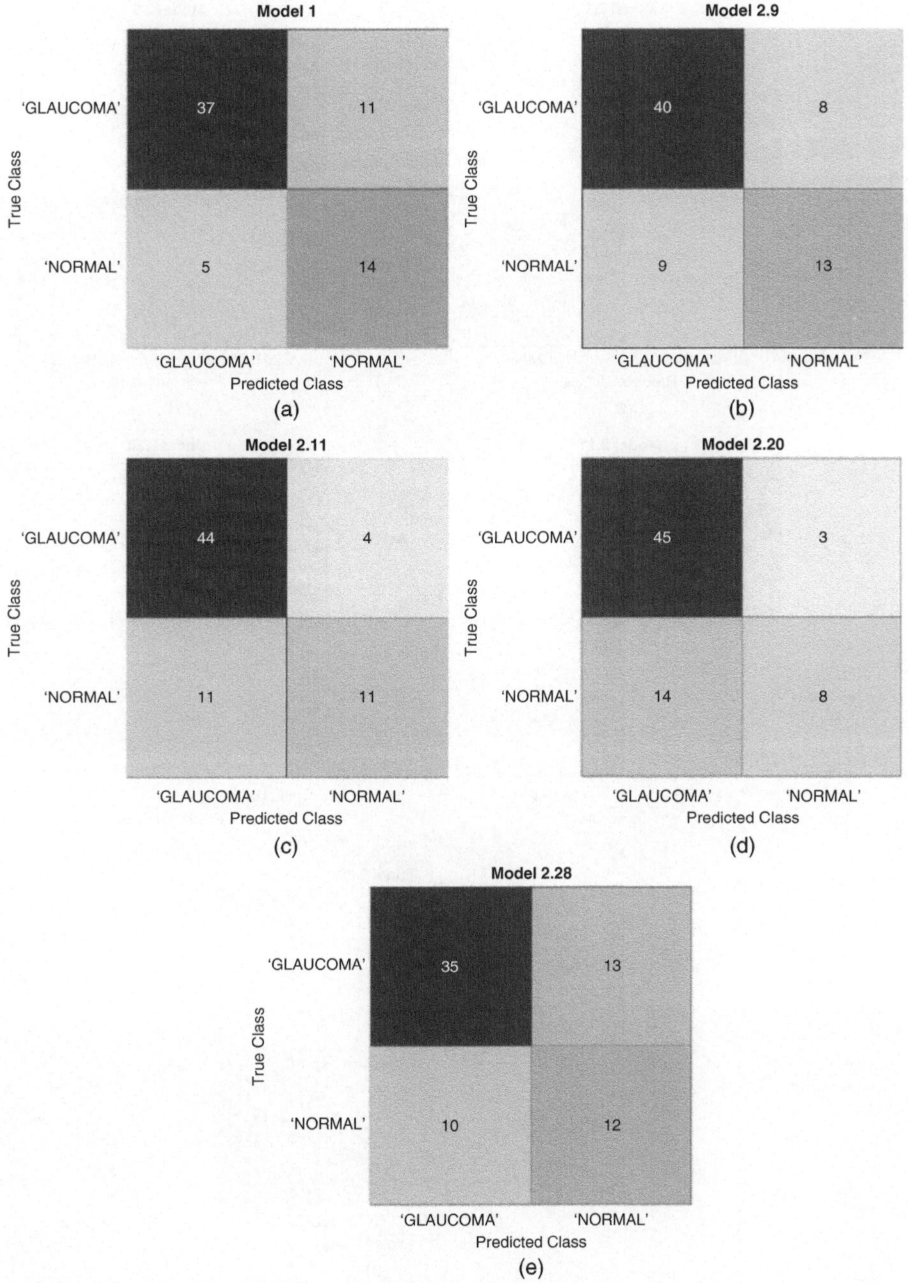

FIGURE 8.11 Confusion matrix achieved for Darknet-53 extracted features of enhanced dataset by classifiers: a) Binary tree b) NAÏVE BAYES c) SVM d) K-NN e) Neural Network.

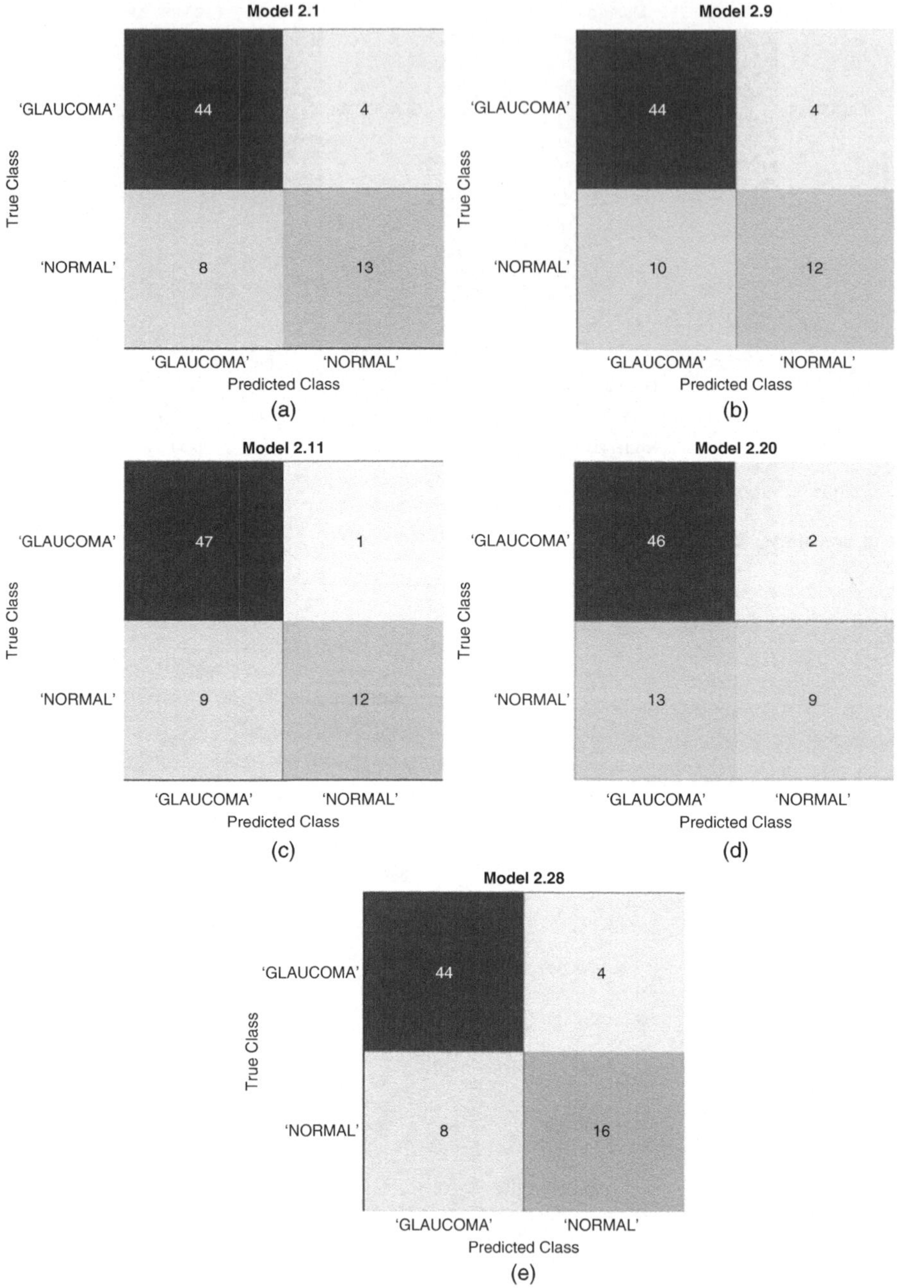

FIGURE 8.12 Confusion matrix achieved for Inception-ResNet-v2 extracted features of enhanced dataset by classifiers: a) Binary tree b) NAÏVE BAYES c) SVM d) K-NN e) Neural Network.

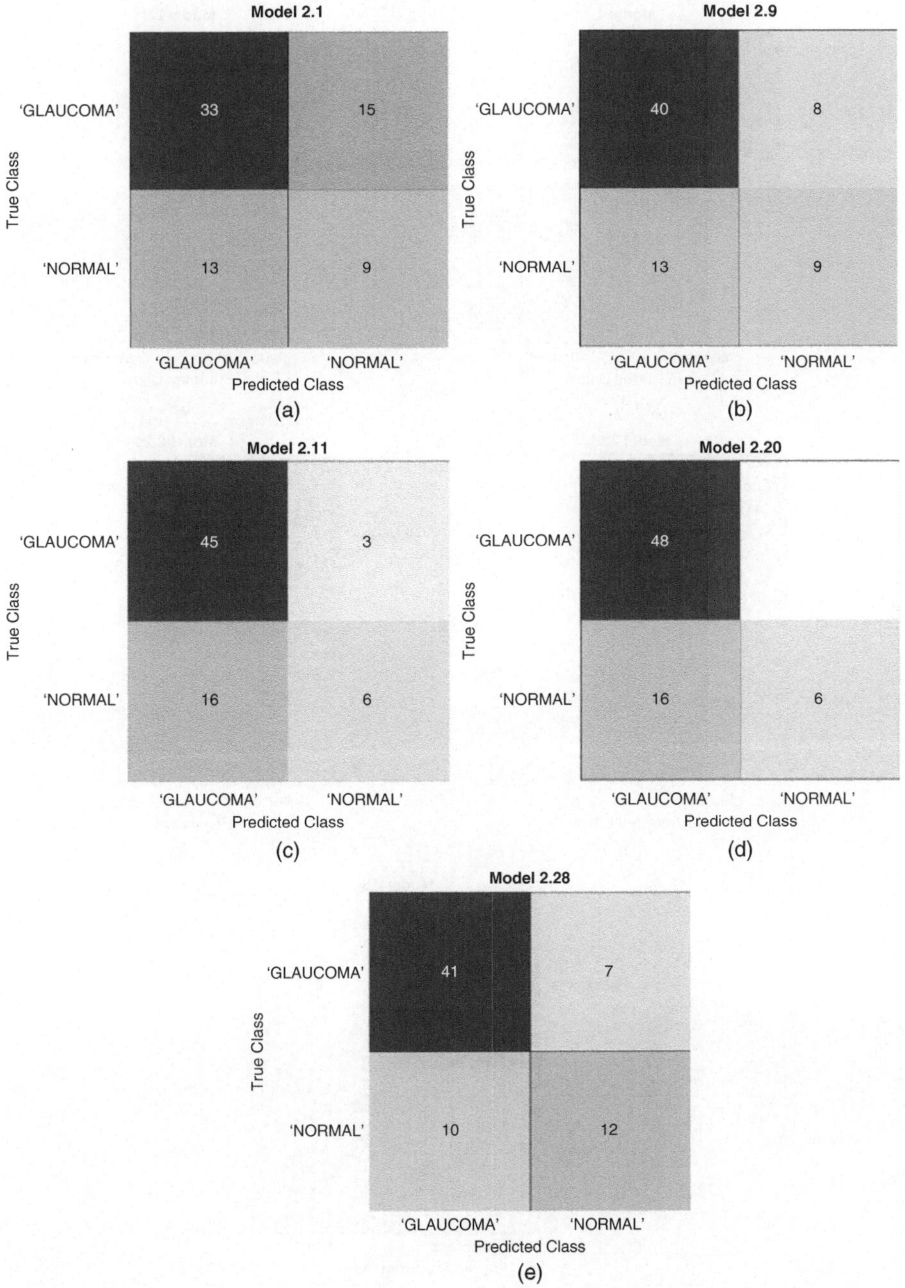

FIGURE 8.13 Confusion matrix obtained for Xception extracted features of enhanced dataset by classifiers: a) Binary tree b) NAÏVE BAYES c) SVM d) K-NN e) Neural Network.

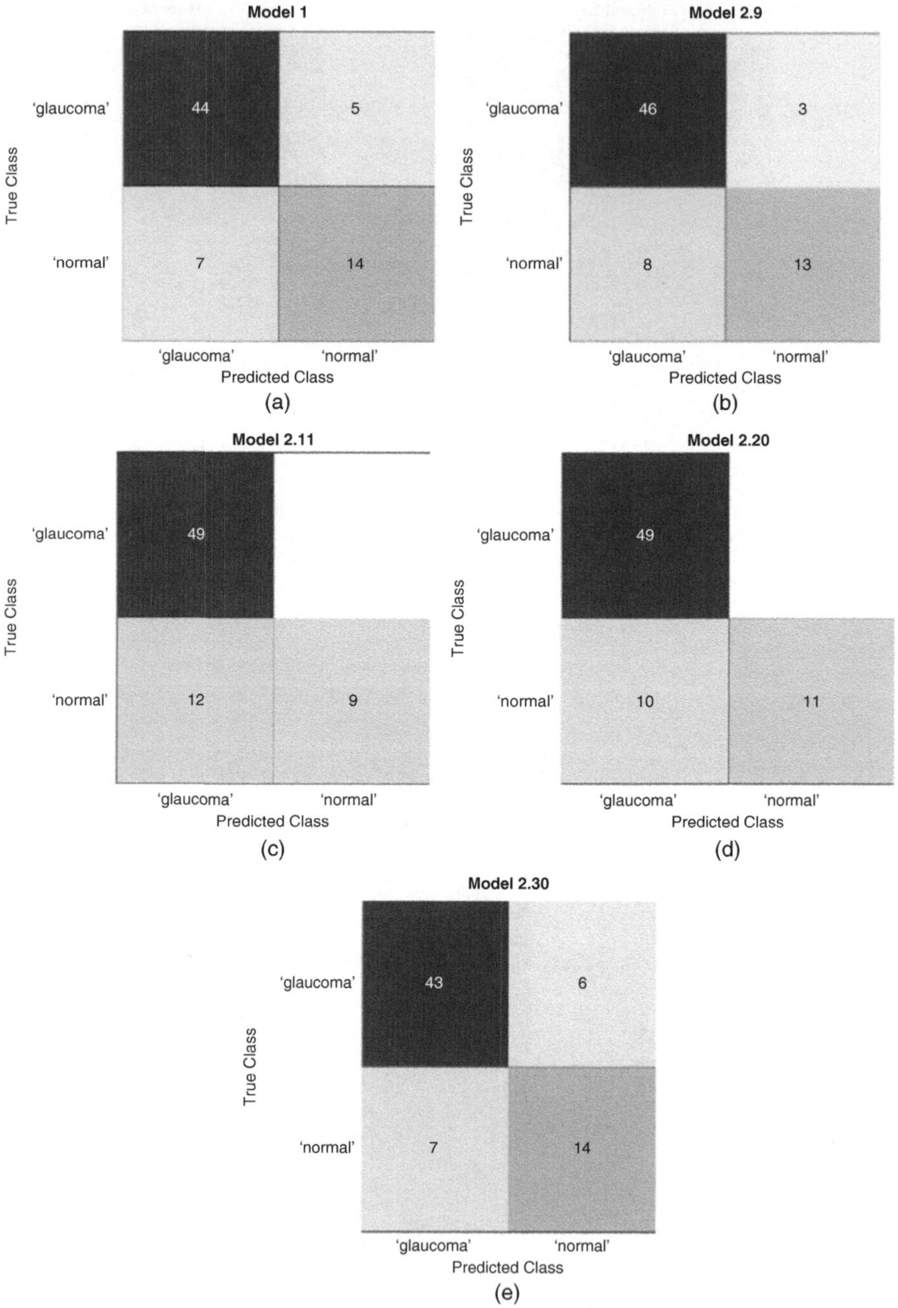

FIGURE 8.14 Confusion matrix obtained for concatenated features of enhanced dataset by classifiers: a) Binary tree b) NAÏVE BAYES c) SVM d) K-NN e) Neural Network.

respectively. It is observed from Table 8.13 that the highest accuracy of 85.71% is achieved for the K-NN classifier.

In this research, by comparing all the models like Binary Tree, Naïve Bayes, SVM, K-NN, Neural Network, the proposed model has achieved better performance in both the training and testing stages by concatenation of features extracted by GoogLeNet, Darknet53, Inception-ResNet-v2, and Xception. The least performance achieved model is neural network has some close performance to the proposed model. Even though the recommended integrated model is delivering higher accuracy, still the limitation is that the model is highly dependent on specific conditions of the given image. The low-light image enhancement method evaluates the illumination of each pixel separately by finding the maximum value in the three colour channels.

8.4 CONCLUSION

This suggested work has a feature concatenation model for fundus image classification on the basis of five individual techniques such as Binary tree, NAÏVE BAYES, SVM, K-NN, and Neural Network. For the improvement of the detection rate, more methods are suggested by concatenating the features of four individual models, GoogLeNet, Darknet53, Inception ResNetv2, and Xception. In the experimental work, DRISHTI-GS dataset is utilized for evaluation, each containing various patterns and features. The detection rate demonstrates that the feature concatenation outperforms each of the individual network, as well as different competitive techniques. The prime contribution of this work is that transfer learning, and feature concatenation are hybridized to achieve better performance fundus image classification though the database is comparatively smaller for the assigned task. Correspondingly, the suggested custom fusion can create a balance between detection rate and efficiency that is vital for automatic fundus classification, and thus help in creating lifelong smart treatment. In further studies

The performance analysis revealed that the suggested model's outcomes are efficient, with the causes for not obtaining optimal outcomes being false positives and false negatives. In the future, this imbalance will be addressed by upgrading the classifier and the efficient feature selection techniques.

REFERENCES

1. "Global estimates on the number of people blind or visually impaired by glaucoma: A meta-analysis from 2000 to 2020." *Eye, 2024*, 1–11.
2. Mansour, R.F. and Al-Marghilnai, A. (2021). Glaucoma detection using novel perceptron based convolutional multi-layer neural network classification. *Multidimensional Systems and Signal Processing*, *32*(4), 1217–1235.
3. Latif, J. et al., (2022). ODGNet: a deep learning model for automated optic disc localization and glaucoma classification using fundus images. *SN Applied Sciences*, *4*(4), p.98.
4. Velpula, V.K. and Sharma, L.D. (2023). Multi-stage glaucoma classification using pre-trained convolutional neural networks and voting-based classifier fusion. *Frontiers in Physiology*, *14*, p.1175881.

5. Joshi, S. et al., (2022). Glaucoma detection using image processing and supervised learning for classification. *Journal of Healthcare Engineering*, *2022*, 2988262. https://doi.org/10.1155/2022/2988262
6. Hervella, Á.S., et al., (2022). End-to-end multi-task learning for simultaneous optic disc and cup segmentation and glaucoma classification in eye fundus images. *Applied Soft Computing*, *116*, p.108347.
7. Thakur, N. and Juneja, M., (2020). Classification of glaucoma using hybrid features with machine learning approaches. *Biomedical Signal Processing and Control*, *62*, p.102137.
8. Tarcoveanu, F. et al., (2022, September). Classification algorithms used in predicting glaucoma progression. In *Healthcare* (Vol. 10, No. 10, p. 1831). MDPI.
9. Sudhan, M.B. Sinthuja, M., Pravinth Raja, S., Amutharaj, J., Charlyn Pushpa Latha, G., Sheeba Rachel, S., … & Waji, Y. A., (2022). Segmentation and classification of glaucoma using U-net with deep learning model. *Journal of Healthcare Engineering*, *2022*, 1601354.
10. Kashyap, R. Nair, R., Gangadharan, S. M. P., Botto-Tobar, M., Farooq, S., & Rizwan, A., (2022, December). Glaucoma detection and classification using improved U-Net Deep Learning Model. In *Healthcare* (Vol. 10, No. 12, p. 2497). MDPI.
11. Shyamalee, T. and Meedeniya, D. (2022). Glaucoma detection with retinal fundus images using segmentation and classification. *Machine Intelligence Research*, *19*(6), 563–580.
12. Ajitha, S. and Judy, M.V., (2020, December). Faster R-CNN classification for the recognition of glaucoma. In *Journal of Physics: Conference Series* (Vol. 1706, No. 1, p. 012170). IOP Publishing.
13. Sonti, K., & Dhuli, R. (2023). A new convolution neural network model "KR-NET" for retinal fundus glaucoma classification. *Optik*, *283*, 170861.
14. Singh, L. K. et al., (2024). Emperor penguin optimization algorithm-and bacterial foraging optimization algorithm-based novel feature selection approach for glaucoma classification from fundus images. *Soft Computing*, *28*(3), 2431–2467.
15. Sivaswamy, J. et al., (2014, April). Drishti-gs: Retinal image dataset for optic nerve head (onh) segmentation. In *2014 IEEE 11th international symposium on biomedical imaging (ISBI)* (pp. 53–56). IEEE.
16. Guo, X. et al., (2016). LIME: Low-light image enhancement via illumination map estimation. *IEEE Transactions on Image Processing*, *26*(2), 982–993.
17. Baldassarre, F., et al., (2017). Deep koalarization: Image colorization using cnns and inception-ResNet-v2. *arXiv preprint arXiv:1712.03400.*
18. Vasavi, S. et al., (2020). Invariant feature-based darknet architecture for moving object classification. *IEEE Sensors Journal*, *21*(10), 11417–11426.
19. Chollet, F., (2017). Xception: Deep learning with depthwise separable convolutions. In *Proceedings of the IEEE conference on computer vision and pattern recognition* (pp. 1251–1258).
20. He, K. et al., (2016). Deep residual learning for image recognition. In *Proceedings of the IEEE conference on computer vision and pattern recognition* (pp. 770–778).

9 Tumor Detection and Classification of Oral Squamous Cell Carcinoma on Histopathological Images utilizing Personalized Transfer Learning Approaches

Singaraju Ramya and R.I. Minu

9.1 INTRODUCTION

OSCC is a kind of cancer that develops in the mucous membrane of the mouth and neck. The sequence 1, 2, and 3 is provided. Based on data compiled by the Global Cancer Observatory (GCO), the number of cases of OSCC worldwide in 2020 amounted to 377,713, with the highest incidence observed in the Asian continent. OSCC exhibits a higher incidence in males compared to females, particularly among middle-aged to elderly individuals of the male gender who are more prone to developing this condition (Tan et al., 2023).

Moreover, there is a notable variation in the geographical distribution of OSCC on a global scale. For instance, OSCC is the most common kind of cancer globally among countries in Southeast Asia. On the other hand, it is the sixteenth most common cancer in Finland (Badwelan et al., 2023). Differences in the degree of exposure to carcinogens, such as tobacco smoke and smokeless versions, maybe the cause of the variance in prevalence around the world (Wang et al., 2023).

The characteristics of oral cancer include a gradual beginning, difficult detection, quick progression, and sometimes complicated therapy and metastasis. The high rates of morbidity and death draw attention to the pressing need for early diagnostic instruments and efficient screening techniques. Currently, the accepted method for identifying OSCC and possibly malignant illnesses (PMDs) is regular oral exams

DOI: 10.1201/9781003503385-9

that include tissue samples in addition to visual and tactile assessments of accessible oral structures. However, this method has certain limitations, such as sampling bias, which can lead to underdiagnosis or misdiagnosis, particularly in cases of multi-focal lesions (Li et al., 2023).

Advancements in the field of artificial intelligence have led to the integration of deep learning (DL) algorithms in computer-aided detection and diagnosis (CAD) systems. CNN has predominantly emerged as the leading approach in the field of medical image analysis. CNNs employ convolutional kernels with small perceptual fields to extract features through weight sharing and local connectivity (Sun et al., 2023).

Using a microscope to do a microscopic biopsy on tissue samples is the traditional approach used to diagnose OSCC (Flügge et al., 2023; Deo et al., 2024). Lower-resolution settings are often used to view histopathological pictures in order to enable a more in-depth analysis of tissue architecture. The identification of cancer cells primarily relies on the examination of cell distribution, cell size and shape, as well as the size and form of the cell nucleus. Prior to conducting surgical procedures, it is imperative to carry out histopathological analysis in order to accurately ascertain the size of the tumour. The diagnostic pathology approach described in this study depends on the expertise of histopathologists for interpretation, a process that can be time-consuming and susceptible to errors, thereby restricting its practical use in clinical settings (Weber et al., 2024).

The key findings of the research study are as follows:

- The extensive use of TL on a diverse range of pre-trained models, including VGG16, VGG19, ResNet50, DenseNet121, InceptionV3, MobileNetV2, Xception, and InceptionResNetV2, for the classification of OSCC images. By freezing the last layer of each neural network and customizing the dense layer with new weights and biases, their ability to recognize OSCC-specific features was improved. Through a detailed evaluation, DenseNet121 was found to be the most precise model for categorizing OSCC images, based on an extensive analysis of classification ACC and multiple performance metrics.
- Additionally, I assessed the computational efficiency by comparing the training and prediction times of each TL model. This comprehensive approach, which balances precision (P) and efficiency, highlights the practical significance of my research in optimizing models for OSCC data analysis, providing valuable insights into both training ACC and computational performance.

9.2 RELATED WORK

This overview of the literature offers a critical evaluation of the recent studies that use AI and computer vision to enhance the diagnosis of cancer of the mouth. This publication synthesizes and analyses important research, methodology, and results in an effort to provide a thorough overview of the developments in the nexus of medical and computer sciences (Zhou et al., 2024).

One significant benefit of AI is its ability to decrease the burden of manually visualizing slides. Additionally, it aids pathologists in expediting decision-making processes with enhanced P. The utilization of computerized image analysis in the examination of tissue slides has the potential to capture information that may be overlooked through conventional slide-viewing methods. In order to achieve early diagnosis, classification, prediction, and specific treatment planning for oral cancer (OC), it is imperative to obtain histological findings that are both precise and accurate (de Chauveron et al., 2024). Several works were published with the detailing of AI in staring detection, prediction and categorization of OSCC.

The effectiveness of TL in the context of binary classification using OSCC images. Specifically, the study aims to compare the performance of fine-tuning existing DL models with a model that is built from scratch (Khanagar et al., 2023). Some of the frozen layers in the DCNN algorithms have to be taken into account throughout the fine-tuning procedure. As a result, training using the OSCC pictures is allowed for half of the model's layers.

The present diagnostic techniques employed for OSCC exhibit certain limitations in terms of their ACC and efficiency, thereby underscoring the necessity for the development of more dependable methodologies (Araújo et al., 2023). The goal of this study is to evaluate the ability of histopathological images to differentiate between epithelium oral tissues and OSCC. A tailored DL model that is EfficientNetB3 was created using 230 patients from a dataset of 1,220 images. Different magnifications of these images are publicly available. The purpose of the model is to differentiate between normal cells and OSCC components through the application of advanced techniques, including data augmentation, regularization, and optimization (Panigrahi et al., 2023).

The present study focuses on the investigation of the OSCC using DL techniques. This research aims to improve the diagnostic process by making it quicker, more affordable, and highly accurate. This work is to offer a comprehensive analysis of different methodologies for the effective identification of carcinogenic cells (Albalawi et al., 2024). A thorough analysis was performed using methodologies like local binary patterns and histogram features to showcase the effectiveness of CNN-based techniques in improving OSCC detection (Ananthakrishnan et al., 2023).

The objective of this study was to create an AI system capable of identifying cellular and structural abnormalities in order to diagnose the complete spectrum of SCC, including well-differentiated SCC with unremarkable cytology (Haq et al., 2023). In order to achieve this objective, training datasets were constructed using broad views of various magnifications, which were intended to simulate the diagnostic approach of a pathologist (Oya et al., 2023).

The CNN model presented in this book has been trained using a dataset including pathology visuals. The model employs a multi-layered approach to extract characteristics and carry out classifying (Afify et al., 2023). The ResNet101 model attained an ACC of 89%, R of 93%, a P of 89%, and a TN of 88%. Ahmed et al., (2023) conducted a study where they created a new meta-heuristic algorithm that combines particle swarm optimization (PSO) with Al-Biruni Earth Radius Optimization (ABERO) techniques to identify cancer (Pereira-Prado et al., 2023).

This technique was trained using an expanded dataset of oral pictures. Instead of using computerized microscopic pictures for assessing the grade of OSCC, Das et al. opted to choose tiny patches from 156 Whole Slide pictures (WSIs) and convert them into digital format at a magnification of 40X. A comparative analysis was carried out between the TL approaches and architectures and the models built from scratch (Pandiar et al., 2023). The findings, with an ACC of 96.51%, showed that CNNs built from the ground up performed better than TL models (Mohan et al., 2023).

This study systematically reviewed various TL models, including ResNet50, DenseNet121, VGG16, InceptionV3, VGG19, MobileNetV2, and InceptionResNetV2. Notably, Dense Net121 exhibited superior classification ACC in comparison to all other models. The DenseNet121 model completed its training process in 32 epochs.

9.3 APPROACH AND TECHNIQUES

The current study focuses on categorizing oral histopathology pictures into two groups using TL and a new CNN model. It highlights the need to include weight and bias modifications to improve performance. The detection procedure occurs in different steps, as shown in Figure 9.1. We collected and pre-processed a collection of histological pictures of OSCC using Gaussian filtering and CLAHE methods, along with data augmentation. We then divided the dataset into training, validation, and testing subsets.

9.3.1 Dataset Collection

The primary work of this study was to classify an oral database into two distinct categories: benign and malignant. We achieved this by utilizing a dataset from a repository that contained samples of both normal oral cavities and OSCC (Deif et al., 2022). The dataset, which can be accessed via the URL "https://data.mendeley.com/datasets/ftmp4cvtmb/1", comprises 1224 total images of the histopathological oral cavity. We categorize these images into two distinct groups. The initial dataset consists of 528 images captured at a magnification of 100×. Among these images, 439 portray instances of "oral cancer", while the remaining 89 images depict normal conditions. The second category comprises a total of 696 images, each magnified at a factor of 400×. We have classified 495 of these images as malignant, indicating the presence of cancerous cells, and 201 as benign, indicating the absence of cancerous cells. Table 9.1 presents a comprehensive breakdown of 1224 images, comprising 290 normal and 934 cancerous instances.

Concurrently, the utilization of datasets is crucial for the advancement of models, and the collection of epithelial biopsy tissue samples took place at SRM Kattankulathur Dental College & Hospital, which is affiliated with the SRM Institute of Science and Technology. The dataset comprises a collection of biopsy images obtained from a hospital, encompassing a total of 96 images. These datasets were integrated with publicly available and real-time datasets. Now the dataset contains a total 1276 images.

9.3.1.1 Ethical Considerations

The research adheres to ethical standards, obtaining necessary approvals and informed consent for the utilization of medical data. Privacy and confidentiality measures are implemented to protect the identities of individuals represented in the OSCC dataset. Here is the ethical clearance number for real-time dataset **8758/IEC/2023**.

9.3.2 Data Splitting

Using the commonly employed train-test split method, we divided the total amount of stained images from Table 9.1 into three categories: train, validation, and test. More specifically, we designate 70% of the total amount for training, and allocate 15% for both validation and testing. The used dataset is further divided into "training

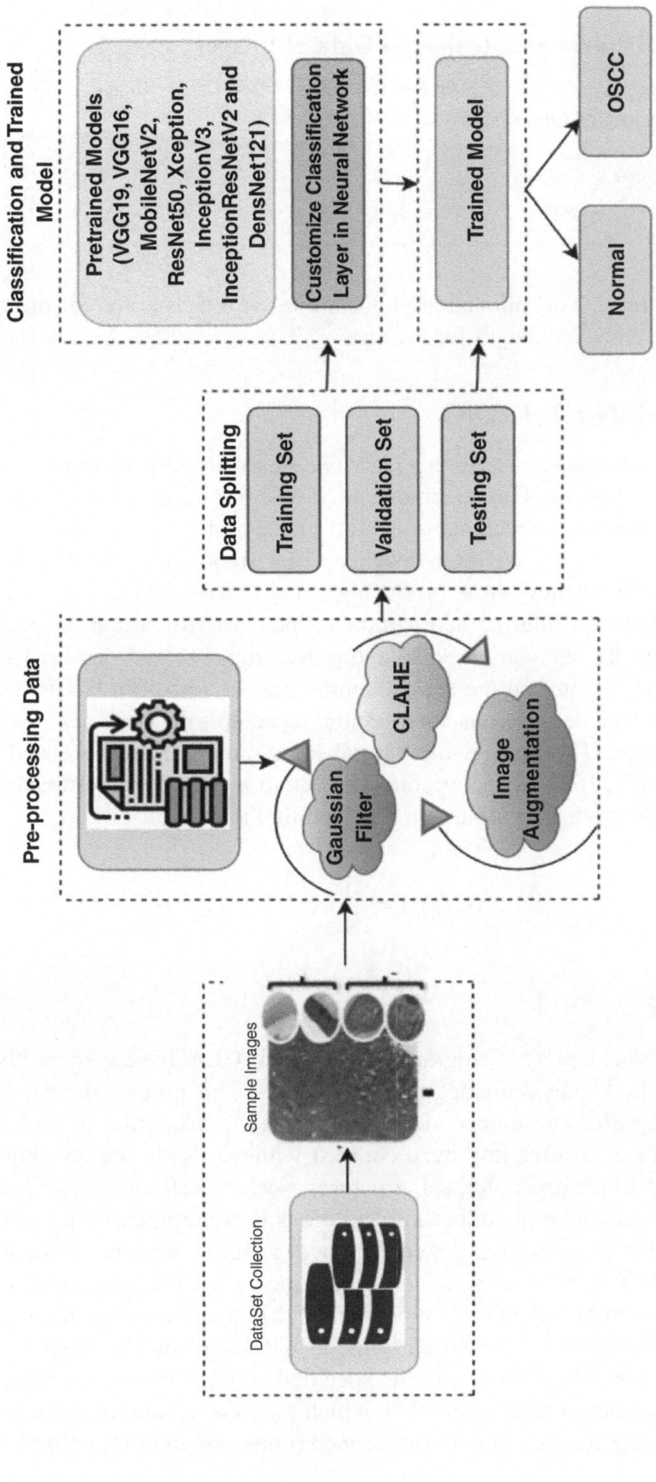

FIGURE 9.1 Overall architecture for proposed work.

TABLE 9.1
Distribution of Public and Real-Time Dataset Images

Type of Category	Total No of Images	Non-Cancer Images	OSCC Images
(4X, 10X, and 40X magnification) Category-1	96	58	36
(400 × magnification) Category-2	695	201	494
(100 × magnification) Category-3	530	89	441

and validation sets". This allocation yields a total of 4955 photos for the train, 120 images for Val, and 126 images for the test.

9.4 GAUSSIAN FILTERING

Histopathological image processing uses Gaussian filtering to reduce noise and enhance image features. This technique involves the image with a Gaussian kernel, which assigns higher weights to central pixels and gradually lower weights to surrounding pixels based on their distance. This smoothing operation effectively suppresses high-frequency noise, producing a more visually pleasing image. In histopathology, Gaussian filtering helps improve the clarity of structures, such as cellular boundaries, by attenuating noise and preserving essential details. Here G (X, Y), where x and y represent the spatial coordinates of a pixel in the image, here, π stands for the mathematical constant Pi, and σ represents the Gaussian distribution's standard deviation. The base of the natural logarithm, denoted by e and approximately equal to 2.71828, is incorporated in Equation 9.1. The coordinates x and y correspond to the spatial location of a pixel within the image.

$$G(X,Y) = \frac{1}{2\pi\sigma} e^{\frac{-X+Y}{2\sigma 2}} \tag{9.1}$$

9.5 CLAHE

Contrast Limited Adaptive Histogram Equalization (CLAHE) enhances histopathological images by locally adjusting pixel intensities. This process divides the image into overlapping tiles and independently equalizes the histogram of each tile. This localized approach ensures improved contrast within specific regions, highlighting intricate details in histopathological structures, such as cell nuclei and boundaries. CLAHE proves effective in addressing variations in staining and illumination, providing a valuable pre-processing step for good, accurate evaluations of images of pathology. Here, *L* represents the lower limit of the contrast enhancement, *U* denotes the upper limit, and *M* is the maximum pixel value in the image. The numerator, *I–L*, quantifies the pixel intensity deviation from the lower limit, and dividing by the range (*U–L*) ensures normalization within the specified contrast limits. We then scale the result by the maximum pixel value (M), which provides a contrast-enhanced image while constraining amplification to the defined limits shown in Equation 9.2.

$$\mathrm{CLAHE}(\mathrm{I}) = \frac{\mathrm{I} - \mathrm{L}}{\mathrm{U} - \mathrm{L}} * \mathrm{M} \tag{9.2}$$

9.6 PERSONALIZED DENSE LAYER IN NEURAL NETWORK

In this book chapter, prominent benchmark models for TL are selected, encompassing VGG16, VGG19, ResNet50, Inception V3, DenseNet121, MobileNetV2, and InceptionResNetV2. Each of these pre-trained models underwent customization through the addition of a flattening layer, transforming the multi-dimensional output into a one-dimensional vector. We incorporated a dense layer with 1024 neurons and ReLU activation to capture intricate correlations within the data. The final layer comprised a dense output layer with six neurons, specifically tuned for the task, employing Soft Max activation to enable effective multi-class classification. Here's a step-by-step procedure to add 1024 neurons to the dense layer of a DenseNet121 model shown in Figure 9.2.

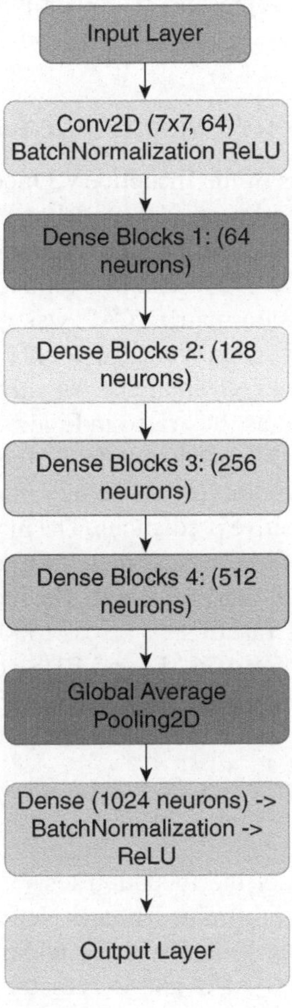

FIGURE 9.2 Customized 1024-neuron dense layer in TL models.

9.7 FINDINGS AND ANALYSIS OF THE TL MODELS UNDER CONSIDERATION

The following paragraphs will evaluate the outcomes of the TL models being examined, and contrast them with the suggested model. In addition, it will include the evaluation criteria and confusion matrices.

9.7.1 Evaluation Metrics

The examination of oral histopathology image categorization produced different classification findings for each DL model. We trained and tested models like InceptionV3, InceptionResNetV2, ResNet50, MobileNetV2, VGG19, VGG16, and DenseNet121 using a dataset of 4000 pictures per class. The classification reports include detailed information on the performance indicators of each model, such as accuracy(ACC), Recall(R), F1-Score(F1-Sc), and Sup. P assesses the model's ACC in predicting good outcomes, whereas R evaluates its capability to identify all positive events. The Sup measure represents the quantity of actual occurrences in each category.

9.7.2 Analysis of InceptionV3 Model Outcomes

We evaluated the effectiveness of the InceptionV3 model on the cancer histopathology dataset using a pre-trained Image Net model as the base. The ResNet50 architecture was utilized and enhanced with an additional Soft Max classifier to separate images into 'Normal' & 'OSCC'. ACC and loss for both training and validation were plotted over epochs. A confusion matrix (CM) was generated for the InceptionV3 model to analyze the findings, displaying the counts of True Positives (TP), False Positives (FP), True Negatives (TN), and False Negatives (FN). The CM showed 700 TN, 34 FP, 30 FN, and 736 TP, as illustrated in Figure 9.3.

The classification report highlights the model's exceptional performance in distinguishing between categories in oral histopathology images. The P scores of 0.96 for both classes underscore the positive predictions. The model's high R scores of 0.96 for both classes indicate its ability to correctly identify true cases. The F1-Sc of 0.96 for both reflects a balanced combination of P and R. The model demonstrates outstanding reliability, with an overall ACC rate of 95% across 1500 instances. The macro average and weighted average of 0.96 for ACC, R, and F1-Sc confirm the model's effectiveness in oral histopathology image categorization, as shown in Table 9.2.

9.7.3 Analysis of the Outcomes Obtained from the InceptionResNetV2 Model

We assessed the performance of the InceptionResNetV2 model on OSCC histopathology images, leveraging a pre-trained Image Net model as the foundation. The ResNet50 architecture was augmented with an additional Soft Max classifier into images 'Normal' and 'OSCC'. ACC and curves for both training and validation were meticulously plotted over epochs, providing insights into the model's learning

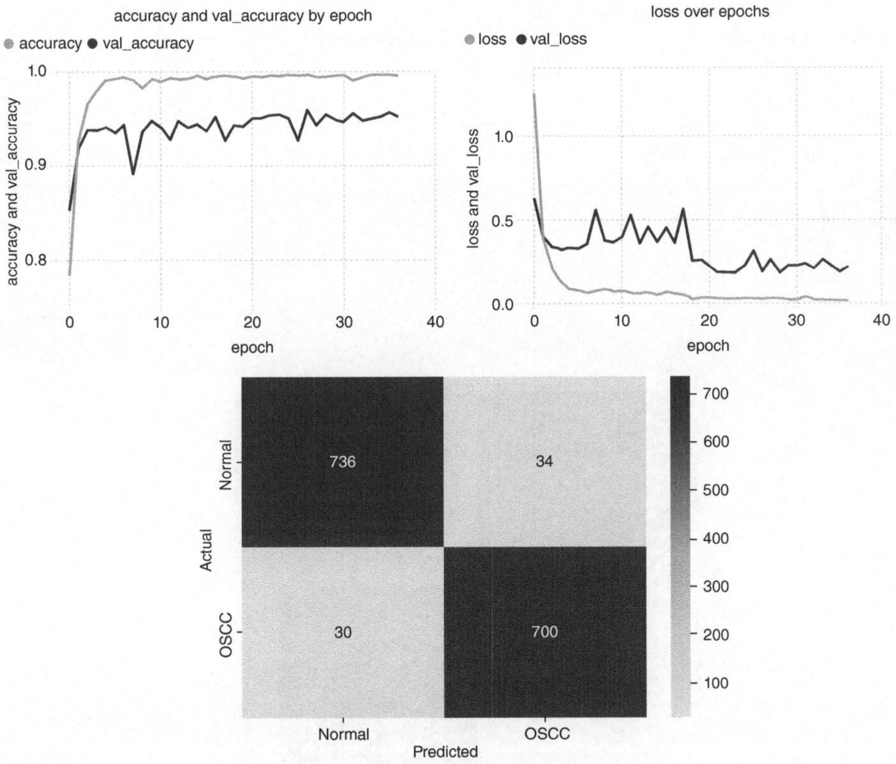

FIGURE 9.3 ACC and Loss plots over epochs and CM of InceptionV3.

TABLE 9.2
Classification Report for InceptionV3_model_4000_images_per_class

Type of Class	P	R	F1-Sc	Sup
normal	0.96	0.96	0.96	770
OSCC	0.95	0.96	0.96	730
ACC	-	-	0.95	1500
Mac Avg	0.96	0.96	0.96	1500
Weig Avg	0.96	0.96	0.96	1500

dynamics. A CM was generated, revealing 702 TN, 40 FP, 28 FN, and 730 TP as detailed in Figure 9.4.

The classification report underscores the InceptionResNetV2 model's strong performance in accurately differentiating between 'Normal' and 'OSCC' classes. P values of 0.96 for 'Normal' and 0.95 for 'OSCC' reflect the model's high ACC in positive predictions. R values of 0.95 for 'Normal' and 0.96 for 'OSCC' highlight the effectiveness of model in correctly identifying true cases. F1-Sc of 0.96 for 'Normal'

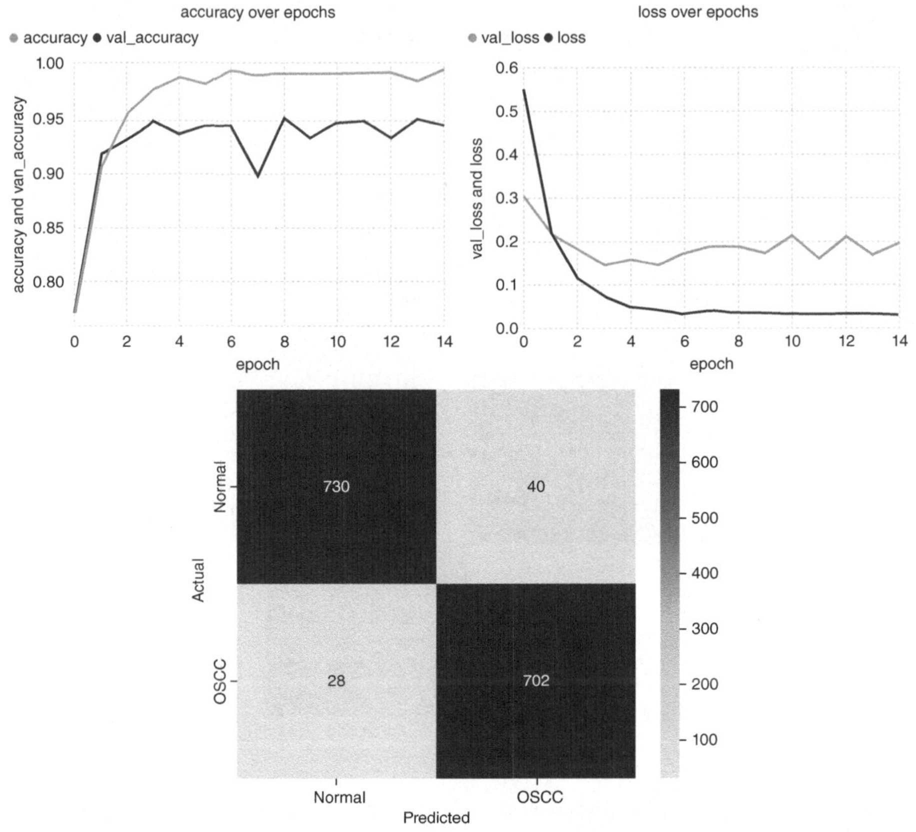

FIGURE 9.4 ACC and loss curve over epochs and CM of InceptionResnetV2 model.

and 0.95 for 'OSCC' illustrate a strong balance between P and R. The model achieved an overall ACC of 95% across 1500 instances, demonstrating its reliability and effectiveness. Table 9.3 further validates the model's consistent performance, with macro and weighted averages of 0.95 for ACC, R, and F1-Sc, affirming its potential for enhancing the ACC and efficiency of OSCC diagnosis in clinical practice.

TABLE 9.3
Classification for InceptionResNetV2_model_ 4000_images_per_class

Type of Class	P	R	F1-Sc	Sup
Normal	0.96	0.95	0.96	770
OSCC	0.95	0.96	0.95	730
ACC	-	-	0.95	1500
Mac Avg	0.95	0.95	0.95	1500
Weig Avg	0.95	0.95	0.95	1500

9.7.4 Results Achieved by the ResNet50 Model

In evaluating the ResNet50 model's performance on histopathological images, a pre-trained Image Net model served as the foundational framework. The ResNet50 architecture was enhanced with an additional Soft Max classifier to enable classification into distinct categories. ACC and loss curves for both training and validation were meticulously plotted over epochs to assess the model's performance. A CM was computed for the ResNet50 model, presenting counts of TP, FP, TN, and FN. The CM revealed 623 TN, 184 FP, 107 FN, and 586 TP, as illustrated in Figure 9.5.

The classification analysis demonstrates that the ResNet50 model performs robustly in oral histopathology image categorization. P scores of 0.85 for 'Normal' and 0.77 for 'OSCC' indicate accurate positive predictions. R values of 0.76 for 'Normal' and 0.81 for 'OSCC' reflect the model's effectiveness in identifying true cases. F1 scores of 0.80 for 'Normal' and 0.85 for 'OSCC' illustrate a strong balance between P and R. The model's reliability is further underscored by an overall ACC of 85% across 1500 instances. The macro average and weighted average of 0.85 for ACC, R, and F1-Sc, as shown in Table 9.4, affirm the model's consistent and reliable performance, highlighting its potential for accurate classification in oral histopathology applications.

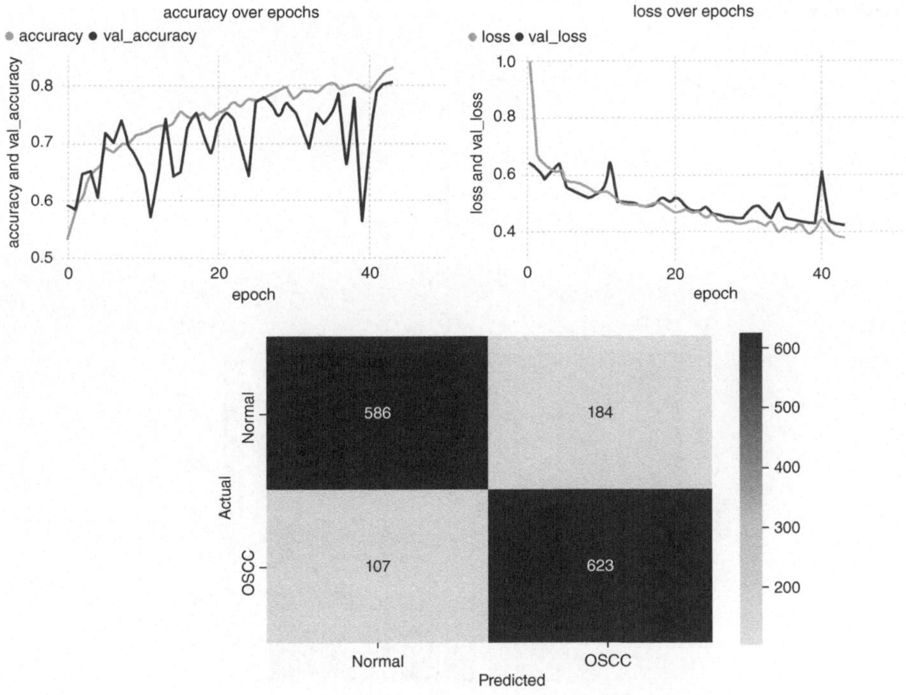

FIGURE 9.5 ACC and Loss plots of training over epochs and CM of Resnet50.

TABLE 9.4
Classification Report for ResNet50_model_ 4000_images_per_class

Type of Class	P	R	F1-Sc	Sup
normal	0.85	0.76	0.80	770
OSCC	0.77	0.81	0.85	730
ACC	-	-	0.85	1500
Mac Avg	0.85	0.85	0.85	1500
Weig Avg	0.85	0.85	0.85	1500

9.7.5 Reviewing the Results Obtained from the MobileNetV2 Model

In assessing the capability of the MobileNetV2 model on the Mendeley histopathological a pre-trained Image Net model was utilized as the basis. The MobileNetV2 was employed, augmented with an additional Soft Max classifier for classifying images into "Normal and OSCC". "Training and validation ACC", as well as loss curves, were plotted over epochs. To further interpret the results, a CM for the model was computed, illustrating counts of "TP, FP, TN, and FN". Notably, the CM revealed 708 TN, 24 FP, 22 FN and 746 TP in Figure 9.6.

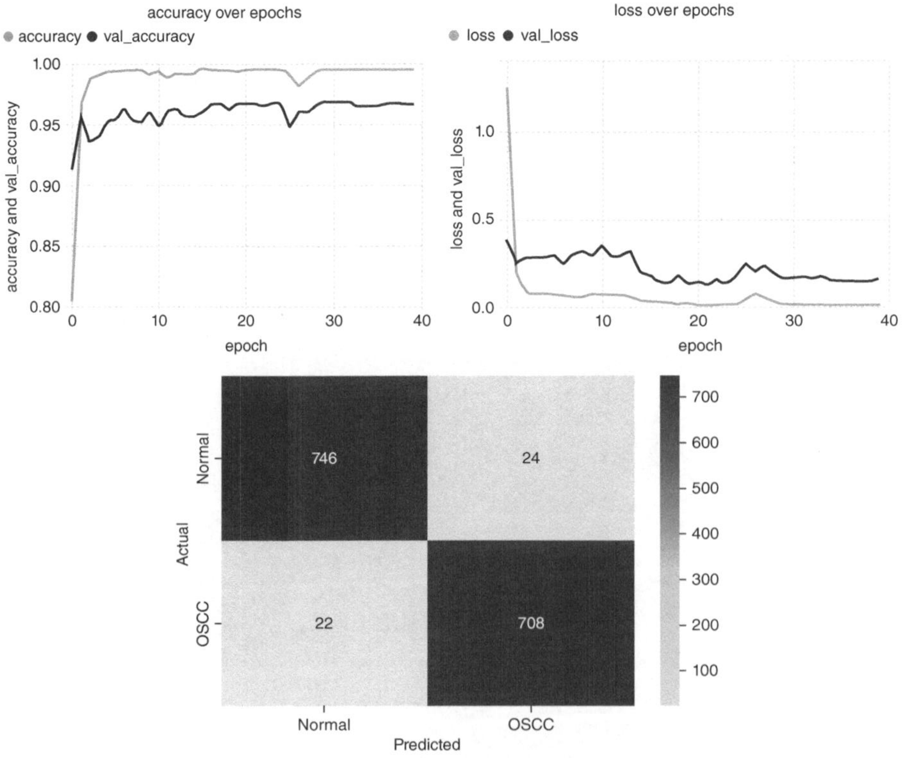

FIGURE 9.6 ACC and Loss plots of training over epochs and CM of MobileNetV2.

TABLE 9.5
Classification Report for MobileNetV2_model_4000_images_per_class

Type of Class	P	R	F1-Sc	Sup
normal	0.97	0.97	0.97	770
OSCC	0.97	0.97	0.97	730
ACC	-	-	0.97	1500
Mac Avg	0.97	0.97	0.97	1500
Weig Avg	0.97	0.97	0.97	1500

The analysis highlights the exceptional performance of the MobileNetV2 model in discriminating among 'Normal' and 'OSCC' classes in oral histopathology images. Both classes have P values of 0.97, indicating accurate positive predictions. The R values of 0.97 for both categories demonstrate the model's successful capacity to catch genuine cases. An F1-Sc of 0.97 for both indicates a balanced performance in terms of ACC and R. The model's great dependability is shown by an overall ACC of 97% over 1500 occurrences. The MobileNetV2 model demonstrates strong and consistent performance in oral histopathology image categorization, with ACC, R, and F1-Sc all averaging at 0.97 in Table 9.5.

9.7.6 Analysis of the Results Generated by the VGG19 Model

In the result of the VGG19 working on the OSCC histopathological images, a pre-trained Image Net model served as the foundation. The VGG19 architecture was employed, augmented with an additional SoftMax classifier for classifying images into "Normal and OSCC" categories. "Training and validation ACC", as well as loss curves, were plotted over epochs. To further interpret the results, a CM for the model was computed, illustrating counts of "TP, FP, TN, and FN". Notably, the CM revealed 623 TN, 184 FP, 107 FN and 586 TP in Figure 9.7.

The classification report for the VGG19 model demonstrates commendable performance in the classification of classes within oral histopathological images. P values of 0.96 ('Normal') and 0.94 ('OSCC') signify accurate positive predictions, while R values of 0.94 ('Normal') and 0.95 ('OSCC') indicate the model's ability to effectively capture true instances. F1-Scores of 0.95 for both 'Normal' and 'OSCC' classes highlight a balanced trade-off between P and R. The overall ACC of 95% across 1500 instances underscores the model's reliability. Consistent Mac Avg and Weig Avg of 0.95 for "P, R, and F1-Sc" of the VGG19 model robust and stable performance in oral histopathological image classification in Table 9.6.

9.7.7 Discussion of VGG16 Model Results

The VGG16 model's performance on the cancer histopathology was evaluated with a pre-trained Image Net model as the base. The VGG16 architecture was used, enhanced with an extra Soft Max classifier to categorize pictures into "Normal and OSCC". ACC and loss curves for training and validation were graphed over epochs.

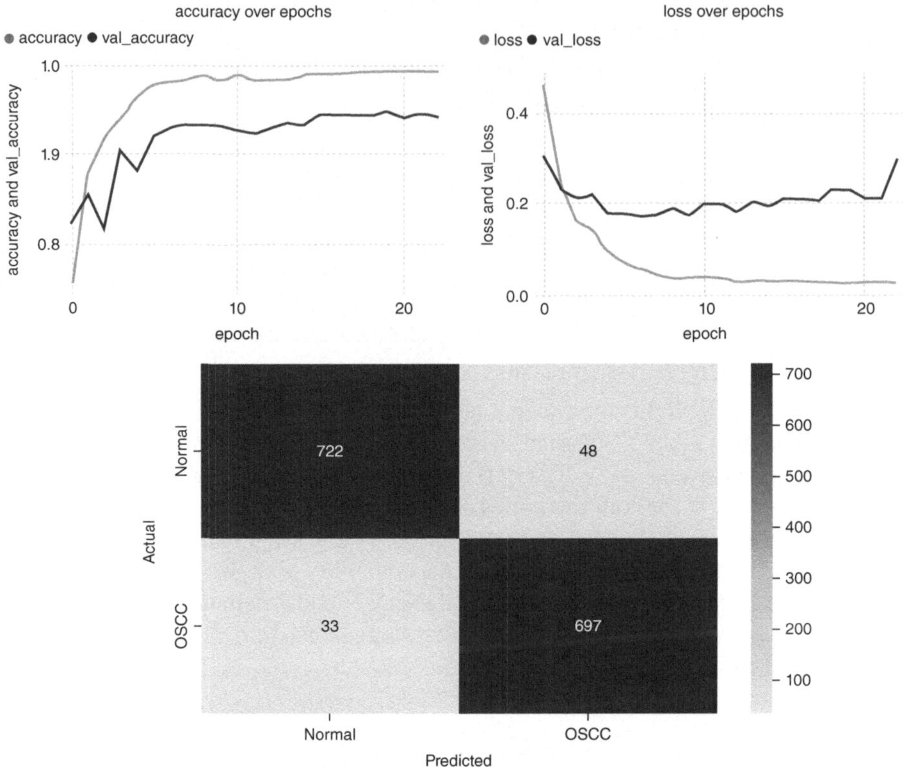

FIGURE 9.7 ACC and Loss plots of training over epochs and CM of VGG19.

TABLE 9.6
Classification Report for VGG19_model_ 4000_images_per_class

Type of Class	P	R	F1-Sc	Sup
normal	0.96	0.94	0.95	770
OSCC	0.94	0.95	0.95	730
ACC	-	-	0.95	1500
Mac Avg	0.95	0.95	0.95	1500
Weig Avg	0.95	0.95	0.95	1500

A CM was calculated to understand the data, showing the counts of "True Positive (TP), False Positive (FP), True Negative (TN), and False Negative (FN)". The CM in Figure 9.8 showed 705 TN, 40 FP, 25 FN and 730 TP.

The classification report for the VGG16 model illustrates exemplary performance in the classification of distinct classes within oral histopathological images. P values

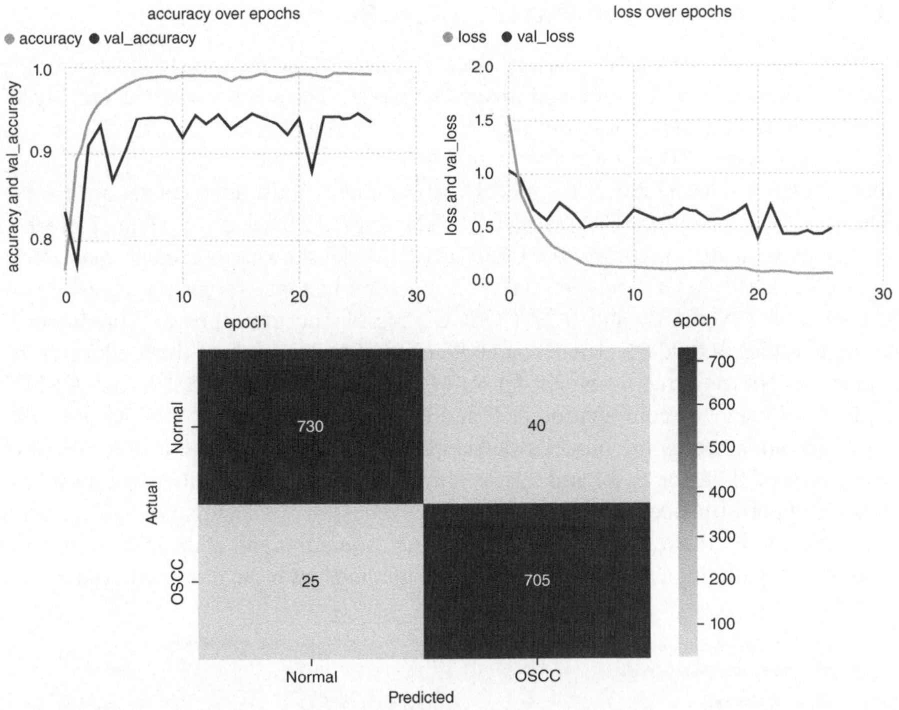

FIGURE 9.8 ACC and Loss plots of training over epochs and CM of VGG16.

of 0.97 ('Normal') and 0.95 ('OSCC') signify accurate positive predictions, while R values of 0.95 ('Normal') and 0.97 ('OSCC') indicate the model's adeptness in capturing true instances. The F1-Scs of 0.96 for both 'Normal' and 'OSCC' classes highlight a harmonious balance between P and R. The overall ACC of 96% across 1500 instances underscores the model's reliability. Consistent Mac Avg and Weig Avg of 0.96 for P, R, and F1-Sc further affirm the VGG16 model's robust and consistent performance in oral histopathological image classification in Table 9.7.

TABLE 9.7
Classification Report for VGG16_model_4000_images_per_class

Type of Class	P	R	F1-Sc	Sup
normal	0.97	0.95	0.96	770
OSCC	0.95	0.97	0.96	730
ACC	-	-	0.96	1500
Mac Avg	0.96	0.96	0.96	1500
Weig Avg	0.96	0.96	0.96	1500

9.7.8 Discussion of DensNet121 Model Results

In the analysis of the DensNet121 quality on the histopathological, the foundation of the model was built upon a pre-trained Image Net model. The architecture was employed, augmented with an additional soft max classifier for dividing images into "Normal & OSCC" categories. "Training and validation ACC", were plotted over epochs. To further interpret the results, a CM for the model was computed, illustrating counts of "TP, FP, TN, and FN". Notably, the CM revealed 718 TN, 25 FP, 12 FN and 745 TP in Figure 9.9.

The classification report for the DensNet121 model showcases exceptional performance in classifying a variety of classes within oral histopathological images. P values of 0.98 ('Normal') and 0.97 ('OSCC') signify accurate positive predictions, while R values of 0.97 ('Normal') and 0.98 ('OSCC') demonstrate the model's proficiency in capturing true instances. F1-Sc of 0.98 for 'Normal' and 0.97 for 'OSCC' highlight a balanced combination of P and R. The overall ACC of 98% across 1500 instances underscores the model's outstanding reliability. Consistent Mac Avg and Weig Avg of 0.98 for P, R, and F1-Sc affirm the DensNet121 model's robust and consistent performance, emphasizing its effectiveness in oral histopathological image classification in Table 9.8. Table 9.9 shows the evaluation and comparative analysis of oral histopathological image classification methods with the proposed system.

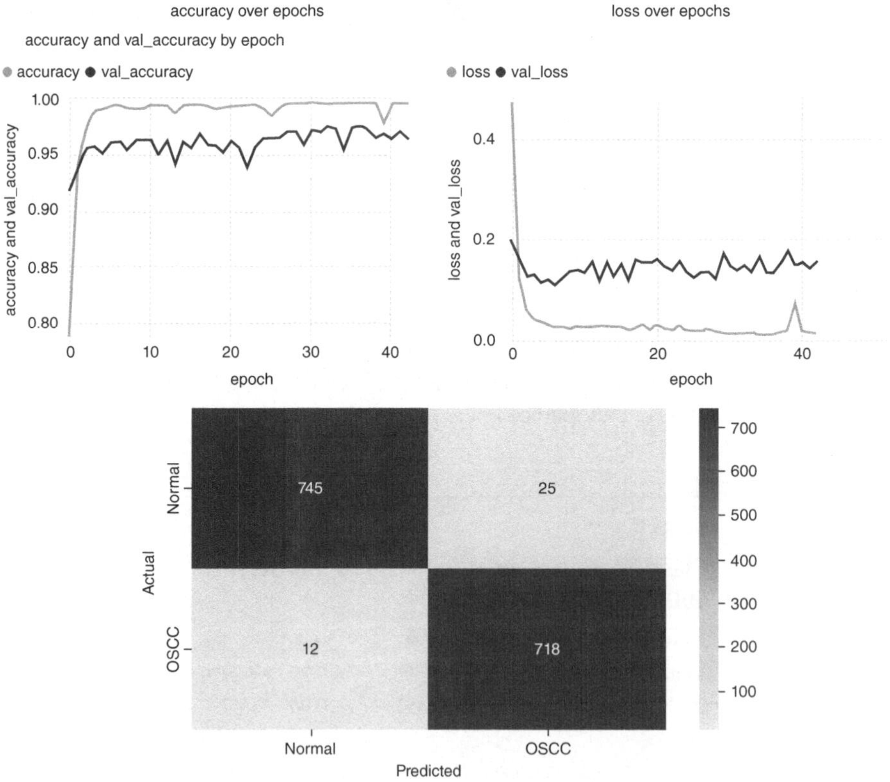

FIGURE 9.9 ACC and Loss plots of training over epochs CM of DenseNet121.

TABLE 9.8
Classification Report for DenseNet121_model_4000_images_per_class

Class Type	P	R	F1-Sc	Sup
normal	0.98	0.97	0.98	770
OSCC	0.97	0.98	0.97	730
ACC	-	-	0.98	1500
Mac Avg	0.98	0.98	0.98	1500
Weig Avg	0.98	0.98	0.98	1500

TABLE 9.9
Evaluation and Comparative Analysis of Oral Histopathological Image Classification Methods with a Proposed System

Existing Approach	Number of Images in Dataset	Type of Images and Features	Methods Used	ACC of Images
(Nanditha B R et al.)	Benign-63 Malignant-269	Image's raw pixel data	Ensemble model (ResNet50 and VGG16)	96.2
(Mohanad A. Deif)	Normal Epithelium of the oral cavity (NEOR) and OSCC	Image's raw pixel dataset	Inception V3 with BPSO	96.3%
(Rahman, A. U. et al.)	Sick (OSCC) 2511 Healthy 2435	Different Rank features from OSCC	Transfer Learning (Alex Net)	96.6%
Proposed TL Customized model	Normal images-316 OSCC images 960	Images of raw pixel data	Densnet121	97.55%

9.8 LIMITATION AND FUTURE WORK

The study focused on comparing pre-trained models for OSCC image classification but did not address cancer grading and staging. Real-time data analysis posed challenges, affecting time efficiency. The model, trained on both public and real-time data, may lack generalization to other clinical environments, as its performance across diverse imaging equipment and protocols is yet to be validated. While the study highlights the limitations of manual screening, no direct comparison with manual methods was made to quantify the AI-driven approach's improvement. Future research should address these limitations to enhance the model's robustness and clinical applicability.

9.9 CONCLUSION

The utilization of automated systems incorporating AI holds great potential for improving the diagnosis and classification of OSCC tumours within the healthcare industry.

The present study undertakes a comparative analysis of different Customized TL methodologies, utilizing feature extraction models including ResNet50, DenseNet121, VGG16, InceptionV3, VGG19, MobileNetV2, and InceptionResNetV2. Distinctive features are extracted from OSCC biopsy images using a DenseNet121 model implemented in a CNN framework, showcasing its strong training capabilities. The results of this study demonstrate a significant achievement in classification ACC, with a training ACC of 99% and a testing ACC of 97.55%, using both public and real-time data. These findings highlight the potential of AI-driven systems to enhance the ACC and efficiency of OSCC tumour classification. This is particularly important as it addresses the limitations of manual screening procedures and the presence of stain artefacts in biopsy tissues. Additional investigation and verification in practical clinical environments are imperative in order to fully comprehend the clinical efficacy of these sophisticated artificial intelligence technologies, ultimately propelling the field of pathology and improving patient results in the field of oncology.

REFERENCES

Afify, H. M., Mohammed, K. K., & Hassanien, A. E. (2023). Novel prediction model on OSCC histopathological images via deep transfer learning combined with Grad-CAM interpretation. *Biomedical Signal Processing and Control*, *83*, 104704.

Ahmed, I. A., Senan, E. M., & Shatnawi, H. S. A. (2023). Analysis of histopathological images for early diagnosis of oral squamous cell carcinoma by hybrid systems based on CNN fusion features. *International Journal of Intelligent Systems*, *2023*(1), 2662719.

Albalawi, E., Thakur, A., Ramakrishna, M. T., Bhatia Khan, S., SankaraNarayanan, S., Almarri, B., & Hadi, T. H. (2024). Oral squamous cell carcinoma detection using EfficientNet on histopathological images. *Frontiers in Medicine*, *10*, 1349336.

Ananthakrishnan, B., Shaik, A., Kumar, S., Narendran, S. O., Mattu, K., & Kavitha, M. S. (2023). Automated detection and classification of oral squamous cell carcinoma using deep neural networks. *Diagnostics*, *13*(5), 918.

Araújo, A. L. D., da Silva, V. M., Kudo, M. S., de Souza, E. S. C., Saldivia-Siracusa, C., Giraldo-Roldán, D., … Moraes, M. C. (2023). Machine learning concepts applied to oral pathology and oral medicine: a convolutional neural networks' approach. *Journal of Oral Pathology & Medicine*, *52*(2), 109–118.

Badwelan, M., Muaddi, H., Ahmed, A., Lee, K. T., & Tran, S. D. (2023). Oral squamous cell carcinoma and concomitant primary tumors, what do we know? A review of the literature. *Current Oncology*, *30*(4), 3721–3734.

de Chauveron, J., Unger, M., Lescaille, G., Wendling, L., Kurtz, C., & Rochefort, J. (2024). Artificial intelligence for oral squamous cell carcinoma detection based on oral photographs: A comprehensive literature review. *Cancer Medicine*, *13*(1), e6822.

Deif, M. A., Attar, H., Amer, A., Elhaty, I. A., Khosravi, M. R., & Solyman, A. A. (2022). Diagnosis of oral squamous cell carcinoma using deep neural networks and binary Particle Swarm optimization on histopathological images: an AIoMT approach. *Computational Intelligence and Neuroscience*, *2022*(1), 6364102.

Deo, B. S., Pal, M., Panigrahi, P. K., & Pradhan, A. (2024). An ensemble deep learning model with empirical wavelet transform feature for oral cancer histopathological image classification. *International Journal of Data Science and Analytics*, 22, 1–18.

Flügge, T., Gaudin, R., Sabatakakis, A., Tröltzsch, D., Heiland, M., van Nistelrooij, N., & Vinayahalingam, S. (2023). Detection of oral squamous cell carcinoma in clinical photographs using a vision transformer. *Scientific Reports*, *13*(1), 2296.

Haq, I. U., Ahmad, M., Assam, M., Ghadi, Y. Y., & Algarni, A. (2023). Unveiling the future of oral squamous cell carcinoma diagnosis: an innovative hybrid AI approach for accurate histopathological image analysis. *IEEE Access*, 11, 2169–3536.

Khanagar, S. B., Alkadi, L., Alghilan, M. A., Kalagi, S., Awawdeh, M., Bijai, L. K., … Singh, O. G. (2023). Application and performance of artificial intelligence (AI) in oral cancer diagnosis and prediction using histopathological images: a systematic review. *Biomedicines*, *11*(6), 1612.

Li, X., Wang, C., Zhang, H., Li, Y., Hou, D., Liu, D., … Jiang, H. (2023). circFNDC3B accelerates vasculature formation and metastasis in oral squamous cell carcinoma. *Cancer Research*, *83*(9), 1459–1475.

Mohan, R., Rama, A., Raja, R. K., Shaik, M. R., Khan, M., Shaik, B., & Rajinikanth, V. (2023). OralNet: fused optimal deep features framework for oral squamous cell carcinoma detection. *Biomolecules*, *13*(7), 1090.

Oya, K., Kokomoto, K., Nozaki, K., & Toyosawa, S. (2023). Oral squamous cell carcinoma diagnosis in digitized histological images using convolutional neural network. *Journal of Dental Sciences*, *18*(1), 322–329.

Pandiar, D., Choudhari, S., & Krishnan, R. P. (2023). Application of InceptionV3, SqueezeNet, and VGG16 convoluted neural networks in the image classification of oral squamous cell carcinoma: A cross-sectional study. *Cureus*, *15*(11). https://doi.org/10.7759/cureus.49108

Panigrahi, S., Nanda, B. S., Bhuyan, R., Kumar, K., Ghosh, S., & Swarnkar, T. (2023). Classifying histopathological images of oral squamous cell carcinoma using deep transfer learning. *Heliyon*, *9*(3), 1–14.

Pereira-Prado, V., Martins-Silveira, F., Sicco, E., Hochmann, J., Isiordia-Espinoza, M. A., González, R. G., … Bologna-Molina, R. (2023). Artificial intelligence for image analysis in oral squamous cell carcinoma: a review. *Diagnostics*, *13*(14), 2416.

Sun, L., Kang, X., Wang, C., Wang, R., Yang, G., Jiang, W., … Sun, S. (2023). Single-cell and spatial dissection of precancerous lesions underlying the initiation process of oral squamous cell carcinoma. *Cell Discovery*, *9*(1), 28.

Tan, Y., Wang, Z., Xu, M., Li, B., Huang, Z., Qin, S., … Huang, C. (2023). Oral squamous cell carcinomas: state of the field and emerging directions. *International Journal of Oral Science*, *15*(1), 44.

Wang, S., Yang, M., Li, R., & Bai, J. (2023). Current advances in noninvasive methods for the diagnosis of oral squamous cell carcinoma: a review. *European Journal of Medical Research*, *28*(1), 53.

Weber, A., Enderle-Ammour, K., Kurowski, K., Metzger, M. C., Poxleitner, P., Werner, M., … Bronsert, P. (2024). AI-Based Detection of Oral Squamous Cell Carcinoma with Raman Histology. *Cancers*, *16*(4), 689.

Zhou, J., Wu, H., Hong, X., Huang, Y., Jia, B., Lu, J., … Wu, T. (2024). A pathology-based diagnosis and prognosis intelligent system for oral squamous cell carcinoma using semi-supervised learning. *Expert Systems with Applications*, *254*, 124242.

10 Artificial Intelligence (AI)-Enabled Diabetic Retinopathy Detection Techniques

Ravi Bhushan Dixit and Chandan Kumar Jha

10.1 INTRODUCTION

In the healthcare domain, the initial detection of any disease is very effective in the treatment and diagnosis aspects. The rapid growth of the digital world and emerging technologies has made human life very comfortable, but on the other side, it has led our world to major challenges that threaten a healthy lifestyle. Due to this, people face many health complications, such as headaches, obesity and hypertension, cardiovascular diseases, eye-related issues, and other metabolic diseases. Diabetes, also known as diabetes mellitus (DM), is a metabolic disease where our body produces insulin irregularly, leading to an increase in the amount of sugar (glucose) in our blood. Our bodies use the hormone insulin to regulate blood sugar levels. Hyperglycemia, or high blood sugar, is a common side effect of untreated diabetes that can cause major injury to the body's system, mainly the blood capillaries and neurons. Diabetic retinopathy (DR) is a common chronic condition caused by diabetes. Diabetic patients who suffer for a long time are at high risk of developing eye disease, which further leads to blindness. Sometimes, retinal vessels swell and leak fluid and blood due to abnormal glucose levels. Therefore, to avoid the risk of permanent blindness, it is very essential to get treatment for DR at an earlier stage. The statistics report by the World Health Organization (WHO) roughly calculated that about 347 patients with diabetes are at high risk of DR, and this is rapidly increasing every year. Rising prevalence of diabetes in Asian nations like China and India will cause these rates to rise even more. In the United States of America (USA), out of 29.1 million people, 40 percent of the total suffer from different stages of DR. The International Diabetic Federation (IDF) conducted a poll and estimates that by the year 2045, there will be about 600 million diabetic patients (Sun et al., 2022). Moreover, based on WHO estimations, 79.4 million Indians will have diabetes by 2030, and an additional 25 million will be at increased risk of getting the disease in the future. Diabetes raises DR risk, which is the primary cause of blindness. Developing countries have a high number of diabetic patients, and there

DOI: 10.1201/9781003503385-10

is a lack of proper equipment for image analysis, which can take a couple of days (Ramachandran et al., 2010). Remote areas lack access to state-of-the-art diagnostic devices, such as fundus cameras. Hence, early detection of DR is necessary to prevent blindness. However, it is challenging to identify it in its initial stages, as DR shows few signs to detect. Generally, ophthalmologists use fundus images for the diagnosis and identification of DR manually. Manual grading or screening of DR using fundus images increases the workload and takes too much time to give the analytical result. Presently, automated DR analysis techniques play an important role in DR diagnosis. It assists experts and doctors in DR detection and saves time. Previously, various AI-enabled DR identification methods have been introduced, such as machine learning, deep learning, ensemble learning, and transfer learning approaches using fundus images. Recently, the convolutional neural network (CNN) has made detection and classification very simple and effective. A hybrid approach has been implemented for automatic DR detection (Ali et al., 2023). Firstly, the model extracts the features using Inceptionv3 and Resnet50 in a parallel manner, and then the extracted features are fed into CNN. In another approach (Kommaraju & Anbarasi, 2024), CNN and residual blocks are applied to detect the severity level of DR using data augmentation techniques to balance the datasets and avoid noise. In Karthika and Durgadevi (2024), the focus is on vessel segmentation using the U-net mechanism, and finally, classification process includes a squeeze and excitation block with Resnet-101. In Wang et al. (2024), the author developed a model for lesion detection using the lesion-aware knowledge distillation method using two datasets: IDRiD and DDR. Presently, the ensemble learning (Bodapati & Balaji, 2024), based approach represents a high level of accuracy for the detection of DR and its classification (Thomas & Jerome, 2024; Bhimavarapu, 2024).

10.2 FACTORS OF DR

As per the report of the WHO, DR mainly occurs in diabetic patients aged between 20 and 74 years. The following attributes may raise the risk of occurring DR: (a) diabetes for a longer period, (b) high cholesterol and blood pressure, (c) patients with poor control of blood glucose (sugar), (d) at the time of pregnancy, (e) regular-smoking. Prior identification of DR is essential to manage the risk of vision loss in diabetic patients. If DR is not detected at the earlier stage, it results in complications in retinal blood vessels. The abnormal growth of new vessels may lead to visual impairment.

10.3 CLASSIFICATION OF DR

Different types of abnormalities and tissue damage are caused by DR, which are termed as lesions. Some common lesions present in DR images are microaneurysms (MA), hemorrhages (HM), soft exudates, and hard exudates (EX). Based on lesions, DR is classified into no DR, mild DR, moderate DR, severe DR, and proliferative DR (Acharya et al., 2016). According to medical standards, DR is categorized into two types: non-proliferative diabetic retinopathy (NPDR) and proliferative diabetic retinopathy (PDR). Further, NPDR is subdivided based on symptoms and its level into

TABLE 10.1
DR Classes and Symptoms

Classes of DR	Characterized Symptoms
Normal	Absent Lesion
Mild	Sign of Microaneurysms
Moderate	More than MA
Severe	Sign of HM, EX, and MA
PDR	Neovascularization

three classes: mild, moderate, and severe (Yonekawa et al., 2020). Different classes of DR with symptoms are mentioned in Table 10.1.

In DR analysis, some basic terminologies are as follows:

- Microaneurysms (MA): retinal vessels become weak and swelled. In this condition, on the surface of the retina, small round red dots appear.
- Hemorrhages (HM): It has a spot size greater than 125 μm and has irregular margins. Spots are found in the internal layer of the retina due to fluid discharge. Hard exudates occur due to leakage of blood plasma, lipids, and protein and appear as yellow patches of variable sizes and shapes on the retina. Soft exudates: It is also called cotton wool spots, where swelling of nerve fibers occurs.
- Neovascularization: the development of novel capillaries occurs due to blockage present in original vessels. Sometimes new vessels rupture, and leakage of blood occurs. In NPDR, accumulation of fluid in subretinal space called exudates, hemorrhages, and microaneurysms are found. In mild NPDR, balloon-like swelling is found, named MA, which causes fluid leakage. In moderate NDPR, there is leakage of fluid and blood that is caused by HM. In severe NPDR, the supply of blood from various vessels of the retina stops, and as a result, new development of blood vessels in the retina occurs. PDR is the next progressive version of NPDR that is characterized by NV.

10.4 FUNDUS IMAGE

Fundus means the part of an eye opposite to the pupil that consists of the optical disc, macula, retinal vasculature, and retina. A specialized camera, which consists of a microscope (low power), is used to capture images. It captures the semi-transparent, retinal tissues associated with layers into a plane in three dimensions. The retinal images captured by the fundus camera may associate noise and discrepancy due to different settings and circumstances such as lighting and environmental effects. Figure 10.1 shows the fundus image of the normal and DR retina. Figure 10.2 shows fundus images of different classes of DR.

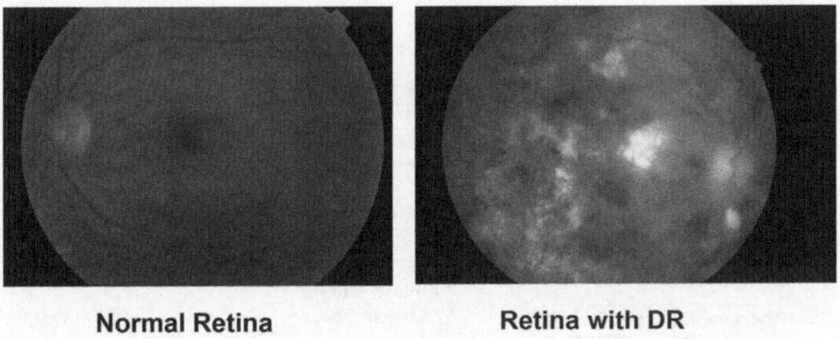

FIGURE 10.1 Normal and DR fundus image.

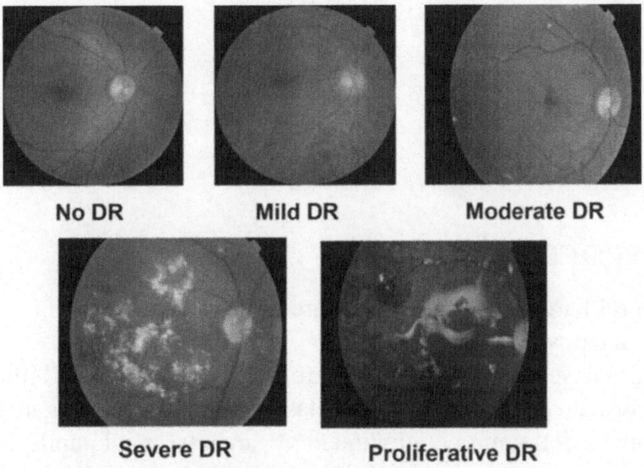

FIGURE 10.2 Fundus images of different DR classes.

10.5 DATASETS

A dataset consists of the records and data in digital form. In artificial intelligence (AI), it is an integral part of data analysis. In DR detection, some publicly available datasets that are widely used are Kaggle EyePACS, DDR, Messidor, DiretDB, E-Optha, IDRid, HRF, and APTOS-2019 (Dubey & Dixit, 2023).

Generally, fundus images of these datasets are classified into five classes: no DR, mild DR, moderate DR, severe DR, and PDR. Several fundus images have different sizes and are captured in different settings of fundus cameras. These images contain noise related to quality, size, and color imbalance. These noises are removed during the pre-processing step. It includes cropping, resizing, filtering, contrast enhancement, and other techniques to increase performance and efficiency. Figure 10.3 shows the proportion of splitting of a dataset into training data, validation data, and test data before feeding into the model.

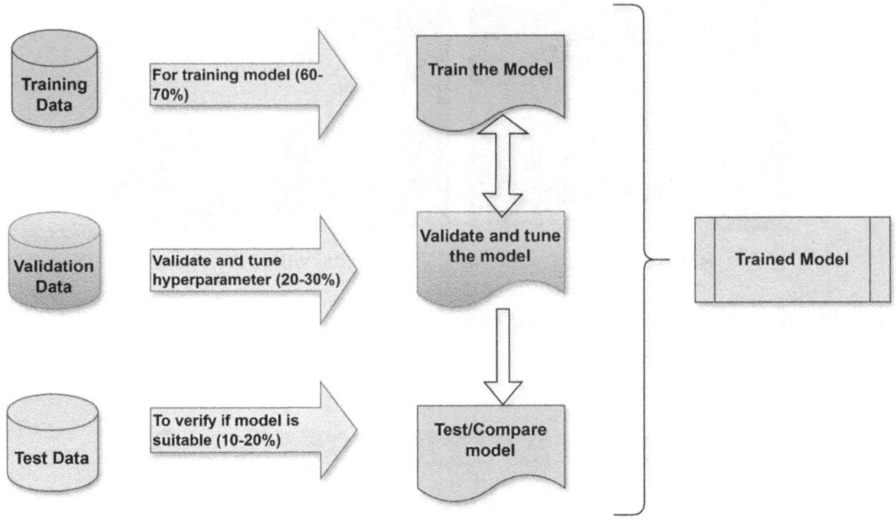

FIGURE 10.3 Dataset splitting.

10.6 PRE-PROCESSING

There are several hardware devices, that are used to capture fundus images, which are often associated with noise.

These images have problems regarding resolution, contrast, and illumination that affect the performance and results of the classification model. In general, some factors such as movement, improper alignment of cameras, small pupils, lighting conditions, and media opacity create problems in image acquisition. For the detailed exploration of features of the image, different pre-processing techniques are required. So we are discussing several techniques related to pre-processing.

- Contrast Enhancement: It is a general pre-processing technique used for highlighting the foreground of the images. For this, histogram equalization, and contrast limited adaptive histogram equalization (CLAHE) are common methods.
- Normalization and Noise removal: It is applied to standardize the image to a certain scale. Z-score normalization and robust scaling are some common normalization techniques.
- Noise removal techniques: It is a method to remove the unwanted variation in the data caused due to some interferences. Different types of filters such as median filter, Wiener filter, Gaussian filter, and non-local are employed according to the requirement and noise characteristics. Color space transformation is another technique used to improve model's efficiency and performance. Color space transformation has specified properties and is appropriate for several applications such as image compression, segmentation, image enhancement, and analysis.

- Size adjustment and cropping: These techniques are implemented to make the image in standard size, aspect ratio, and proper resolution as per requirement. Some other pre-processing techniques includes vessel enhancement, thresholding, and morphological operations (analysis related to image dimension and structure using a mathematical approach).
- Augmentation: It includes geometric transformations such as shifting, rescaling, shearing, flipping, and color augmentation as implemented in Pires et al. (2019). It is used to increase robustness and accuracy and to balance the datasets. Recently, for the generation of realistic synthetic images, generative adversial network (GANs) are used (Wang et al., 2024). GANs are the emerging subclass of AI in the medical healthcare field and deliver successful results in various applications.

10.7 METHODOLOGIES INVOLVED IN DR DETECTION

Machine learning (ML): In this technique, a specific program is given to perform a task and it is assumed that the machine has learned from experience. While executing the task it improves its performance by gaining more and more from previous experience. Further machines make decisions and predict based on data. Frequent problems such as classification, regression, and clustering are widely solved by the ML approach. The different approaches of ML techniques are supervised learning, unsupervised learning, and semi-supervised learning. Supervised learning denotes training of labeled data, which means data, is tagged with appropriate answers. Support vector machine (SVM) is a powerful supervised learning technique used for classification purposes. SVM creates a line, which is called a hyperplane (best decision line) in n-dimensional space to divide data points into distinct classes. Support vectors are the data points that are closest to the hyperplane and have an impact on it. With the help of support vectors, we maximize the margin of the classifier. The sum of positive hyperplane and negative hyperplane is termed as the margin. Figure 10.4 shows the details of the SVM.

Deep Learning (DL): DL is a subpart of AI, which includes the layers of nonlinear processing stages for feature extraction and DR classification. It is widely used in medical healthcare in image analysis, texts, and sound for the classification purpose, detection, and diagnosis of diseases. DL-based techniques are very effective and achieve higher accuracy in automatic DR detection using fundus images because this approach automatically extracts the features, unlike ML techniques.

DL models are trained using labeled datasets and employed in neural networks that contain many layers. The algorithms involved in the model are hierarchical with increasing complexity. CNN is a widely used and very effective learning method for image classification and feature extraction. It identifies features related to DR using mathematical parameters for specified summation and convolution 12 (Shaban et al., 2020). It eliminates the manual feature extraction and automatically detects the features from DR images. CNN architecture mainly consists of three

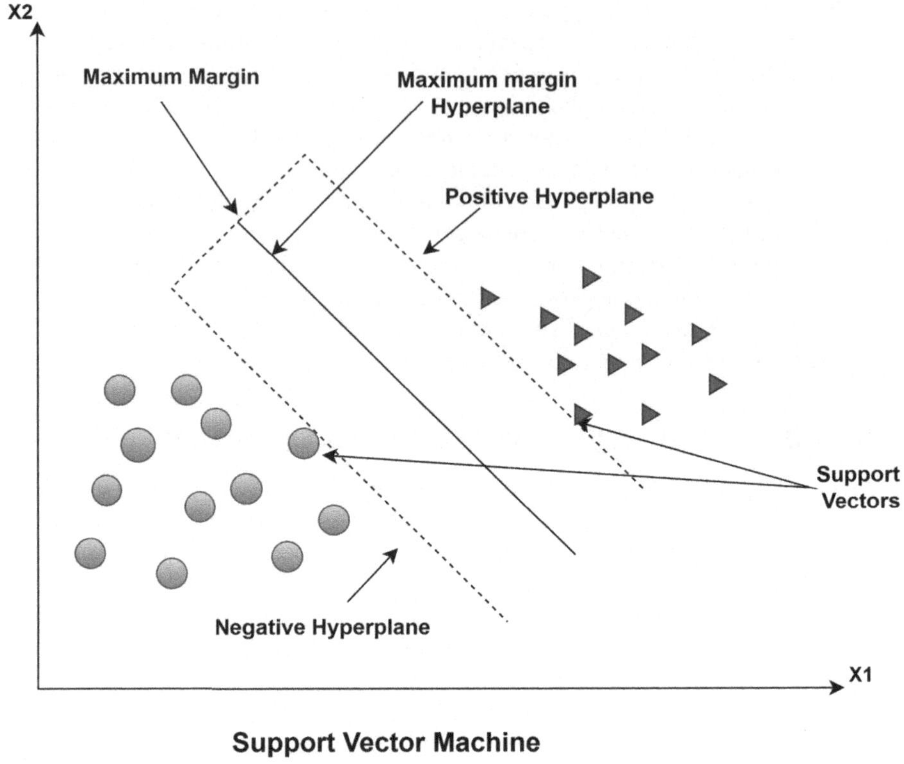

FIGURE 10.4 Support vector machine.

layers: Figure 10.5 showing the different layers present in CNN: the convolution, the pooling, and the fully connected layers. Several architectures of CNN involve training, validation, and testing on large datasets (ImageNet) consisting of labeled images and their classes.

10.7.1 Mathematics of Convolution Neural Network

In the convolution method, there is a combination of two different or the same data. Firstly, this operation takes input, then a convolutional filter is applied, and further we get feature-mapped output.

It can be understood easily by going through Table 10.2(a) and Table 10.2(b). Let us understand convolution using two matrices, p, and q, of one dimension where p = [1, 5, 3, 1, 2, 5] and q = [3, 2, 1]. Convolution involves the multiplication of arrays element-wise and the sum of the product to form a new array that represents p*q.

The next three elements from the p matrix are multiplied by elements present in the q matrix, and the product is added.

The above process continues till the convolution operation is over. Now keeping the above example in mind, our main concern is how CNN recognizes images: Let us understand briefly that starting from the first layer of CNN is the convolution layer, which is the initial step for feature extraction using several filters that perform

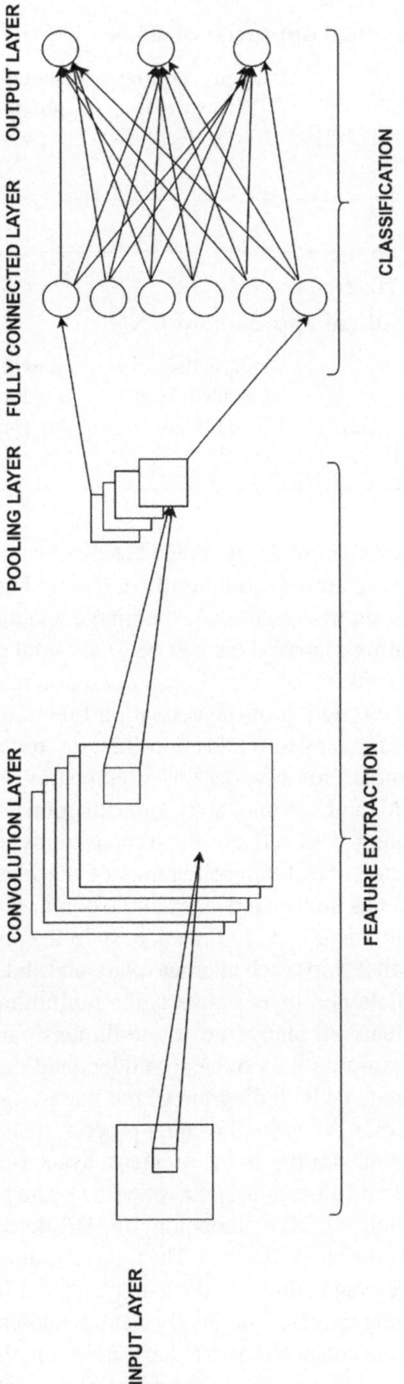

FIGURE 10.5 Different layers of CNN.

TABLE 10.2(a)
Mathematical approach of CNN

p*q	Multiply the arrays elementwise	Sum the product
P = [1, 5, 3, 1, 2, 5]	[3, 10, 3]	p*q = [16]
q = [3, 2, 1]		

TABLE 10.2(b)
Mathematical approach of CNN

p*q	Multiply the arrays element wise	Sum the product
P = [1, 5, 3, 1, 2, 5]	[3, 10, 3]	p*q = [16]
q = [3, 2, 1]	[15, 6, 1]	p*q = [22]

convolution operations. As we know, every image has pixel values. We consider 6×6 images whose pixel values are arranged randomly at 0 or 1. There is also a kernel of dimension 3×3. This filter matrix slides over the image, calculates the dot product, and gets the convolved feature matrix. This can be easily understood in Figure 10.5, in which a stepwise demonstration of convolution operation is mentioned.

Activation Function: The function of the activation function is to send the output of nodes in one layer to the next layer. It adds non-linearity to the network and learns complex patterns and features. Some widely used activation functions are rectified linear unit (ReLU), sigmoid, and softmax activation functions.

Pooling Layer: The pooling layer reduces the dimension by down-sampling operation. It utilizes filters to detect the different features of the images, such as corners, edges, patches, and body. Let us understand an example of a max pooling layer in detail using a matrix block diagram mentioned in Figure 10.6. In the diagram, the term stride 2 is used, which means the filter skips each alternate place and slides two pixels at a time.

Flattening Layer: The flattened layer converts the multidimensional output from the pooling layer (pooled featured maps) into a one-dimensional vector.

Considering the given example we can easily understand this layer as mentioned in Figure 10.7 shows the matrix block diagram of the flattening operation.

Fully Connected Layer (FC): After the flattening process, this FC layer is introduced to connect every neuron and all neurons in the previous layers as mentioned previously. Finally, the output is found and further it is classified according to extracted features. Figure 10.8 shows the generalized DL methodology for DR detection techniques using fundus image is explained by the block diagram. The figure illustrates the following steps: Image acquisition, pre-processing of images, data augmentation (if needed), training of datasets, validation, and testing process, and finally classification including performance evaluation. Recently, AI advancement has assisted researchers in thinking about different approaches for DR detection, and as a result, the adaptation of new methodologies has been introduced such as hybrid models, ensemble models, and so on (Figure 10.9).

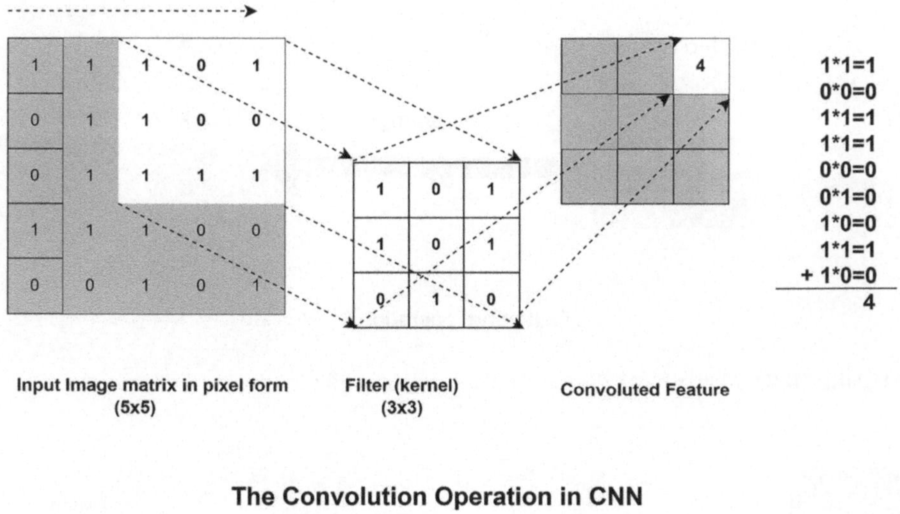

FIGURE 10.6 Convolution operation in CNN.

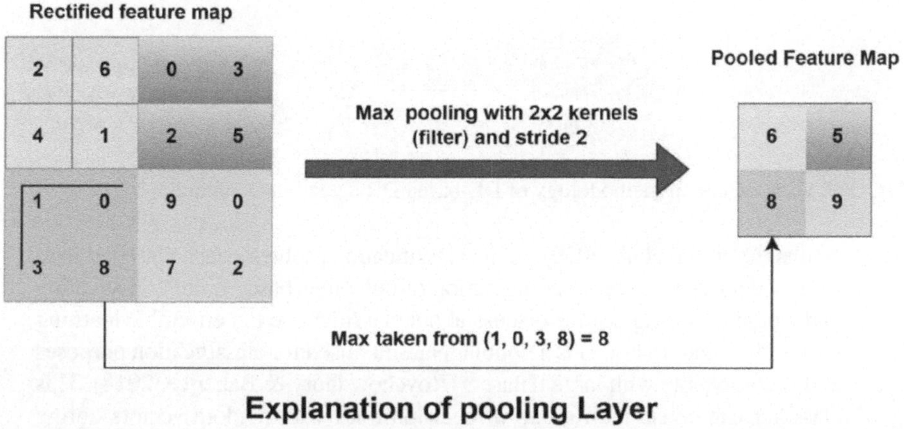

FIGURE 10.7 Matrix block diagram of pooling layer.

In a hybrid model, there is a combination of different models, and in an ensemble approach, there is combination of various methods, and through voting, the desired output is found.

Ensemble Learning: Ensemble learning is another recent topic of research in AI that refers to the combination of multiple models to provide predictive results in classification. This method tries to improve the overall functionality of the model and reduce errors in generalization. These techniques comprise averaging, stacking, bagging, boosting, and voting. For DR classification ensemble learning combined with several classifiers demonstrated powerful

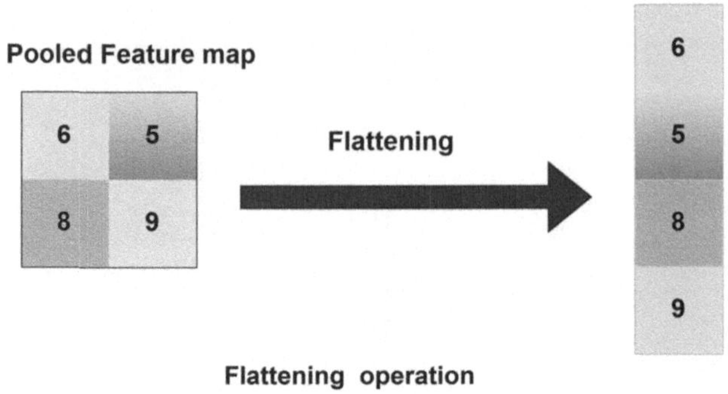

FIGURE 10.8 Matrix block diagram of flattening operation.

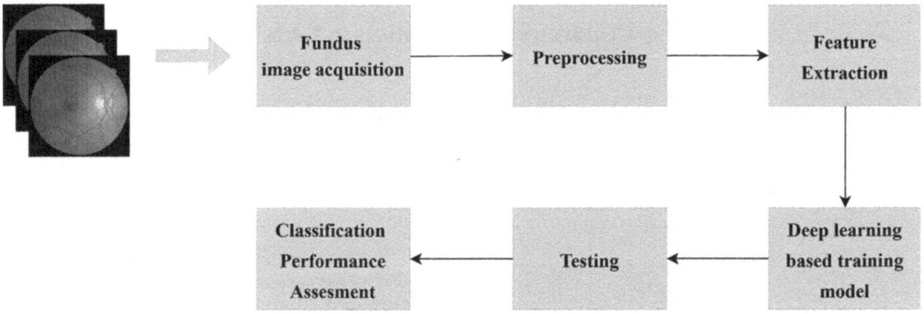

FIGURE 10.9 General methodology of DL-based DR detection technique.

results (Qummar et al., 2019). In the classification problem, each classifier executes the prediction and final prediction of outcomes based on majority voting and weighted voting. Let us discuss about classifier used in ensemble learning approach: Random Forest is a popular classifier used for classification purposes and is compatible with large datasets (Roychowdhury & Banerjee, 2018). This classifier can construct a group of decision trees with random vectors during training time (Somasundaram & Alli 2017). Ada-Boost is another popular classifier used in the ensemble learning approach, which is used for linear classification (Washburn, 2020). It combines a large number of relatively weak and low-accurate rules to produce a highly accurate prediction rule. It is also called adaptive boosting, which has improved accuracy and takes less execution time.

10.8 PERFORMANCE EVALUATION

From the recent research report, it has been found that the CNN model has executed remarkable results related to DR detection in the AI field. The performance and efficiency of the model are evaluated on different matrices such as sensitivity, accuracy, specificity, precision, F1 score, kappa score (Chilukoti et al., 2022), receiver operating curve (ROC), and many more. Before determining the value of the mentioned parameters, we have to calculate the confusion matrix. Confusion Matrix is a table used to determine the assessment of the classification executed by the model. The table based on the model's prediction matrix displays the accurate and inaccurate samples. True positive (TP), true negative (TN), false positive (FP), and false negative (FN) analyses are represented by it. Whereas TN indicates that the model successfully predicts a negative sample, TP indicates that the model accurately predicts a positive sample. A model that predicts a positive class incorrectly is represented by FP, meaning that the sample actually belongs to a negative class, but the model predicts a positive. A model that mispredicts a negative sample but the sample is actually positive is represented by FN.

10.9 CNN BASE MODEL IMPLEMENTATION FOR DR DETECTION (SAMPLE MODEL)

In this section, using the APTOS-2019 public dataset, a basic CNN model is used for Fundus image categorization and feature extraction. The first step involves the dataset distribution, which explains the splitting of the dataset into training, validation, and testing. Out of 3662 images from the APTOS-2019 dataset, 2523 images were used for training purposes, 549 for validation purposes, and for testing purposes 550 images. The CNN base model implementation and performance evaluation are done in Python language using computer vision, and tensorflow with keras. The basic Python code implementation in the CNN model is discussed in Table 10.3.

TABLE 10.3
Shows the Base CNN Model Code Written in Python

```
import tensorflow as tf
from tensorflow.keras import layers, models
# Define the CNN model
def create_cnn_model():
 model = models.Sequential([
 layers.Conv2D(32,(3,3),activation='relu',input_shape=
   (28,28,1)),
 layers.MaxPooling2D((2, 2)),
 layers.Conv2D(64, (3, 3), activation='relu'),
 layers.MaxPooling2D((2, 2)),
 layers.Conv2D(64, (3, 3), activation='relu')
 ])
 model.add(layers.Flatten())
 model.add(layers.Dense(64, activation='relu'))
 model.add(layers.Dense(10, activation='softmax')) #
  Assuming a classification task with 10 classes
 return model
# Create an instance of the CNN model
cnn_model = create_cnn_model()
# Compile the model
cnn_model.compile(optimizer='adam',
 loss='sparse_categorical_crossentropy',
 metrics=['accuracy'])
# Display the model architecture
cnn_model.summary()
```

10.10 RESULTS AND DISCUSSION

The CNN-based method has been applied for DR detection and its classification. The performance evaluation is based on accuracy, precision, sensitivity, F1- score, and Kappa score, which are mentioned in Table 10.4.

These performance matrices are calculated from the confusion matrix, which is shown in Figure 10.10. The implemented CNN model showed average performance because there is a need to adopt appropriate pre-processing techniques. Some

TABLE 10.4
Classification Performance of the CNN Model

Accuracy	**0.5418**
Precision	0.5169
Recall (Sensitivity)	0.5418
F1-Score	0.5230
Specificity	0.3161
Cohen' Kappa	0.2860

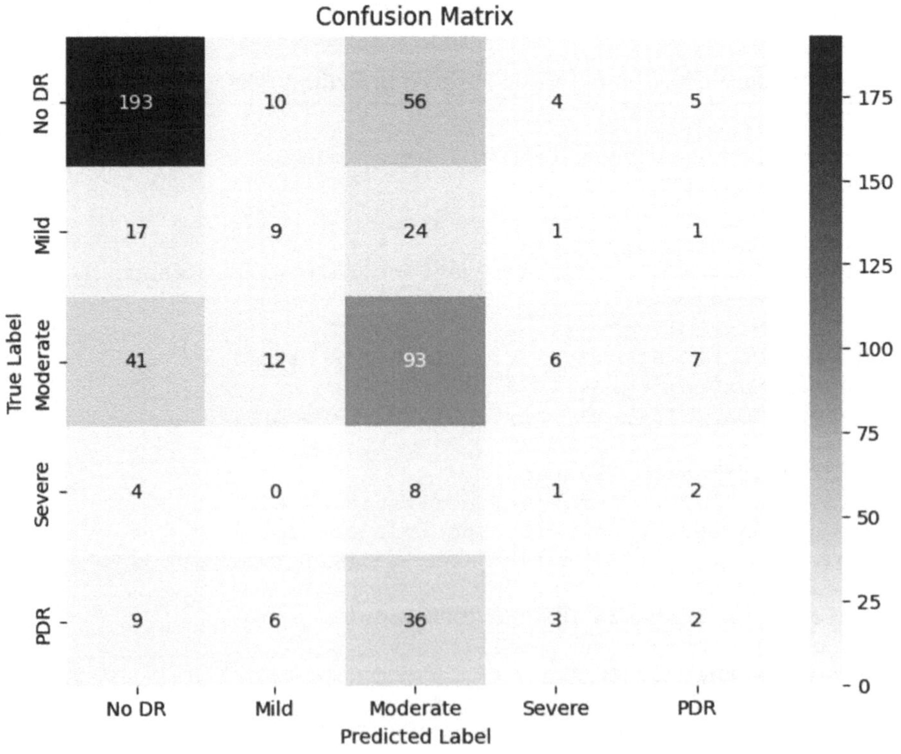

FIGURE 10.10 Confusion Matrix of the CNN-based model.

pre-processing techniques (as discussed in the earlier section) can be used to remove noise and to get better quality of fundus images. Generally, unbalanced and poor-quality of datasets always affect the training process, and performance and make the model very complex.

The data augmentation techniques include color and brightness augmentation, rotating, shifting, rescaling, and flipping of the images are implemented performance enhancement as used in Sarao et al. (2020). Also, the implementation of GANs for image synthesis can be used to balance the data (Zheng et al., 2018). The implementation of modified algorithms, or AI-enabled techniques, needs to be considered to improve performance and its efficiency. The performance of the model can be increased by the development of a simple, efficient algorithm for DR detection.

10.11 CONCLUSION: AI AND HEALTHCARE INTEGRATION

DR has become a prevalent complication leading to damaged retina and finally to vision impairment. Early detection saves and prevents the eye, which is possible using computer vision, which is a subset of AI.

The integration of AI into clinical practice, especially DL, has executed effective results in DR detection to treat patients efficiently (Grauslund, 2022). The efficient progressive report has been executed from the adoption of the ML approach to DL over the past decades. Ensemble and hybrid techniques have also brought the way for more accurate, reliable, and efficient treatment and diagnosis. These AI-enabled techniques evolve and become integrated into practical healthcare systems. However, certain constraints regarding performance, reliability, transparency, and robustness need to be checked out before healthcare integration. The variation regarding data collection, the consistency of the model's performance, and the coding environment (MATLAB or Python) need to be noted during the detection of disease. The experts, ophthalmologists, and clinical operators need to consider the results and output predicted by the model. The overall conclusion is that AI applications have designed a way for more precise and accurate diagnoses of DR, but they still need credibility from experts and ophthalmologists or doctors. Some challenges, such as model complexity, training time, overfitting, and vanishing gradient, are yet to be solved.

In the future, there is a need to develop innovative pre-processing and data augmentation algorithms to make the model efficient and more accurate. In addition, the number of DR patients is increasing day by day, and it is a very complex task to extract severe features from fundus images and difficult to implement lesion-based segmentation technique. Hence, there is extreme requirement of AI-based techniques for the detection and classification of DR to avoid the burden of experts and ophthalmologists.

REFERENCES

Acharya, U. R., Mookiah, M. R. K., Koh, J. E., Tan, J. H., Bhandary, S. V., Rao, A. K., … Laude, A. (2016). Automated screening system for retinal health using bi-dimensional empirical mode decomposition and integrated index. *Computers in Biology and Medicine*, *75*, 54–62.

Ali, G., Dastgir, A., Iqbal, M. W., Anwar, M., & Faheem, M. (2023). A hybrid convolutional neural network model for automatic diabetic retinopathy classification from fundus images. *IEEE Journal of Translational Engineering in Health and Medicine*, *11*, 341–350.

Bhimavarapu, U. (2024). Enhanced convolution neural network and improved SVM to detect and classify diabetic retinopathy. *Multimedia Tools and Applications*, 83, 70321–70342.

Bodapati, J. D., & Balaji, B. B. (2024). Self-adaptive stacking ensemble approach with attention based deep neural network models for diabetic retinopathy severity prediction. *Multimedia Tools and Applications*, *83*(1), 1083–1102.

Chilukoti, S. V., Maida, A. S., & Hei, X. (2022). Diabetic retinopathy detection using transfer learning from pre-trained convolutional neural network models. *IEEE Journal of Biomedical and Health Informatics*, *20*, 1–10.

Dubey, S., & Dixit, M. (2023). Recent developments on computer aided systems for diagnosis of diabetic retinopathy: a review. *Multimedia Tools and Applications*, *82*(10), 14471–14525.

Grauslund, J. (2022). Diabetic retinopathy screening in the emerging era of artificial intelligence. *Diabetologia*, *65*(9), 1415–1423.

Karthika, S., & Durgadevi, M. (2024). Improved ResNet_101 assisted attentional global transformer network for automated detection and classification of diabetic retinopathy disease. *Biomedical Signal Processing and Control*, *88*, 105674.

Kommaraju, R., & Anbarasi, M. S. (2024). Diabetic retinopathy detection using convolutional neural network with residual blocks. *Biomedical Signal Processing and Control*, *87*, 105494.

Pires, R., Avila, S., Wainer, J., Valle, E., Abramoff, M. D., & Rocha, A. (2019). A data-driven approach to referable diabetic retinopathy detection. *Artificial Intelligence in Medicine*, *96*, 93–106.

Qummar, S., Khan, F. G., Shah, S., Khan, A., Shamshirband, S., Rehman, Z. U., … Jadoon, W. (2019). A deep learning ensemble approach for diabetic retinopathy detection. *IEEE Access*, *7*, 150530–150539.

Ramachandran, A., Ma, R. C. W., & Snehalatha, C. (2010). Diabetes in asia. *The Lancet*, *375*(9712), 408–418.

Roychowdhury, A., & Banerjee, S. (2018). Random forests in the classification of diabetic retinopathy retinal images. In *Advanced Computational and Communication Paradigms: Proceedings of International Conference on ICACCP 2017, Volume 1* (pp. 168–176). Springer Singapore.

Sarao, V., Veritti, D., & Lanzetta, P. (2020). Automated diabetic retinopathy detection with two different retinal imaging devices using artificial intelligence: a comparison study. *Graefe's Archive for Clinical and Experimental Ophthalmology*, *258*, 2647–2654.

Shaban, M., Ogur, Z., Mahmoud, A., Switala, A., Shalaby, A., Abu Khalifeh, H., … El-Baz, A. S. (2020). A convolutional neural network for the screening and staging of diabetic retinopathy. *Plos one*, *15*(6), e0233514.

Somasundaram, S. K., & Alli, P. (2017). A machine learning ensemble classifier for early prediction of diabetic retinopathy. *Journal of Medical Systems*, *41*, 1–12.

Sun, H., Saeedi, P., Karuranga, S., Pinkepank, M., Ogurtsova, K., Duncan, B. B., … Magliano, D. J. (2022). IDF Diabetes Atlas: Global, regional and country-level diabetes prevalence estimates for 2021 and projections for 2045. *Diabetes Research and Clinical Practice*, *183*, 109119.

Thomas, N. M., & Jerome, S. A. (2024). Diabetic retinopathy detection using EADBSC and improved dilated ensemble CNN-based classification. *Multimedia Tools and Applications*, *83*(11), 33573–33595

Wang, Y., Hou, Q., Cao, P., Yang, J., & R. Zaiane (2024). Lesion-aware knowledge distillation for diabetic retinopathy lesion segmentation. *Applied Intelligence*, *54*(2), 1937–1956.

Washburn, P. S. (2020). Investigation of severity level of diabetic retinopathy using adaboost classifier algorithm. *Materials Today: Proceedings*, *33*, 3037–3042.

Yonekawa, Y., Modi, Y. S., Kim, L. A., Skondra, D., Kim, J. E., & Wykoff, C. C. (2020). American Society of Retina Specialists clinical practice guidelines: management of nonproliferative and proliferative diabetic retinopathy without diabetic macular edema. *Journal of Vitreoretinal Diseases*, *4*(2), 125–135.

Zheng, R., Liu, L., Zhang, S., Zheng, C., Bunyak, F., Xu, R., … Sun, M. (2018). Detection of exudates in fundus photographs with imbalanced learning using conditional generative adversarial network. *Biomedical Optics Express*, *9*(10), 4863–4878.

11 Artificial Intelligence and Machine Learning in Radiology

Benefits, Drawbacks and Prospects

Aditya Shah, Anagha Brahmajosyula, Varnika Gupta and Bhag Chand Jain

11.1 INTRODUCTION

Artificial intelligence (AI) is a simulation of computerised algorithms to disjoin complicated data. The application of AI in the medical profession rises in tandem with the complexity of data in the healthcare industry. The most favourable use of AI in clinical diagnosis is diagnostic imaging. Excellent accuracy and sensitivity for spotting small radiographic abnormalities have been shown by the investigations done by AI computer-aided diagnostics (CAD) (Oren et al., 2020a, 2020b).

The first effective telemedicine application worldwide was teleradiology, which led to the globalisation of radiology (Mun & Turner, 1999). An integrated diagnostic system combining diagnostic imaging, clinical pathology, and imaging can provide the clinician a clear diagnosis, reducing the need for serial procedures and enabling on-site diagnosis (Mun et al., 2021).

11.2 EVOLUTION IN TECHNOLOGY AND REPORTING STANDARDS

Since the idea of AI in imaging was first proposed in the 1960s, although early attempts were constrained by the available technology of the day. The development of CAD software and ANN (Artificial Neural Networks) in the 1980s signalled the beginning of the broad adoption of AI in radiology reporting (Fazal et al., 2018). Numerous medical applications, notably in the field of medical imaging, have been made possible by the introduction of deep neural networks as a modern AI method. These AI applications must continue to be based on the core principles of science and the publication of scientific research (Chartrand et al., 2017).

 DOI: 10.1201/9781003503385-11

Detection is the primary topic of study in diagnostic imaging. In the 1980s, researchers began creating CAD systems. Imaging techniques like Computed Tomography (CT), Magnetic Resonance Imaging (MRI), and mammography were subjected to conventional machine learning (ML) methods. Despite significant scientific effort, the actual clinical applications did not seem viable. The results of numerous important trials show that, at best, CAD has not been beneficial (Lakhani et al., 2018) and, at worst, that it has reduced radiological accuracy (Rastgarpour & Shanbehzadeh, 2011), increasing recall and biopsy rates (Roth, 2018; Tang et al., 2018).

11.3 CURRENT ROLE

AI is not a single technology, but rather it is a collection of technologies that have immediate relevance and high importance to health care.

11.3.1 Machine Learning

It is a statistical tool used to fit different models to data. The ML commonly applied in health care is supervised learning, as shown in Figure 11.1, where for a given training data set, the output variable is known. Here, the prediction of the treatment protocol of a patient is based on different patient attributes and treatment context. Neural network is next type of ML—it's been used for categorisation such as finding the risk of a disease for the patient. Deep learning (DL) is a NNN having many levels of features or variables that predict outcomes (Oren et al., 2020a, 2020b).

The application of AI-based technologies is viewed as a viable strategy to boost clinical effectiveness in diagnostic imaging, enhance the readability of findings, and support decision-making for the identification and prevention of diseases. CNN has had maximum success in medical imaging as it has been made based on the visual

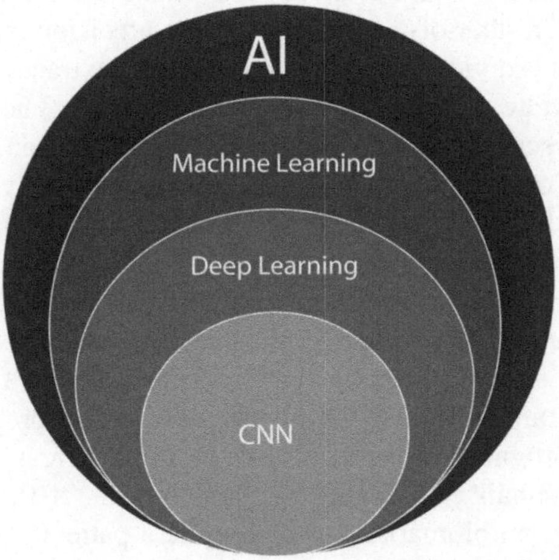

FIGURE 11.1 Diagrammatic representation of AI, machine learning, deep learning, and convolutional neural networks.

cortex of the brain, which explains its extensive use in medical imaging for image identification (Berbís et al., 2021).

11.3.2 Deep Learning

It has so far shown significant advancements in the study field above conventional ML. To forecast the risk of lung cancer, Ardila et al. devised an algorithm that analyses a patient's past and present CT volumes (Ardila et al., 2019). On 6716 cases from the national lung cancer screening study, the model performed at a state-of-the-art level (94.4% area under the curve), and it also did well on an independent clinical validation set of 1139 cases. According to cancer.gov, there are various risks associated with low-dose CT screening compared to conventional screening, including radiation exposure, overdiagnosis, difficulties with the diagnostic process, false-positive tests, and complications with diagnostic evaluation. A 67% overdiagnosis rate was estimated. Additionally, radiation exposure increases the likelihood of developing lung cancer or other cancers in later life. Diagnoses powered by AI decreased these risks (Litjens et al., 2017).

To analyse radiological imagery, DL algorithms are becoming the method of choice (Litjens et al., 2017). All kinds of diagnostic imaging techniques like PET, MRI, CT, and USG, as well as various tasks like tumour identification, segmentation, disease prediction, etc., are covered under this. Research has shown that DL and AI methods perform better than more conventional ML algorithms (Paul et al., 2016). DL gets its understanding from many image examples. It can be completed much more quickly because it only requires carefully selected data and associated metadata, unlike domain expertise, which usually takes years to develop (Hosny et al., 2018). It is predicted that AI will continue to dominate image research in radiology due to the recent success of AI/DL in this field as well as the fact that traditional AI has shown plateauing performance in recent years and requires preset characteristics.

Radiomics is one of the most advanced AI applications in the world of healthcare imaging research and a state-of-the-art approach to precision medicine (Baumann et al., 2016). Radiomics is divided into two steps. Feature extraction is the initial phase. It is possible to integrate pictures from several modalities. The areas of interest are divided using image segmentation methods. Features will then be extracted following segmentation. Common characteristics include tumour volume, shape, pixel intensity, density, and geometric data. In the second stage, mathematical models are built using the retrieved data to decode the tumour's phenotype and forecast how it will respond to treatment. Successful outcome forecasting can offer useful data for precise treatment planning. For instance, the histology and age of many lung cancer patients may be very similar (Arimura et al., 2019). Different treatment plans might be considered if radiomics can use the picture data to interpret the phenotypic and forecast the patient prognosis or survival time before the treatment. This is referred to as precision or personalised medicine (Baumann et al., 2016). Precision medicine has historically relied on biomarkers to determine a patient's specific prognosis or subtype, which typically needed an intrusive biopsy.

A radiomic signature was created by Aerts et al. and evaluated using separate lung data. It demonstrated how radiomics can be applied to various cancer types.

Significant correlations between the radiomic characteristics and gene-expression patterns were also demonstrated by the authors (Aerts et al., 2014). Some researchers used PET pictures, PET/CT scans, or PET/MRI to do radiomics modelling (Ohri et al., 2016; Naqa, 2014). Lung cancer applications were the most common. Applications for head and neck (Marcu et al., 2019). and prostate (Perez-Lopez et al., 2019) malignancies are also available. Reasonable prediction power has been attained by all these models. Radiology has now become a global phenomenon with its use as the first well-accepted and successful application of telemedicine.

11.4 USE OF AI IN MEDICAL IMAGING

For this, several questions have to be kept in mind while training any software for image-based detection: What are the objects visible in the image? What is the precise location of the object in the image? Is the image satisfactory for the purpose of determining a diagnosis? What is the problem identified with the object detected in the image?

The answers to all these questions lie in the domains of classification, segmentation, navigation, and quality assessment for the purpose of accurate clinical diagnosis, as shown in Figure 11.2. Any AI tools used for the purpose of medical imaging should satisfy all these critical requirements to be used for the purpose of making any clinical diagnosis. Figure 11.3 shows the branches in which AI medical imaging is most used.

FIGURE 11.2 A typical clinical workflow.

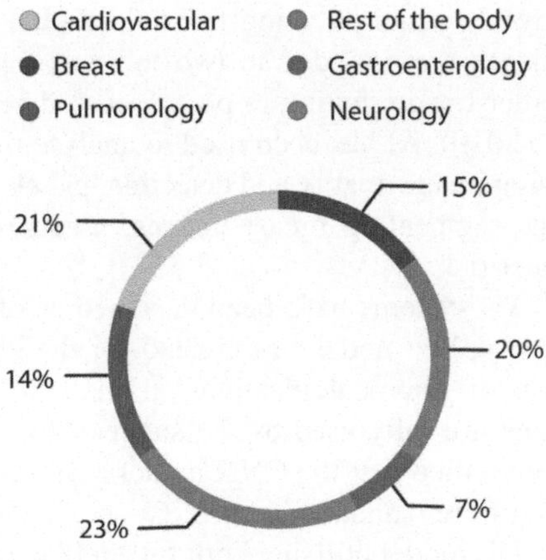

FIGURE 11.3 Branches in which AI medical imaging is most used.

11.4.1 Neurology

As neurology involves extensive use of various imaging modalities like CT and MRI and a significant amount of time and capital is spent in performing these procedures, integration of AI into this process can enable effective optimisation. As AI also could accurately detect and diagnose various lesions entirely without or with minimal use of contrast material, it can help in cost-cutting and preventing the occurrence of hypersensitivity reactions that are traditionally encountered. MIMneuro® (MIM software, Cleveland, OH) (Nishihara et al., 2011), is another FDA-approved AI tool that arranges images obtained through PET into a built-in atlas. This software can quantify the amyloid deposition in the neural tissue by analysis of FDG PET scans of the brain and amyloid PET studies in patients with neurodegenerative conditions and helps in differentiating it from conditions like Alzheimer's. It also calculates whether any organic changes can be considered statistically significant through its region-based analysis with Z-score tables and SUVR statistics.

11.4.2 Cardiovascular Imaging

Echocardiography is one of the most used imaging modalities in cardiovascular studies. Application of DL into echocardiographic assessment will enable the diagnosis of various cardiovascular diseases with high rates of precision and improve diagnostic accuracy, which can normally be interpreted only by physicians with advanced cardiology training. One front where utilisation of AI in echocardiography can prove to be beneficial is the field of valvular heart diseases.

11.4.3 Breast

Mammography is indeed a non-invasive method for detecting that has low pain, is simple to use, has excellent resolution, and has good reproducibility. Age or body form are not restrictions on the stored image, which can be compared before and after. Doctors cannot palpate all breast lumps, but mammography can find them and accurately distinguish between benign lesions and dangerous malignancies. Mammograms are currently acquired using full-field digital mammography (DM) equipment, and the images are provided in two formats: one for processing (raw imaging data) and another for presenting (a postprocessed version of the raw data) (Parvathavarthini et al., 2019). AI has been used to analyse mammography pictures with a focus on improving image quality and detecting and classifying breast masses and microcalcifications, segmenting breast masses, assessing breast density, and determining breast cancer risk.

Different types of CAD systems have been designed as of late to find calcifications in mammograms. A CNN model was created for the identification, examination, and categorisation of microcalcifications in mammography pictures using filtered deep features that are fully used by the suggested CNN structure for traditional descriptors. They verified that the CNN model performed better at extracting images than features that were manually created (Cai et al., 2019).

In addition, a hybrid DL model utilising both full-field mammography and traditional risk factors was developed. They found that compared to the Tyrer-Cusick model, which is already in use in clinical practice, it was more accurate (Yala et al., 2019). As a result, AI more accurately forecasts breast cancer risk than other techniques, which in turn can help to lower the incidence of breast cancer. AI—in particular, DL—performs exceptionally well in tasks involving medical image processing. With its benefits of quick computation, high reproducibility, and lack of tiredness, AI can give physicians unbiased, useful information while lightening their workload and lowering the incidence of incorrect and missing diagnoses. There is now a lot of study being done on the CAD system for breast cancer screening. These systems can identify and categorise breast lesions from mammography, MRI, USG, and other imaging tests; they can also forecast the risk of breast cancer and BD; evaluate treatment efficacy and prognosis; and extract characteristics from the lesions.

While the introduction of AI has often been depicted as a struggle between humans and machines, its true potential will only be realised when it is applied in a way that combines technological prowess and human skill, with an interface that maximises that synthesis and allows for iterative feedback. Traditional CAD fell short of expectations for several reasons, one of which is probably the absence of this harmonisation and feedback.

There are several processes in the breast imaging workflow that is split into four stages: prescreening, screening, diagnostic, and treatment, as shown in Figure 11.4.

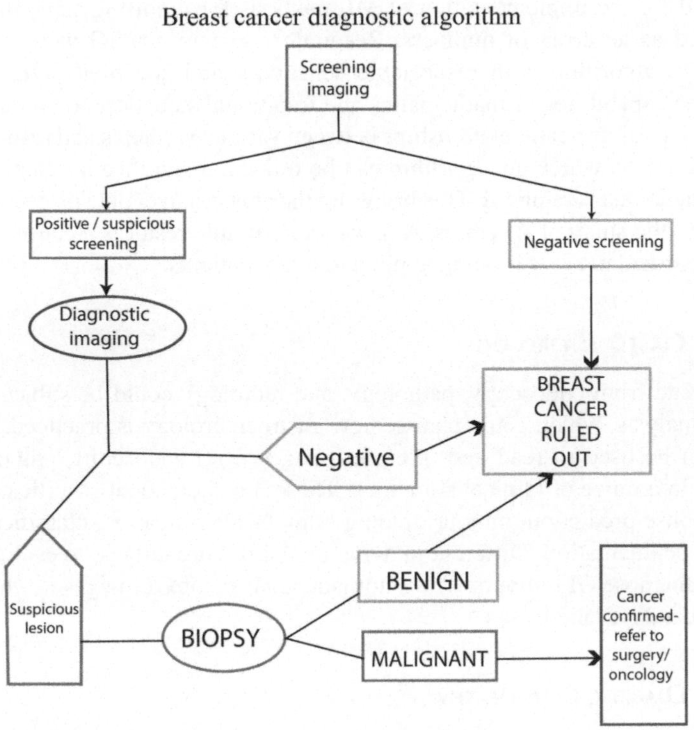

FIGURE 11.4 Processes involved in breast cancer diagnosis.

A thorough comprehension of these decision-making processes can act as a road map for the potential integration of AI technology into the breast imaging procedure.

11.4.4 Pulmonology

Cytopathology has recently been a field where AI has been used in pulmonology. During an endobronchial ultrasound transbronchial needle aspiration procedure, an AI model made up of an open-sourced CNN was able to identify on-site cytology smears. By putting this theory into practice, bronchoscopists could anticipate the final histologic diagnosis in addition to knowing that they had sampled the target lesion. Bronchoscopic images' original red, green, and blue pattern was changed to a hue saturation value texture in a small sample of lung cancer patients. These bronchoscopic images were used to identify different lung cancer subtypes using a CAD method (Feng et al., 2018). In order to expedite a pathologist's histologic diagnosis and subsequent curative therapy, the subgroup of patients who are classified as malignant by ML and DL algorithms would benefit from the application of AI during bronchoscopy.

A comprehensive evaluation of parameters relating to sleep quality is done using polysomnography (PSG), which involves measurements of a broad variety of physiological signals. A position statement on this topic of sleep medicine has also been published by the American Academy of Sleep Medicine. These electrical signals are well-suited for the implementation of ML methods for reporting since they can be represented as an array of numbers. Respiratory events in PSG were categorised using a DL algorithm with respectable sensitivity and specificity (IEEE, 2021). Beyond the capabilities of mathematics and traditional statistics, AI can understand a wide variety of intricate relationships between various variables and results. To create a database on which an algorithm can be trained, a significant quantity of individual patient data is required. This brings up the concern over data protection, which gave rise to the study of AI ethics. A flawed algorithmic result is a cause for serious concern, particularly if it is being applied to many patients.

11.4.5 Gastroenterology

Imaging data from endoscopy, pathology, and radiology could be subject to deep-learning analysis, which could change how gastroenterology is practiced. ML techniques can be used to read and interpret images from endoscopy, pathology, and radiology in a range of clinical situations. These include patient stratification, treatment response prediction, tumour grading, tumour identification, classification, and automatic segmentation. Different imaging modalities are utilised to evaluate the GI tract and diagnose GI tumours. The automatic analysis of GI images is where ML is most frequently applied.

11.4.6 Diabetic Retinopathy

Diabetic retinopathy (DR) is the most common complication that occurs in patients with type-2 Diabetes Mellitus, and it mainly occurs due to pathological changes in the retinal vasculature ranging from intraretinal haemorrhages to neovascularisation. The spectrum of DR mainly involves either proliferative changes in the retina, non-proliferative changes in the retina, or diabetic macular oedema (DME). DR is usually asymptomatic in the early stages, and by the time it is clinically detected, irreversible visual dysfunction usually occurs. Thus, it is imperative to detect any underlying pathology as early as possible to significantly improve the disease prognosis.

In real-world DR screening, a minor proportion of label errors can significantly affect how well DL algorithms function. In the future, research and real-world applications of AI-based DR-screening algorithms should focus on reducing and fixing label errors (Wang et al., 2024). With the advent of AI, it has become possible to detect early changes of DR and DME, age-related macular degeneration, retinopathy of prematurity, and glaucoma.

11.4.7 Dermatology

The utilisation of AI in dermatology has expanded over the last few years from being just focused on the detection of skin cancers like Melanoma initially. An algorithm using CNN performed better in correctly diagnosing melanoma than the majority of 58 dermatologists tested, with a median area under the receiver operating characteristic curve of 0.86 compared with 0.79, $P < 0.01$ (Haenssle et al., 2018).

The Primiero et al. approach outlines how to build an extensive dataset for ML that includes patient-level metadata, sequential-TATA binding protein, lesion categorisation, and phenotypic data. The study's goal is to present a comprehensive strategy for AI-driven CAD tools that aid in melanoma early detection (Primiero et al., 2024).

The presence of any skin markings in dermoscopic images significantly increased the chances of a false predictive rate of a nevus as a melanoma when diagnosed by the CNN (Winkler et al., 2019). Thus, utilisation of CNN in AI requires the acquisition of high-quality dermoscopic images without the presence of any skin markings that might hamper its diagnostic efficiency.

11.4.8 Orthopaedic Imaging

AI is used in orthopaedic radiography in areas like fracture detection, age, osteoporosis, and implant categorisation, as well as alignment assessment and implant placement. In addition to developed algorithms that can calculate the Cobb angle using surface topography before employing radiography and three-dimensional imaging, AI is employed in the assessment and quantification of the curvature of the spine in scoliosis, detecting vertebral fractures or disc herniation.

The DL CNN Model had a highly successful outcome when used for the interpretation of AP shoulder radiographs for the detection and classification of proximal humerus fractures. However, CNN was found to have poor diagnostic accuracy for the detection of 3-part fractures, which were consistently misinterpreted by the AI tool (Lee & Chung, 2022).

A DL model was created to accurately identify bone tumours on knee radiographs, and it outperformed novice radiologists in this regard. DL model has the ability to decrease missed diagnoses and misread diagnoses in a shorter amount of time and may assist general practitioners or radiologists with less experience in identifying possible bone tumours on radiographs (Xu et al., 2024).

11.4.9 Obstetrics and Gynaecology

The main use of AI in obstetrics lies in its benefit of recognising the exact location and determining foetal structures. Prediction of exact gestational age during any month of pregnancy is also an added benefit of training AI tools using repetitive ultrasonographic imaging. As prenatal ultrasonography is of prime importance for the early detection of any chromosomal or genetic abnormalities, structural abnormalities of the fetus as early diagnosis will aid in performing any corrective interventions or even termination of pregnancy to prevent future complications that might compromise not only the foetal quality of life but also that of the mother.

Anthropometric assessment of foetal structures has an important role for predicting foetal survival rates at the various parameters used for this purpose, including CRL (Crown Rump Length), HC (Head Circumference), and FL (Femur Length), to name a few. As this requires identification by a skilled sonographer, automation of this process can certainly enable provision of a high quality of obstetric care even in the rural setup with scarce resources.

In recent times, the application of AI in the detection of various craniocerebral malformations in the fetus has also increased. The automated systems could select the correct plane for performing foetal measurements in equivalence to the results obtained by experienced sonographers due to the recent advances in the algorithms used in such systems (Grandjean et al., 2018).

11.5 PROS/CONS

In AI imaging investigations, lesion identification is often used to define outcome assessment; however, it ignores the biological aggressiveness and nature of a lesion, which could result in an imprecise representation of AI performance. Furthermore, the addition of non-patient-focused radiographic and pathological endpoints may improve projected sensitivity at the cost of a higher rate of false positives and possible overdiagnosis by detecting subtle alterations that may be symptomatic of preclinical or indolent disease. It is assumed that an increase of AI will lead to an automation of jobs and therefore displacement of the workforce however other studies say that other factors, such as the cost of automation technology, would limit job loss. It seems that there would be many occupational, medical, ethical, and technological changes occurring with an increase in the use of AI in healthcare.

It has been demonstrated that using AI software to assist physicians improves their performance compared to using AI or humans alone. This could be used as a tool for training, particularly for junior doctors with less expertise, as well as in clinical practice to improve the quality of diagnosis and speed up the diagnosis.

11.6 FUTURE PROSPECTS

AI will significantly affect the healthcare solutions available in the future. It manifests as ML. While early attempts to prescribe treatment and diagnosis have been challenging, AI will eventually become proficient in those areas as well. Given the rapid developments in AI for imaging analysis, it seems likely that most radiology and pathology photos will soon be evaluated by a computer.

Not whether AI will be beneficial or not, but rather how to guarantee its adoption in standard clinical practice, is the largest challenge facing many healthcare industries. AI will be used in clinical practice more extensively within 10 years, after which it will be used somewhat after five years. Furthermore, it's becoming clearer that AI technology will assist clinicians in patient care rather than completely replace them. Doctors may eventually lean towards roles and schedules that leverage uniquely human skills like empathy, reasoning, and comprehensive integration.

The purpose of AI in healthcare should be to utilise the benefits of both humans and robots because they each have unique strengths. Computers can "see" information that humans are unable to by processing it quickly and at speeds that far beyond human vision. Machines are excellent at identifying patterns, even when there are vast amounts of data and complicated correlations. As a result, their predicting abilities are enhanced. Contrarily, humans can combine many types of facts. With little information, we can draw conclusions and find solutions to a wide range of issues. Humans can take context into account, adjust to local practise norms or other peculiar circumstances, establish collaborative relationships with referring providers and patients, and communicate effectively with them. The massive collection of unorganised data that makes up the state of medical data today can be used by humans to derive value and meaning.

11.7 ACCEPTANCE OF AI AMONG MEDICAL PROFESSIONALS

The present practical clinical experience of radiologists using technologies driven by AI was investigated through a survey of 690 members of the European Society of Radiology in January 2022. Of these, 276 radiologists had actual clinical experience using an AI-based algorithm, and they served as the foundation for this work. As per this survey, only 92 (13.3%) radiologists were willing to utilise AI tools in their regular clinical practice. This study clearly demonstrated that despite the numerous applications of AI for various clinical scenarios, including the emergency setting, practical application of AI into the regular clinical practice is still far-fetched. Additionally, the market will continue to be driven in the upcoming years by advancements in imaging technology and an increase in government efforts. Figure 11.5 shows that the AI medical imaging market size to hit $11.78 billion by 2033 (Research, 2023).

Another reason for the industry's quick expansion is the continual developments in imaging technology, such as CAD. Increasing prevalence of several chronic illnesses like cancer and cardiovascular disorders as well as the growing demand for improved imaging solutions that integrate AI. However, it is anticipated that across all modalities, MRI will expand at the quickest rate between 2021 and 2030. The development of AI-based MRI medical imaging solutions by both large market players and niche vendors is another factor driving this category's overall market growth.

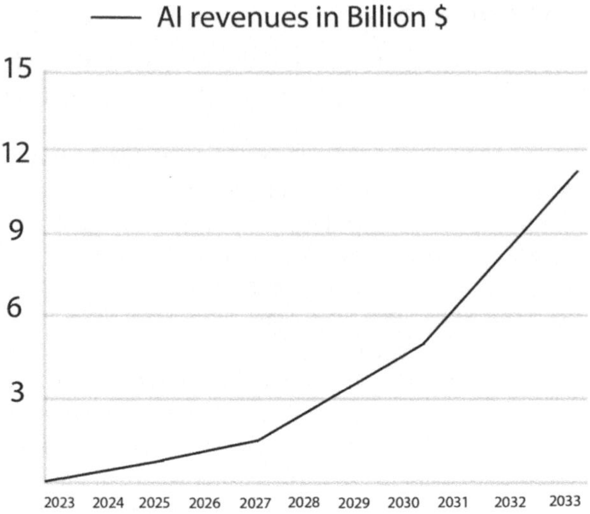

FIGURE 11.5 AI medical imaging market size.

11.8 RECOMMENDATIONS, LIMITATIONS, AND FUTURE RESEARCH

According to our analysis, the healthcare sector should invest in these technologies in order to benefit from the aforementioned advantages. They might collaborate with IT companies, create these technologies on their own, and offer advantages to medical experts that would ultimately benefit the general public. Despite covering a lot of ground, the report doesn't take stakeholders' perspectives into account. A study could be done on this. Future studies could also look into how medical professionals behave or whether they plan to adopt AI products.

11.9 AUTHOR CONTRIBUTIONS

AS: Conceptualization, Data curation, Formal analysis, Methodology, Project administration, Resources, Supervision, Validation, Visualization, Writing – original draft, Writing – review & editing. AB: Data curation, Formal analysis, Methodology, Validation, Writing – original draft, Writing – review & editing. VG: Data curation, Formal analysis, Methodology, Validation, Writing – original draft, Writing – review & editing. BJ: Data curation, Formal analysis, Methodology, Validation, Writing – original draft, Writing – review & editing.

REFERENCES

Aerts, H. J., Velazquez, E. R., Leijenaar, R. T., Parmar, C., Grossmann, P., Carvalho, S., Bussink, J., Monshouwer, R., Haibe-Kains, B., Rietveld, D., Hoebers, F., Rietbergen, M. M., Leemans, C. R., Dekker, A., Quackenbush, J., Gillies, R. J., & Lambin, P. (2014). Decoding tumour phenotype by noninvasive imaging using a quantitative radiomics approach. *Nature Communications*, 5, 4006. https://doi.org/10.1038/ncomms5006

Ardila, D., Kiraly, A. P., Bharadwaj, S., Choi, B., Reicher, J. J., Peng, L., Tse, D., Etemadi, M., Ye, W., Corrado, G., Naidich, D. P., & Shetty, S. (2019). End-to-end lung cancer screening with three-dimensional deep learning on low-dose chest computed tomography. *Nature Medicine*, 25(6), 954–961. https://doi.org/10.1038/s41591-019-0447-x

Arimura, H., Soufi, M., Kamezawa, H., Ninomiya, K., & Yamada, M. (2019). Radiomics with artificial intelligence for precision medicine in radiation therapy. *Journal of Radiation Research*, 60(1), 150–157. https://doi.org/10.1093/jrr/rry077

Baumann, M., Krause, M., Overgaard, J., Debus, J., Bentzen, S. M., Daartz, J., Richter, C., Zips, D., & Bortfeld, T. (2016). Radiation oncology in the era of precision medicine. *Nature Reviews. Cancer*, 16(4), 234–249. https://doi.org/10.1038/nrc.2016.18

Berbís, M. A., Aneiros-Fernández, J., Mendoza Olivares, F. J., Nava, E., & Luna, A. (2021). Role of artificial intelligence in multidisciplinary imaging diagnosis of gastrointestinal diseases. *World Journal of Gastroenterology*, 27(27), 4395–4412. https://doi.org/10.3748/wjg.v27.i27.4395

Cai, H., Huang, Q., Rong, W., Song, Y., Li, J., Wang, J., Chen, J., & Li, L. (2019). Breast Microcalcification Diagnosis Using Deep Convolutional Neural Network from Digital Mammograms. *Computational and Mathematical Methods in Medicine*, 2019, 1–10. https://doi.org/10.1155/2019/2717454

Chartrand, G., Cheng, P. M., Vorontsov, E., Drozdzal, M., Turcotte, S., Pal, C. J., Kadoury, S., & Tang, A. (2017). Deep Learning: A Primer for Radiologists. *Radiographics*, 37(7), 2113–2131. https://doi.org/10.1148/rg.2017170077

Fazal, M. I., Patel, M. E., Tye, J., & Gupta, Y. (2018). The past, present and future role of artificial intelligence in imaging. *European Journal of Radiology*, 105, 246–250. https://doi.org/10.1016/j.ejrad.2018.06.020

Feng, P., Lin, Y., & Lo, C. (2018). A machine learning texture model for classifying lung cancer subtypes using preliminary bronchoscopic findings. *Medical Physics*, 45(12), 5509–5514. https://doi.org/10.1002/mp.13241

Grandjean, G. A., Hossu, G., Bertholdt, C., Noble, P., Morel, O., & Grangé, G. (2018). Artificial intelligence assistance for fetal head biometry: Assessment of automated measurement software. *Diagnostic and Interventional Imaging*, 99(11), 709–716. https://doi.org/10.1016/j.diii.2018.08.001

Haenssle, H., Fink, C., Schneiderbauer, R., Toberer, F., Buhl, T., Blum, A., Kalloo, A., Hassen, A. B. H., Thomas, L., Enk, A., Uhlmann, L., Alt, C., Arenbergerova, M., Bakos, R., Baltzer, A., Bertlich, I., Blum, A., Bokor-Billmann, T., Bowling, J., … Zalaudek, I. (2018). Man against machine: diagnostic performance of a deep learning convolutional neural network for dermoscopic melanoma recognition in comparison to 58 dermatologists. *Annals of Oncology*, 29(8), 1836–1842. https://doi.org/10.1093/annonc/mdy166

Hosny, A., Parmar, C., Quackenbush, J., Schwartz, L. H., & Aerts, H. J. W. L. (2018). Artificial intelligence in radiology. *Nature Reviews. Cancer*, 18(8), 500–510. https://doi.org/10.1038/s41568-018-0016-5

IEEE. (2021, April 1). Automatic Sleep Data Scoring by Artificial Intelligence: A Pilot Study in Thai Population. IEEE Conference Publication | IEEE Xplore. https://ieeexplore.ieee.org/document/9426262

Lakhani, P., Prater, A. B., Hutson, R. K., Andriole, K. P., Dreyer, K. J., Morey, J., Prevedello, L. M., Clark, T. J., Geis, J. R., Itri, J. N., & Hawkins, C. M. (2018). Machine Learning in Radiology: Applications Beyond Image Interpretation. *Journal of the American College of Radiology*, 15(2), 350–359. https://doi.org/10.1016/j.jacr.2017.09.044

Lee, J., & Chung, S. W. (2022). Deep Learning for Orthopedic Disease Based on Medical Image Analysis: Present and Future. *Applied Sciences*, 12(2), 681. https://doi.org/10.3390/app12020681

Litjens, G., Kooi, T., Bejnordi, B. E., Setio, A. A. A., Ciompi, F., Ghafoorian, M., van der Laak, J. A. W. M., van Ginneken, B., & Sánchez, C. I. (2017). A survey on deep learning in medical image analysis. *Medical Image Analysis*, 42, 60–88. https://doi.org/10.1016/j.media.2017.07.005

Marcu, L. G., Boyd, C., & Bezak, E. (2019). Feeding the Data Monster: Data Science in Head and Neck Cancer for Personalized Therapy. *Journal of the American College of Radiology: JACR*, 16(12), 1695–1701. https://doi.org/10.1016/j.jacr.2019.05.045

Mun, S. K., & Turner, J. W. (1999). Telemedicine: emerging e-medicine. *Annual Review of Biomedical Engineering*, 1, 589–610. https://doi.org/10.1146/annurev.bioeng.1.1.589

Mun, S. K., Wong, K. H., Lo, S. C. B., Li, Y., & Bayarsaikhan, S. (2021). Artificial Intelligence for the Future Radiology Diagnostic Service. *Frontiers in Molecular Biosciences*, 7. https://doi.org/10.3389/fmolb.2020.614258

Naqa, I. E. (2014). The role of quantitative PET in predicting cancer treatment outcomes. *Clinical and Translational Imaging*, 2(4), 305–320. https://doi.org/10.1007/s40336-014-0063-1

Nishihara, M., Sasayama, T., Kudo, H., & Kohmura, E. (2011). Morbidity of stereotactic biopsy for intracranial lesions. *The Kobe Journal of Medical Sciences*, 56(4), E148–E153.

Ohri, N., Duan, F., Snyder, B. S., Wei, B., Machtay, M., Alavi, A., Siegel, B. A., Johnson, D. W., Bradley, J. D., DeNittis, A., Werner-Wasik, M., & El Naqa, I. (2016). Pretreatment 18F-FDG PET Textural Features in Locally Advanced Non-Small Cell Lung Cancer: Secondary Analysis of ACRIN 6668/RTOG 0235. *Journal of Nuclear Medicine: Official Publication, Society of Nuclear Medicine*, 57(6), 842–848. https://doi.org/10.2967/jnumed.115.166934

Oren, O., Gersh, B. J., & Bhatt, D. L. (2020a). Artificial intelligence in medical imaging: switching from radiographic pathological data to clinically meaningful endpoints. *The Lancet Digital Health*, 2(9), e486–e488. https://doi.org/10.1016/s2589-7500(20)30160-6

Oren, O., Gersh, B. J., & Bhatt, D. L. (2020b). Artificial intelligence in medical imaging: switching from radiographic pathological data to clinically meaningful endpoints. *The Lancet Digital Health*, 2(9), e486–e488. https://doi.org/10.1016/s2589-7500(20)30160-6

Parvathavarthini, S., Karthikeyani, V. N., & Shanthi, S. (2019). Breast Cancer detection using crow search optimization based intuitionistic fuzzy clustering with neighborhood attraction. *Asian Pacific Journal of Cancer Prevention*, 20(1), 157–165. https://doi.org/10.31557/apjcp.2019.20.1.157

Paul, R., Hawkins, S. H., Balagurunathan, Y., Schabath, M. B., Gillies, R. J., Hall, L. O., & Goldgof, D. B. (2016). Deep feature transfer learning in combination with traditional features predicts survival among patients with lung adenocarcinoma. *Tomography (Ann Arbor, Mich.)*, 2(4), 388–395. https://doi.org/10.18383/j.tom.2016.00211

Perez-Lopez, R., Tunariu, N., Padhani, A. R., Oyen, W. J. G., Fanti, S., Vargas, H. A., Omlin, A., Morris, M. J., de Bono, J., & Koh, D. M. (2019). Imaging diagnosis and follow-up of advanced prostate cancer: clinical perspectives and state of the art. *Radiology*, 292(2), 273–286. https://doi.org/10.1148/radiol.2019181931

Primiero, C. A., Betz-Stablein, B., Ascott, N., D'Alessandro, B., Gaborit, S., Fricker, P., Goldsteen, A., González-Villà, S., Lee, K., Nazari, S., Nguyen, H., Ntouskos, V., Pahde, F., Pataki, B. E., Quintana, J., Puig, S., Rezze, G. G., Garcia, R., Soyer, H. P., & Malvehy, J. (2024). A protocol for annotation of total body photography for machine learning to analyze skin phenotype and lesion classification. *Frontiers in Medicine*, 11. https://doi.org/10.3389/fmed.2024.1380984

Rastgarpour, M., & Shanbehzadeh, J. (2011, March). Application of AI techniques in medical image segmentation and novel categorization of available methods and tools. In *Proceedings of the international multiconference of engineers and computer scientists* (Vol. 1, pp. 16-18).

Research, P. (2023, December 4). AI in medical imaging market size to hit USD 11.76 Bn By 2033. https://www.precedenceresearch.com/ai-in-medical-imaging-market

Roth, H. R. (2018). Deep learning and its application to medical image segmentation. *Medical Imaging Technology*, 36, 63–71. [Google Scholar]

Tang, X., Wang, B., & Rong, Y. (2018). Artificial intelligence will reduce the need for clinical medical physicists. *Journal of Applied Clinical Medical Physics*, 19(1), 6–9. https://doi.org/10.1002/acm2.12244

Wang, Y., Han, X., Li, C., Luo, L., Yin, Q., Zhang, J., Peng, G., Shi, D., & He, M. (2024). Impact of gold-standard label errors on evaluating performance of deep learning models in diabetic retinopathy screening: Nationwide real-world validation study. *Journal of Medical Internet Research*, 26, e52506. https://doi.org/10.2196/52506

Winkler, J. K., Fink, C., Toberer, F., Enk, A., Deinlein, T., Hofmann-Wellenhof, R., Thomas, L., Lallas, A., Blum, A., Stolz, W., & Haenssle, H. A. (2019). Association between surgical skin markings in dermoscopic images and diagnostic performance of a deep learning convolutional neural network for melanoma recognition. *JAMA Dermatology*, 155(10), 1135. https://doi.org/10.1001/jamadermatol.2019.1735

Xu, D., Li, B., Liu, W., Wei, D., Long, X., Huang, T., Lin, H., Cao, K., Zhong, S., Shao, J., Huang, B., Diao, X. F., & Gao, Z. (2024). Deep learning-based detection of primary bone tumors around the knee joint on radiographs: a multicenter study. *Quantitative Imaging in Medicine and Surgery*, 14(8), 5420–5433. https://doi.org/10.21037/qims-23-1743

Yala, A., Lehman, C., Schuster, T., Portnoi, T., & Barzilay, R. (2019). A Deep Learning Mammography-based Model for Improved Breast Cancer Risk Prediction. *Radiology*, 292(1), 60–66. https://doi.org/10.1148/radiol.2019182716

12 Unlocking Effective Applications of Artificial Intelligence for Healthcare Management Systems

Shreyan Saha and Esha Saha

12.1 INTRODUCTION

Healthcare is one of the significant sectors all around the globe. In recent times, the increasingly challenging situation for the healthcare systems is to provide affordable and quality healthcare. Creating effective and efficient healthcare systems has been a top priority for healthcare policymakers due to the constant increase in healthcare spending and concurrently rising demand for healthcare services (Saha & Rathore, 2024). The health sector in India is expanding and modernizing at a CAGR of about 16%. In India, health spending accounts for barely 4% of GDP (the total of public and private spending), compared to a global average of 9.9%. The total amount spent by the government makes up 1.4% of GDP, whereas the global average is 6% (www.dfat.gov.au). The management aspect of healthcare systems has recently come under increased scrutiny. Healthcare management systems include various functions, including operations, marketing, finance, and human resource management. Among the various functions of healthcare management, operations management in healthcare includes streamlining patient flow processes, managing inventories of medicines and medical equipment and other health products, scheduling patient appointments, allocating beds and other resources, and providing quality treatment and care at affordable cost (Saha & Ray, 2019). It ensures executing a highly focused strategy and organizational change enabled by various analytical tools, techniques, and programs. Operations management is necessary for healthcare systems to provide quality services to patients. This can be accomplished by reducing costs and improving the healthcare facilities at hospitals. Healthcare managers regularly use operations management techniques for improving the healthcare service quality and reducing service costs simultaneously (Jha et al., 2016). Further, marketing management in healthcare systems helps hospitals to establish connections with patients and nurture the customer base for an extended period. Healthcare marketing includes communicating and delivering health-related information. It primarily focuses on understanding the attitudes of patients, which leads them to make perceptions about a particular healthcare service provider. The marketing strategy of a healthcare service provider attracts potential patients by letting them know why the

 DOI: 10.1201/9781003503385-12

treatment they provide is the best in the market. Apart from that, healthcare financial management includes all the financial activities necessary to keep healthcare institutions solvent and operate and deliver patient care effectively and efficiently. Financial management in healthcare focuses on cash, capital, costs, and control. Generating revenue, detecting fraud, financial evaluation, planning, mitigating risk, budgeting, forecasting, and complying with regulations are the main financial management activities in healthcare management systems. There are important ramifications for public health, equity, and growth from the health financing transformation (Fan & Savedoff, 2014). Finally, human resource management in the healthcare sector is another important function in healthcare management that is required to deliver medical services effectively and efficiently to achieve satisfaction among patients (Elarabi & Johari, 2014). Human resource departments in healthcare organizations perform functions like recruiting, hiring, advising senior management on compensation, etc. Apart from these, healthcare human resource managers are also responsible for managing a high employee turnover rate, looking after employees' physical and mental health, monitoring certification compliance, and determining success based on the number of patients and their satisfaction levels. Building a sustainable work culture is also the responsibility of healthcare human resource managers to attract new talents and engage existing employees.

Recent years have seen a tremendous advancement in Artificial Intelligence (AI) and its applications. Hospitals that have a substantial market share are more susceptible to AI adoption (Pham et al., 2024). In this study, we cover the recent AI applications in the healthcare sector. More specifically, this study systematically reviews the effective models and applications of AI from the perspective of healthcare operations, marketing, finance, and human resource. Prior studies observed that AI possesses an extensive array of potential to change healthcare systems, going beyond only clinical care. AI can assist in streamlining business processes throughout the healthcare industry, from operations and finance to marketing and human resource management. The first instance when AI was involved in medicine was in the early 1950s. At that time, physicians made attempts to improve diagnoses using computers (Secinaro et al., 2021). Emotional value, functional value, optimism, innovativeness, and personal involvement positively affect physicians' intentions to adopt AI-assisted medical equipment (Hsieh, 2023). AI techniques in the healthcare sector include machine learning methods, modern deep learning, natural language processing, etc. (Jiang et al., 2017). AI technology can raise the effectiveness of a healthcare facility by keeping administrative workflow smooth, providing virtual nursing assistants, detecting dosage errors, making surgeries less invasive, preventing fraud, etc.

In the case of operations management in healthcare, AI can enable effective scheduling for both scheduled appointments and emergencies and thus reduce unnecessary waiting time. AI-enabled scheduling tools help book appointments faster in suggested time windows. AI tools can alert the staff about unscheduled appointments. In recent years, a new simulation methodology has gained popularity in healthcare management systems, which is agent-based modeling. In the case of dispatching mobile healthcare workers, travel time can be reduced, and on-time arrivals can be ensured by using AI technology. AI algorithms, which are flexible and capable of adapting to intricate patterns, could be ideal for solving complex healthcare operations management problems (Pianykh et al., 2020). In the case of the healthcare supply chain, the critical success factors are technological, institutional, environmental, human, and organizational dimensions. Among these four factors, technological factors are the most critical factor that influences AI adoption in the healthcare supply chain in India (Kumar et al., 2023a). Consumers' perceived risk influences the effect of innovation loci on the adoption of medical AI by consumers. Consumers are more likely to consume peripheral products than core products, which use AI (Huang et al., 2023). In the healthcare setting, a customer relationship management system is referred to as an application of healthcare information technology that supports patient-centric care ideals (Dastjerdi et al., 2023). In the healthcare industry, patients expect clinical skills and competence as primary requirements. The usage of AI-enabled CRM systems can meet such expectations. AI-enabled customer services have the potential to generate capabilities for improved performance in the healthcare sector (Kumar et al., 2023b). AI is also transforming healthcare marketing by providing personalized patient experiences, enabling data-driven decision-making, enhancing patient outreach, using predictive analytics, etc. Now, AI-powered chatbots are available all the time. This facility has reduced administrative costs and made data collection more accessible. Many AI-enabled models anticipate financial costs depending on the disease severity. Robotic process automation can enable AI applications in healthcare finance by streamlining data-gathering. It can combine billing data from various sources and perform monthly account reconciliations, which is labor- and time-intensive. AI can also help in managing health insurance claims. In healthcare institutes, AI methods can be applied to introduce adaptable, sophisticated fraud detection systems that can detect possible financial fraud schemes. AI has the capability to eradicate the human resources crisis in the healthcare sector by enabling decision-making, facilitating diagnostics, etc. (Meskó et al., 2018). By using AI tools, healthcare human resource managers can reduce the hiring time and increase the staff retention rate and employee engagement. AI can respond automatically in real time. This will enable both employees and applicants to get replies instantly. Thus, chatbots can help the healthcare administration by reducing the workload of repetitive tasks. AI can help human resource managers by identifying applicants' profiles and matching them with the available positions to get the most suitable candidates. AI can also evaluate employees' training needs by tracking existing and new hires' data. In the healthcare sector, working together, humans and AI can help medical professionals, address the shortage of trained healthcare personnel and enhance service quality. Overall, of late, there has been a growth in works related to AI. Further, it is being seen that different challenging functions of healthcare management can be solved by the implementation of AI. This has motivated us to further explore this area of research. Specifically, we aim to critically review and analyze the existing AI applications that can support healthcare management systems from the perspective of healthcare operations, marketing, finance, and human resources. In the case of AI governance and AI education, safe and effective adoption of AI is required in the healthcare industry (Stogiannos et al., 2024). The main requirements for successful AI implementation in clinical settings are promoting knowledge about AI, infrastructure, finance and resources, data accessibility, accurate and consistent data, organizational cooperation, proper regulatory framework, and implementation strategies (Marco-Ruiz et al., 2024). Transforming the entire healthcare system into a digitalized one is a challenging task. The main barriers to this transformation are risk barriers, value barriers, legal barriers, and tradition barriers (Kumari et al., 2024). During the adoption of AI in the healthcare ecosystem, resistance usually occurs from both patients and healthcare professionals. It has been observed that during the pre-adoption stage, physicians resist the implementation of AI, and patients reject AI-enabled healthcare services. Patients usually trust human physicians when they are between AI and human physicians. During the post-adoption stage, it has been seen that physicians disagree with AI advice and use AI less frequently. In this stage, patients' perceptions of AI are not positive and tend to exhibit less compliance with AI recommendations (Yang et al., 2024). To address the above-mentioned research issues, this chapter addresses the following research questions: RQ1: What are the applications of AI in healthcare management systems, specifically from the perspective of healthcare operations, marketing, finance, and human resource management? RQ2: What are the existing modeling approaches for solving problems in the domain of AI applications in healthcare management systems? RQ3: What is the roadmap for adopting and diffusing AI technology in healthcare management systems?

The main contribution of this review can be summarized as follows:

- This study systematically reviews the effective models and applications of AI from the perspective of healthcare operations, marketing, finance, and human resource.
- This review identifies the several research problems around AI applications in healthcare management systems. Based on the identified research problems, the review classifies different modeling approaches. The review also discusses the key findings of the existing research works in the related field.
- Critical appraisal of existing research work in the related field is presented, which identifies some noteworthy research issues.
- A roadmap is developed to add essential elements to the existing literature on AI applications in healthcare management systems. The proposed roadmap will guide researchers and practitioners dealing with the adoption and diffusion of AI to improve the system.
- Lastly, the review paper recommends some important future research directions in the field of AI adoption in healthcare management systems. The adoption and diffusion of AI-enabled healthcare management systems will improve the productivity of hospitals, which will result in greater satisfaction among patients.

12.2 LITERATURE REVIEW

Many studies have been carried out in the last few years by the researchers and practitioners on AI applications in the healthcare sector. We pilot a systematic review on AI applications, specifically, in the healthcare management systems. We critically appraised the existing AI applications, analyzed, and classified them based on AI applications in healthcare operations, marketing, finance, and human resources. The set of reviews of existing studies is derived from peer-reviewed journal articles. Numerous databases, including ScienceDirect, ResearchGate, and Scopus with keywords such as 'healthcare operations', 'healthcare marketing', 'healthcare finance', 'healthcare human resources', in combination with 'artificial intelligence' are used. As seen in Table 12.1, there are a significant number of papers reviewed in the domain of AI applications in healthcare management, viz., healthcare operations, marketing,

TABLE 12.1
Review of Related Literature

	References	Research Problem	Method Used	Key Findings
AI applications in healthcare operations	Ala et al. (2024)	Enhancing the standard of treatment based on AI.	Metaheuristics	92.5% accuracy obtained.
	Kassem et al. (2024)	Adoption of AI-based clinical decision support systems.	Machine learning models	Innovative AI-based method for clinical decision support is developed.
	Almutairi and Olatunji (2024)	Patient appointment no-shows.	Machine learning models	Predictive model for appointment no-shows is developed.
	Niu et al. (2024)	Patient disease prediction.	Machine learning models	Patient disease risk prediction using clustering method is proposed.
	Kumar et al. (2023b)	Adopting AI in healthcare supply chain.	Empirical (qualitative)	Technological factors impact AI adoption in the healthcare supply chain.
	Bertl et al. (2023)	Exploring barriers and facilitators for AI-based digital decision support systems in healthcare.	Empirical (qualitative)	Framework considering disease, data, and technology is developed.
	Bag et al. (2023)	Exploring antecedents of big data analytics and AI in omnichannel health care processes.	Empirical (quantitative)	Managerial factors improve the capacity of healthcare institutions.
	Abadie et al. (2023)	AI adoption for omnichannel integration quality in healthcare.	Empirical (quantitative)	Strategies such as translating organizational resources into capabilities are recommended.
	Damoah et al. (2021)	Exploring AI-based drones in the healthcare supply chain.	Empirical (qualitative)	AI-enhanced medical drones contribute significantly to Ghana's healthcare supply chain and sustainable development goals.
	Dastjerdi et al. (2023)	Adoption of AI-based customer relationship management systems in the healthcare sector.	Multicriteria decision-making	Government, hospital size, security, management support, and employee training are significant factors for adoption.

AI applications in healthcare marketing	Latinovic and Chatterjee (2022)	AI-powered solutions in a B2B contexts in healthcare.	Conceptual	AI delivers economic and relational customer value in B2B context in healthcare.
	Leone et al. (2021)	Understanding how AI supports healthcare organizations in co-creating value.	Empirical (qualitative)	Framework with value co-creation and patient journey is developed.
	Uzir et al. (2021)	Exploring usage of AI-enabled products for patient monitoring.	Empirical (quantitative)	Service quality, product quality, and perceived convenience affect user experience and trust.
	Higgins and Madai (2020)	Adoption of AI-based biomedical products.	Review	Recommended procedures for AI in healthcare product development.
	Ramezani et al. (2023)	Optimizing healthcare financing systems.	Review	AI significantly affects health finance governance, income generation, pooling, and strategic purchasing.
AI applications in healthcare finance	Ali Mohamad et al. (2023)	Identifying the impact of AI on the competitive advantage of healthcare organizations.	Empirical (qualitative)	Primary outcomes of implementing AI in healthcare organizations are clinical, financial, and technological.
	Birzhandi and Cho (2023)	Focusing on the application of fairness techniques in healthcare, organizational justice, and finance.	Review	Discriminations are identified and comprehensively discussed.
	Sachan et al. (2021)	Addressing uncertainty in AI-enabled decisions in health care and finance.	Machine learning models	Proving one's capacity for managing uncertainty and how it affects the explainability of actual financial and medical data.
	Hua et al. (2023)	Factors affecting medical imaging experts' acceptance of artificial intelligence.	Review	User factors, system usage factors, and socio-organizational-cultural factors are identified.

(*Continued*)

Table 12.1 (Continiued)

	References	Research Problem	Method Used	Key Findings
AI applications in healthcare human resource management	Rouhani et al. (2024)	Developing human resources management model using AI in a healthcare context.	Machine learning models	92% accuracy is obtained.
	Rebelo et al. (2023)	Verifying to what extent AI impacts mental healthcare workers' tasks.	Review	AI has an impact on mental health professionals' tasks by offering assistance.
	Shahzad et al. (2023)	Impact of AI on human resource functions in healthcare systems.	Empirical (quantitative)	Through social media impact, technical understanding, and individual creativity, AI influences human resource functions.
	Li et al. (2023)	Exploring the impact of AI in healthcare sector on human resource strategies and hospital performance.	Empirical (qualitative)	AI can improve human resource performance in terms of employee engagement and assignment of tasks.
	Gupta et al. (2021)	Estimating the prevalence of burnout among healthcare workers.	Empirical (quantitative)	AI-enabled model for predicting stress and burnout among healthcare workers.
	Meskó et al. (2018)	Solving human resource problems in healthcare using AI.	Empirical (qualitative)	AI will not replace caregivers; however, those who utilize AI may replace those who do not use AI.

finance, and human resources. In this systematic review, an attempt has been made to examine the research problems, methodologies used, and the key findings related to AI applications in healthcare management. The methods used are further classified based on the conceptual, review, empirical studies (qualitative, quantitative, and mixed), and mathematical (i.e., optimization methods (metaheuristics), machine learning (ML) methods, and multicriterial decision-making (MCDM) approaches). The following research gaps are identified from the review of literature:

- AI applications in healthcare management systems is an emerging domain; however, to the best of our knowledge, there are no research works that have classified the applications of AI based on the functional areas of healthcare management systems such as AI applications in healthcare operations, healthcare marketing, healthcare finance, and human resource management.
- Besides, from our review of literature, it is observed that research works in the area of AI applications in healthcare finance are very limited.
- Further, the mathematical models to solve the challenging problems related to AI applications in healthcare management systems are very limited.
- Finally, to the best of our knowledge, there are no studies that provided an overall roadmap for the adoption and diffusion of AI technology in healthcare management systems. As AI applications in healthcare management systems are a new phenomenon in this area, it requires understanding the entire healthcare management system, identifying the problems and challenges in the adoption of AI applications, collecting opinions from the stakeholders (patients, physicians, and hospital managers), etc. Hence, a detailed roadmap will be very beneficial.

12.3 RESULTS AND DISCUSSION

We identified from the review that around 25 number of research centered on using AI in various healthcare management functions like healthcare operations, marketing, finance, and human resources (refer to Figure 12.1).

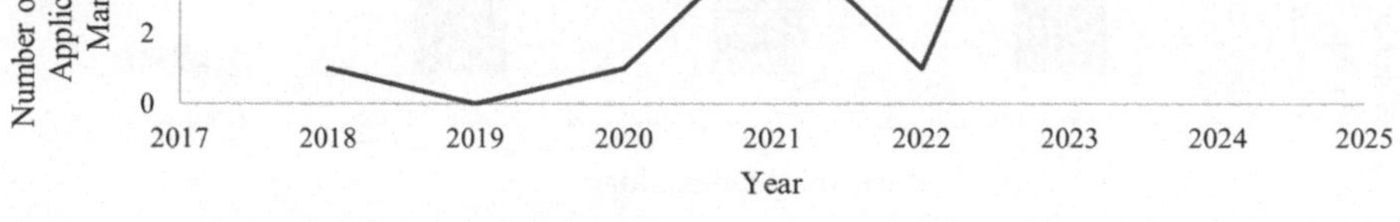

FIGURE 12.1 Number of research papers on AI applications in healthcare management over the years.

Around nine research centered on using AI in operations management, five studies focused on applications of AI in marketing management, four research centered on using AI in financial management, and seven research centered on using AI in human resource management (refer to Figure 12.2).

The review also classifies the solution approaches, such as mathematical and empirical models (refer to Figure 12.3).

Besides, the review classifies the challenging problems in healthcare management systems that can be solved by the application of AI, like disease risk prediction, clinical decision-making, healthcare supply chain management, smart healthcare systems, omnichannel healthcare processes, new healthcare product development, healthcare value co-creation, customer relationship management, optimizing healthcare financing, stress management among healthcare workers, and many more (Johnson et al., 2021; Wang & Preininger, 2019; Gupta et al., 2021; Bag et al., 2023; Uzir et al., 2021; Ramezani et al., 2023). The AI-enabled system has the potential to

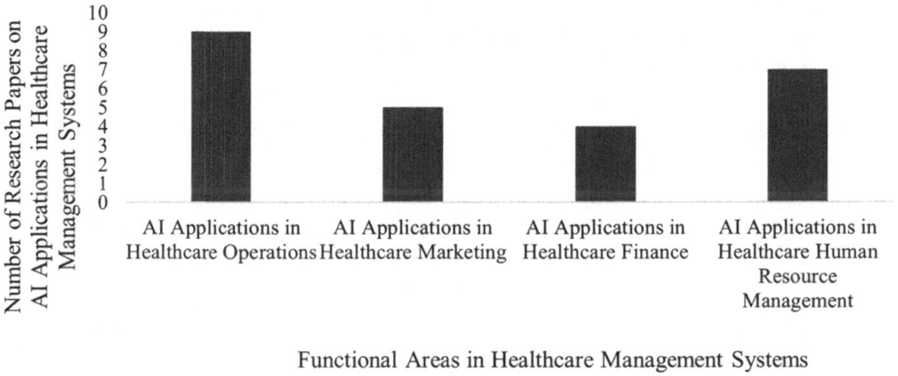

FIGURE 12.2 Number of research papers on AI applications specific to operations, marketing, finance and human resource management.

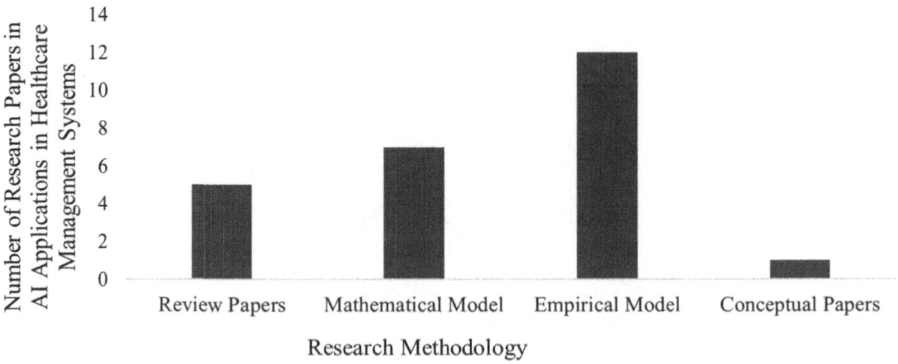

FIGURE 12.3 Number of review papers, mathematical and empirical works on AI applications in healthcare management.

assist doctors in making everyday clinical decisions (Niu et al., 2024). Prior studies observed that AI has a wide range of potential to change healthcare, going beyond only clinical care. AI can assist in streamlining business processes throughout the healthcare industry, from operations, finance, marketing to human resource management. Companies in the biopharmaceutical and medical technology sectors can employ AI solutions to streamline healthcare operations, including the global HC supply chain. Medical inventory automation can be utilized to handle forecasting, planning, managing stock-outs, overstocks, and expirations; automate the stocking and fulfillment operations; and meet the required patient demand ontime. The impact of AI is also being seen in healthcare marketing. Predictive analytics powered by AI can estimate future patient acquisition costs. The chatbot is one of the more personalized implementations of AI technology that can assist healthcare marketers by boosting website engagement and pointing potential patients to online resources, thereby enhancing the patient experience. Additionally, AI could help marketing teams produce concise and understandable content for emails or presentations to healthcare practitioners. Interestingly, customer relationship management systems aid healthcare organizations in managing relationships with patients. An AI-enabled customer relationship management system will help healthcare organizations analyze large volumes of patient data in a moment, resulting in informed decisions made by the staff (Dastjerdi et al., 2023). A linear relationship exists between AI-enabled customer relationship management system capability, customer service flexibility, and service innovation. Healthcare financial management is significantly impacted by AI in several ways. Pooling, strategic purchasing, income raising, and governance can improve performance when AI technology assists their activities. If healthcare organizations adopt AI tools and use their applications, the susceptible groups will face fewer trials and get benefits from an advanced healthcare finance system (Ramezani et al., 2023; Sachan et al., 2021). Besides, AI technology can improve the work in healthcare finance through robotic process automation, which can streamline repetitive processes like merging billing data from several sources or carrying out labor- and time-intensive monthly account reconciliations. Medical insurance automation can also be used to improve policy management, claim processing, and regulatory compliance. Finally, AI may help with the healthcare industry's human resource management. AI can assist in managing human resources in the healthcare industry, including recruiting potential healthcare workforce. Besides, AI can free up time for typical tasks in the healthcare industry, like administrative work or taking notes, allowing doctors and nurses to spend more time with patients. AI has the capability of raising ethical standards in healthcare organizations. AI-enabled human resource management systems in healthcare organizations can boost the ecosystem through social media influence, individual creativity, and technological understanding (Shahzad et al., 2023). Perceived risks can affect the link between technological familiarity and human resource functions. Human resource practitioners and policymakers in healthcare organizations can use AI technology to optimize hospital performance. Human resources in healthcare organizations can provide a sustainable competitive advantage. Healthcare workers are not devoid of emotions, and in a healthy workplace condition, their performance can improve. AI can detect the emotions of healthcare workers from a large dataset of facial images. Emotion

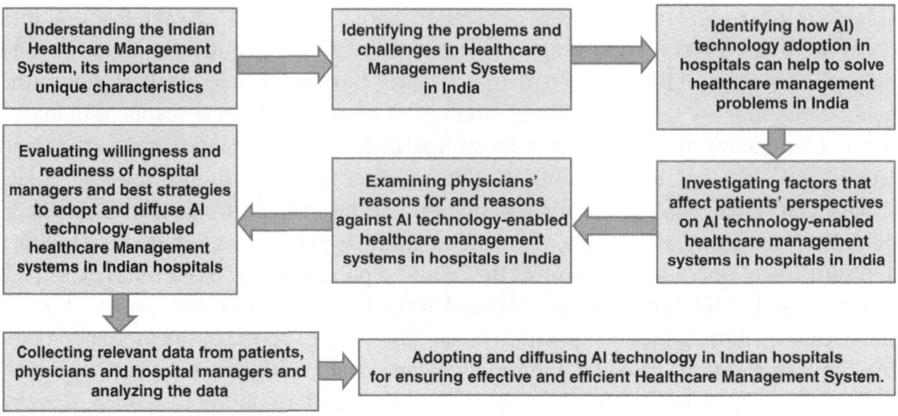

FIGURE 12.4 Roadmap for AI technology adoption in healthcare systems.

recognition in human resource management can significantly impact work performance in the healthcare industry (Rouhani et al., 2024). Overall, through this extensive review, this study reveals the useful considerations for building the next generation of healthcare using AI that have the potential to significantly advance the healthcare sector. A roadmap for adoption of AI technology in healthcare systems is proposed in Figure 12.4.

12.4 CONCLUDING REMARKS AND FUTURE RESEARCH DIRECTIONS

This review study considers articles on AI applications in healthcare management systems and identifies several elements necessary for the implementation of AI in healthcare operations, marketing, finance, and human resource management. Specifically, healthcare omnichannel systems is an important area for future research. Further, the impact of sustainable innovation, resource efficiency, supply chain planning, process optimization, supply chain risk management, supply chain agility, and closed-loop service models in the healthcare industry may be considered for future research. Optimizing telemedicine and remote patient monitoring for chronic diseases can be another future avenue.

Interestingly, identifying cultural and contextual factors across different countries that have the capability to impact the relationship between AI-enabled technology used in the healthcare sector and various human resource functions is a probable pathway for doing future research. Other future directions for healthcare human resources research include investigating AI's applications for tasks like treatment prescription and documentation, assessing the effectiveness of AI-enabled systems against humans in a hybrid setting, investigating AI-supported mental healthcare, and gauging the effects of AI-driven therapy systems, and examining the fallout from deploying AI technologies in real-world settings. Finally, integrating AI and the Internet of Things, analytics, and blockchain technology may further improve the healthcare management systems and the healthcare services offered to patients.

REFERENCES

Abadie, A., Roux, M., Chowdhury, S., & Dey, P. (2023). Interlinking organisational resources, AI adoption and omnichannel integration quality in Ghana's healthcare supply chain. *Journal of Business Research*, *162*, 113866.

Ala, A., Simic, V., Pamucar, D., & Bacanin, N. (2024). Enhancing patient information performance in internet of things-based smart healthcare system: Hybrid artificial intelligence and optimization approaches. *Engineering Applications of Artificial Intelligence*, *131*, 107889.

Ali Mohamad, T., Bastone, A., Bernhard, F., & Schiavone, F. (2023). How artificial intelligence impacts the competitive position of healthcare organizations. *Journal of Organizational Change Management*, *36*(8), 49–70.

Almutairi, T. H., & Olatunji, S. O. (2024). The utilization of AI in healthcare to predict no-shows for dental appointments: A case study conducted in Saudi Arabia. *Informatics in Medicine Unlocked*, *46*, 101472.

Bag, S., Dhamija, P., Singh, R. K., Rahman, M. S., & Sreedharan, V. R. (2023). Big data analytics and artificial intelligence technologies based collaborative platform empowering absorptive capacity in health care supply chain: An empirical study. *Journal of Business Research*, *154*, 113315.

Bertl, M., Ross, P., & Draheim, D. (2023). Systematic AI support for decision-making in the healthcare sector: Obstacles and success factors. *Health Policy and Technology*, *12*(3), 100748.

Birzhandi, P., & Cho, Y. S. (2023). Application of fairness to healthcare, organizational justice, and finance: A survey. *Expert Systems with Applications*, *216*, 119465.

Damoah, I. S., Ayakwah, A., & Tingbani, I. (2021). Artificial intelligence (AI)-enhanced medical drones in the healthcare supply chain (HSC) for sustainability development: A case study. *Journal of Cleaner Production*, *328*, 129598.

Dastjerdi, M., Keramati, A., & Keramati, N. (2023). A novel framework for investigating organizational adoption of AI-integrated CRM systems in the healthcare sector; using a hybrid fuzzy decision-making approach. *Telematics and Informatics Reports*, *11*, 100078.

Elarabi, H. M., & Johari, F. (2014). The impact of human resources management on healthcare quality. *Asian Journal of Management Sciences & Education*, *3*(1), 13–22.

Fan, V. Y., & Savedoff, W. D. (2014). The health financing transition: a conceptual framework and empirical evidence. *Social Science & Medicine*, *105*, 112–121.

Gupta, M. D., Bansal, A., Sarkar, P. G., Girish, M. P., Jha, M., Yusuf, J., … Gupta, A. (2021). Design and rationale of an intelligent algorithm to detect BuRnoUt in HeaLthcare workers in COVID era using ECG and artificiaL intelligence: The BRUCEE-LI study. *Indian Heart Journal*, *73*(1), 109–113.

Higgins, D., & Madai, V. I. (2020). From bit to bedside: a practical framework for artificial intelligence product development in healthcare. *Advanced Intelligent Systems*, *2*(10), 2000052.

Hsieh, P. J. (2023). Determinants of physicians' intention to use AI-assisted diagnosis: An integrated readiness perspective. *Computers in Human Behavior*, *147*, 107868.

Hua, D., Petrina, N., Young, N., Cho, J. G., & Poon, S. K. (2023). Understanding the factors influencing acceptability of AI in medical imaging domains among healthcare professionals: A scoping review. *Artificial Intelligence in Medicine*, 30, 102698.

Huang, X., Wu, X., Cao, X., & Wu, J. (2023). The effect of medical artificial intelligence innovation locus on consumer adoption of new products. *Technological Forecasting and Social Change*, *197*, 122902.

Jha, R. K., Sahay, B. S., & Charan, P. (2016). Healthcare operations management: a structured literature review. *Decision*, *43*(3), 259–279.

Jiang, F., Jiang, Y., Zhi, H., Dong, Y., Li, H., Ma, S., … Wang, Y. (2017). Artificial intelligence in healthcare: past, present and future. *Stroke and Vascular Neurology*, *2*(4). https://doi.org/10.1136/svn-2017-000101

Johnson, K. B., Wei, W. Q., Weeraratne, D., Frisse, M. E., Misulis, K., Rhee, K., ... Snowdon, J. L. (2021). Precision medicine, AI, and the future of personalized health care. *Clinical and Translational Science*, *14*(1), 86–93.

Kassem, K., Sperti, M., Cavallo, A., Vergani, A. M., Fassino, D., Moz, M., ... Deriu, M. A. (2024). An innovative artificial intelligence-based method to compress complex models into explainable, model-agnostic and reduced decision support systems with application to healthcare (NEAR). *Artificial Intelligence in Medicine*, *151*, 102841.

Kumar, A., Mani, V., Jain, V., Gupta, H., & Venkatesh, V. G. (2023a). Managing healthcare supply chain through artificial intelligence (AI): A study of critical success factors. *Computers & Industrial Engineering*, *175*, 108815.

Kumar, P., Sharma, S. K., & Dutot, V. (2023b). Artificial intelligence (AI)-enabled CRM capability in healthcare: The impact on service innovation. *International Journal of Information Management*, *69*, 102598.

Kumari, P., Shankar, A., Behl, A., Pereira, V., Yahiaoui, D., Laker, B., ... Arya, V. (2024). Investigating the barriers towards adoption and implementation of open innovation in healthcare. *Technological Forecasting and Social Change*, *200*, 123100.

Latinovic, Z., & Chatterjee, S. C. (2022). Achieving the promise of AI and ML in delivering economic and relational customer value in B2B. *Journal of Business Research*, *144*, 966–974.

Leone, D., Schiavone, F., Appio, F. P., & Chiao, B. (2021). How does artificial intelligence enable and enhance value co-creation in industrial markets? An exploratory case study in the healthcare ecosystem. *Journal of Business Research*, *129*, 849–859.

Li, P., Bastone, A., Mohamad, T. A., & Schiavone, F. (2023). How does artificial intelligence impact human resources performance. evidence from a healthcare institution in the United Arab Emirates. *Journal of Innovation & Knowledge*, *8*(2), 100340.

Marco-Ruiz, L., Hernández, M. Á. T., Ngo, P. D., Makhlysheva, A., Svenning, T. O., Dyb, K., ... Tayefi, M. (2024). A multinational study on artificial intelligence adoption: Clinical implementers' perspectives. *International Journal of Medical Informatics*, *184*, 105377.

Meskó, B., Hetényi, G., & Győrffy, Z. (2018). Will artificial intelligence solve the human resource crisis in healthcare?. *BMC Health Services Research*, *18*, 1–4.

Niu, S., Yin, Q., Ma, J., Song, Y., Xu, Y., Bai, L., ... Yang, X. (2024). Enhancing healthcare decision support through explainable AI models for risk prediction. *Decision Support Systems*, *181*, 114228.

Pham, P., Zhang, H., Gao, W., & Zhu, X. (2024). Determinants and performance outcomes of artificial intelligence adoption: Evidence from US Hospitals. *Journal of Business Research*, *172*, 114402.

Pianykh, O. S., Guitron, S., Parke, D., Zhang, C., Pandharipande, P., Brink, J., & Rosenthal, D. (2020). Improving healthcare operations management with machine learning. *Nature Machine Intelligence*, *2*(5), 266–273.

Ramezani, M., Takian, A., Bakhtiari, A., Rabiee, H. R., Fazaeli, A. A., & Sazgarnejad, S. (2023). The application of artificial intelligence in health financing: a scoping review. *Cost Effectiveness and Resource Allocation*, *21*(1), 83.

Rebelo, A. D., Verboom, D. E., dos Santos, N. R., & de Graaf, J. W. (2023). The impact of artificial intelligence on the tasks of mental healthcare workers: A scoping review. *Computers in Human Behavior: Artificial Humans*, 30, 100008.

Rouhani, S., Rezvani, M., & Madadi, Y. (2024). Human Resource Management Through Artificial Intelligence Model in the Healthcare. *Qeios*. https://doi.org/10.32388/3936al

Sachan, S., Almaghrabi, F., Yang, J. B., & Xu, D. L. (2021). Evidential reasoning for preprocessing uncertain categorical data for trustworthy decisions: An application on healthcare and finance. *Expert Systems with Applications*, *185*, 115597.

Saha, E., & Rathore, P. (2024). The impact of healthcare 4.0 technologies on healthcare supply chain performance: Extending the organizational information processing theory. *Technological Forecasting and Social Change*, *201*, 123256.

Saha, E., & Ray, P. K. (2019). Patient condition-based medicine inventory management in healthcare systems. *IISE Transactions on Healthcare Systems Engineering*, *9*(3), 299–312.

Secinaro, S., Calandra, D., Secinaro, A., Muthurangu, V., & Biancone, P. (2021). The role of artificial intelligence in healthcare: A structured literature review. *BMC Medical Informatics and Decision Making*, *21*, 1–23.

Shahzad, M. F., Xu, S., Naveed, W., Nusrat, S., & Zahid, I. (2023). Investigating the impact of artificial intelligence on human resource functions in the health sector of China: A mediated moderation model. *Heliyon*, *9*(11), 20.

Stogiannos, N., Litosseliti, L., O'Regan, T., Scurr, E., Barnes, A., Kumar, A., … Malamateniou, C. (2024). Black box no more: A cross-sectional multi-disciplinary survey for exploring governance and guiding adoption of AI in medical imaging and radiotherapy in the UK. *International Journal of Medical Informatics*, *186*, 105423.

Uzir, M. U. H., Al Halbusi, H., Lim, R., Jerin, I., Hamid, A. B. A., Ramayah, T., & Haque, A. (2021). Applied Artificial Intelligence and user satisfaction: Smartwatch usage for healthcare in Bangladesh during COVID-19. *Technology in Society*, *67*, 101780.

Wang, F., & Preininger, A. (2019). AI in health: state of the art, challenges, and future directions. *Yearbook of medical informatics*, *28*(01), 016–026.

Yang, Y., Ngai, E. W., & Wang, L. (2024). Resistance to artificial intelligence in health care: literature review, conceptual framework, and research agenda. *Information & Management*, 61, 103961.

13 Transformative Synergy
Revolutionizing Healthcare Accounting Information Systems with AI

Hrishikesh Desai

13.1 INTRODUCTION

In an email conversation with the administrator of a large acute-care hospital in the state of Arkansas, USA, the administrator told me – "*we have built an entire AI Team to look at how we will use it moving forward within our system*". The healthcare industry has always faced significant challenges in maintaining financial stability while delivering high-quality patient care (American Hospital Association, 2023). Central to this challenge is Revenue Cycle Management (RCM), a complex process that involves appointment scheduling, patient registration, claims generation, billing, and payment collection (Atluri & Thummisetti, 2023). Each stage presents unique challenges and opportunities for improvement through the application of generative Artificial Intelligence (AI).

Based on an analysis of the Management Discussion and Analysis (MD&A) section of the 10-K annual reports of 14 publicly listed firms in the United States in the Standard Industrial Classification (SIC) code 8062 (General Medical and Surgical Hospitals), relevant RCM processes were identified. Firms' 10-K annual reports are widely used by stakeholders to understand how firms' business models evolve in response to the external environment (Desai, 2022). Appointment scheduling is an important component of RCM that can significantly impact patient satisfaction and revenue generation (Pazoki & Samarghandi, 2021). Generative AI can streamline the appointment scheduling process by utilizing natural language processing (NLP) and machine learning algorithms. AI-powered chatbots can interact with patients to schedule appointments, provide information about available time slots, send automated reminders, and even reschedule appointments if necessary.

When a patient arrives at a healthcare facility, the registration process involves capturing demographic information, insurance details, and medical history. Generative AI can automate this process by extracting relevant information from patient documents, such as insurance cards and ID proofs, using optical character recognition (OCR) and NLP techniques. After a patient receives medical services, the healthcare provider generates a claim to bill the insurance company or the patient (Derricks, 2021). Generative AI can automate the claims generation process by analyzing the patient's medical records, procedure codes (standardized codes used to identify and

DOI: 10.1201/9781003503385-13

describe the specific medical services, procedures, and treatments provided to a patient), and insurance policies to create accurate and compliant claims.[1] The billing process involves generating invoices, sending statements to patients, and following up on outstanding balances (Chandawarkar et al., 2024). Generative AI can streamline this process by automatically generating personalized invoices based on patient data and treatment history. AI can also assist in payment collection by predicting payment trends, identifying high-risk accounts, and recommending optimal payment plans.

There are seven scenarios discussed in this chapter detailing how generative AI such as ChatGPT or Claude can significantly improve hospital RCM processes by integrating with their Electronic Health Records (EHR) and RCM systems, assist with healthcare data analytics, and help with healthcare fraud detection, prevention, and investigations. This chapter makes several key contributions to the understanding and application of generative AI in healthcare accounting information systems. The core contributions are summarized below:

- *Comprehensive Framework*: Presents a framework for integrating generative AI into healthcare RCM through detailed scenarios, covering all major aspects from appointment scheduling to fraud detection.
- *AI-EHR Integration*: Explores the important aspect of integrating AI systems with existing HER and RCM systems, addressing technical and operational considerations.
- *Data Analytics Insights*: Demonstrates how generative AI can be used effectively for advanced healthcare data analytics, enabling predictive modeling.
- *Fraud Detection Framework*: Outlines an approach to using AI for healthcare fraud detection and prevention to ensure financial integrity in healthcare organizations.
- *Algorithms*: Explores three key algorithms that might prove effective in addressing critical RCM challenges.
- *API Architecture and Data Flow*: Outlines the key components of this architecture for seamless flow of data between AI and legacy systems.
- *AI System Training and Validation*: Offers insights into key processes (e.g., data preparation/training) used in developing robust AI models in healthcare accounting information systems (AIS).
- *Challenges and Solutions*: Identifies key challenges in implementing AI in healthcare settings and proposes practical solutions based on the technology's potential and limitations.
- *Future Directions*: Offers insights into the future of healthcare AIS, highlighting areas for further research and development in AI applications.
- *Ethical Considerations*: Addresses important ethical considerations in the use of AI in healthcare finance, including data privacy, security, and the need for human oversight.

13.2 SCENARIOS: GENERATIVE AI AND HOSPITAL RCM SYSTEMS

The flowchart in Figure 13.1, built using the Mermaidv10.9.1 Live Editor, illustrates the RCM process in healthcare, highlighting where AI interventions are applied. The

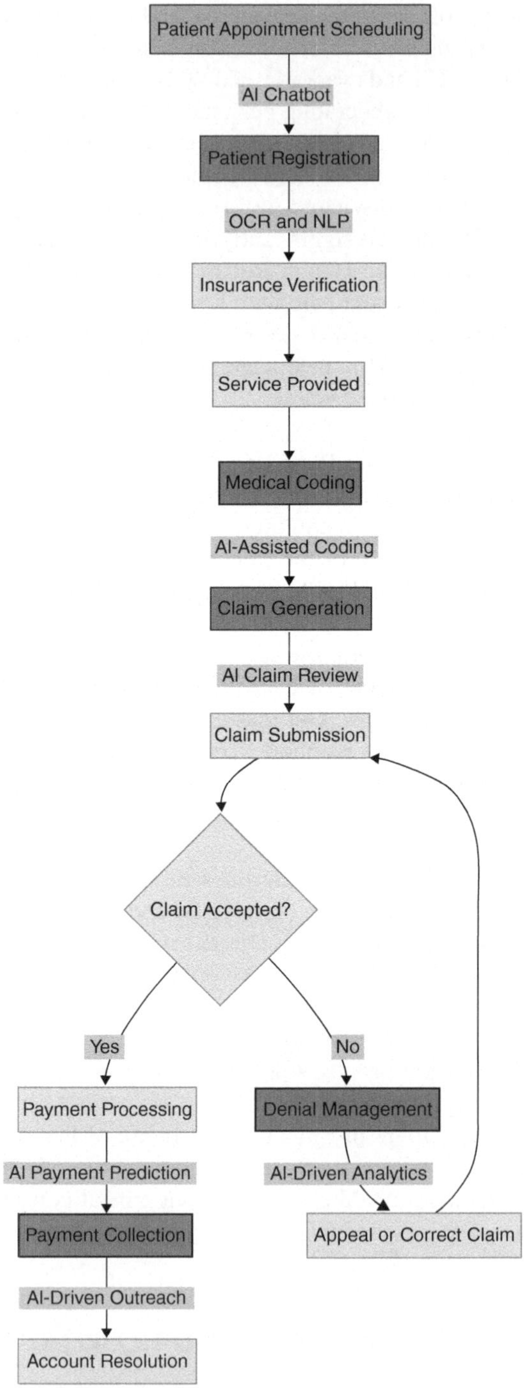

FIGURE 13.1 Revenue Cycle Management (RCM) Process Flow (self-created).

process begins with patient appointment scheduling, facilitated by AI chatbots, followed by patient registration using OCR and NLP technologies. After insurance verification and service provision, AI assists in medical coding and claim generation. The claims then undergo AI-powered review before submission. If a claim is accepted, it moves to payment processing, where AI predicts payment patterns. For denied claims, AI-driven analytics support the denial management and appeal process. The cycle concludes with payment collection, supported by AI-driven outreach, leading to final account resolution. The following scenarios in this chapter summarize this AI-augmented RCM process by detailing the problems in the traditional processes, AI-powered solutions, and the outcomes with AI integration.

13.2.1 Scenario I: AI-Powered Appointment Scheduling

Problems:

- Long wait times; Frequent no-shows; Patient dissatisfaction due to scheduling issues

AI Solutions:

- AI-powered chatbot for patient interaction
- Generative AI for schedule optimization; Analysis of historical appointment data

Outcomes:

- Reduced average wait times; Increased patient satisfaction
- Better resource allocation; Reduced medical staff overtime; Reduced no-shows
- More efficient handling of complex cases

13.2.2 Scenario II: AI-Powered Patient Registration

Problems:

- Long wait times in the Emergency Department (ED)
- High volume of patients; Registration errors due to manual data entry

AI Solutions:

- Generative AI system integrated with EHR; AI-powered chatbot for patient assistance
- OCR for document scanning
- NLP for data interpretation

Outcomes:

- Reduced manual data entry errors; Improved accuracy of patient records
- Reduced workload on registration staff; More efficient completion of registration forms
- Shortened wait times; Improved patient satisfaction

13.2.3 Scenario III: AI-Powered Claims Generation

Problems:

- Claims denials; Revenue loss due to incorrect coding; Incomplete documentation

AI Solutions:

- Generative AI system for automated claims generation
- AI analysis of operative reports; Prediction of claim denial likelihood

Outcomes:

- Reduction in manual coding errors; Increased staff productivity; Time savings for billing staff
- Increased compliance with payer policies; Increase in first-pass claim acceptance rates
- Reduction in claim rejections; Improved revenue

13.2.4 Scenario IV: AI-Powered Billing

Problems:

- Delayed payments; High accounts receivable
- Patient dissatisfaction due to confusing billing statements

AI Solutions:

- Generative AI system for payment collection and patient billing
- AI analysis of historical payment data
- AI-driven chatbot for patient portal and billing website

Outcomes:

- Proactive engagement with high-risk patients; Increased patient portal usage
- Personalized payment solutions; Reduction in accounts receivable; Higher patient collections
- Improved patient engagement and satisfaction; Lower claim denials; Better clean claim rates
- Reduction in billing-related customer service calls; Streamlined billing process

13.2.5 Scenario V: AI-Powered Payment Collection

Problems:

- Challenges with patient collections; Delayed payments
- Patient confusion about treatment costs and insurance coverage

AI Solutions:

- Generative AI system for payment collection and patient communication
- AI analysis of historical payment data
- Natural Language Generation (NLG) for personalized outreach messages

Outcomes:

- Automated and personalized outreach to high-risk patients; Improved patient engagement
- Increased likelihood of payment plan enrollment or upfront payments; Reduced receivables
- Reduced working capital tied up & admin costs for insurance verification/payment processing

13.2.6 Scenario VI: AI-Powered Healthcare Data Analytics

Problems:

- Financial challenges due to increasing costs; Declining reimbursements
- Inefficiencies in resource allocation

AI Solutions:

- Generative AI system for financial data analysis
- AI-powered predictive models for financial forecasting

Outcomes:

- Identification of high-profit margin procedures; Improved cash flow management
- Detection of seasonal variations in patient volumes; Real-time financial risk alerts
- Discovery of payer-specific payment patterns; Optimized resource allocation
- Accurate revenue and expense forecasts; Identification of cost-saving opportunities

13.2.7 Scenario VII: AI-Powered Healthcare Fraud Detection and Prevention

Problems:

- Increase in fraudulent activities (upcoding, unbundling, phantom billing); Financial losses
- Regulatory scrutiny

AI Solutions:

- Generative AI system for fraud detection and prevention; AI-powered risk scoring
- Real-time transaction analysis; AI analysis of historical financial data

Outcomes:

- Significant reduction in fraudulent activities; Prevention of financial losses
- Real-time fraud detection capabilities; Strengthened anti-fraud controls
- Prompt investigation and addressing of fraudulent activities; Fraud deterrence
- Improved compliance with regulatory requirements; Avoidance of penalties

13.3 MACHINE LEARNING ALGORITHMS IN HEALTHCARE RCM

The application of machine learning algorithms in healthcare RCM has significantly enhanced predictive capabilities and decision-making processes. This section explores three key algorithms that can prove effective in addressing critical RCM challenges: Random Forest for predicting patient no-shows, Gradient Boosting for claims denial prediction, and Neural Networks for fraud detection.

13.3.1 Random Forest for Predicting Patient No-Shows

Random Forest, an ensemble learning method, has the potential for remarkable efficacy in predicting patient no-shows, a persistent issue that impacts healthcare providers' efficiency and revenue (Parmar et al., 2019). Its key features include: handling both categorical and numerical data; resistance to overfitting due to averaging of uncorrelated trees; and providing feature importance rankings (Mafarja et al., 2023). In the context of predicting no-shows, a Random Forest model might consider features such as Patient demographics (age, gender, socioeconomic status); Appointment characteristics (day of week, time of day, specialty); Patient history (previous no-shows, cancellations); and External factors (weather conditions, public holidays). The model output is a probability score for each scheduled appointment, indicating the likelihood of a no-show. The following sample code in Python sets up a basic Random Forest model to predict the probability of patient no-shows, which can be used to manage appointment scheduling more effectively.

```
from sklearn.ensemble import RandomForestClassifier
from sklearn.model_selection import train_test_split
# Assume X is our feature set and y is our target (no-show or not)
X_train, X_test, y_train, y_test = train_test_split(X, y,
  test_size=0.2, random_state=42)
rf_model = RandomForestClassifier(n_estimators=100, max_
  depth=10, random_state=42)
rf_model.fit(X_train, y_train)
# Predict probabilities
no_show_probabilities = rf_model.predict_proba(X_test)[:, 1]
```

13.3.2 Gradient Boosting for Claims Denial Prediction

Gradient Boosting, particularly implementations like XGBoost or LightGBM, has proven effective in predicting insurance claim denials, allowing healthcare providers to proactively address potential issues (Bentéjac et al., 2021). Its key features are: High predictive accuracy; ability to handle non-linear relationships well; and robustness to outliers and missing data (Guo, et al., 2023). For predicting claim denials, a Gradient Boosting model might consider: Claim characteristics (procedure codes, diagnosis codes, billed amount); Patient information (insurance type, coverage details); Provider information (specialty, historical denial rates); and Payer-specific factors (historical denial patterns by payer). The model output is typically a probability of claim denial, allowing billing departments to prioritize claims for review or additional documentation before submission. The following sample code in Python sets up such a model using XGBoost to predict the probability of claim denials.

```
from xgboost import XGBClassifier
from sklearn.model_selection import train_test_split
# Assume X is our feature set and y is our target (claim
  denied or not)
X_train, X_test, y_train, y_test = train_test_split(X, y,
  test_size=0.2, random_state=42)
xgb_model = XGBClassifier(learning_rate=0.1, n_
  estimators=1000, max_depth=5, random_state=42)
xgb_model.fit(X_train, y_train)
# Predict probabilities
denial_probabilities = xgb_model.predict_proba(X_test)[:, 1]
```

13.3.3 Neural Networks for Fraud Detection

Deep Neural Networks, with their ability to capture complex patterns, have an important role to play in detecting fraudulent activities in healthcare billing. Neural Networks consist of interconnected layers of nodes (neurons) that process and transmit information (Sharifani & Amini, 2023; Taye, 2023). Its key features are: The ability to learn highly complex, non-linear relationships; adaptability to various types of input data (structured, text, images); and capable of automatic feature extraction. In healthcare fraud detection, a Neural Network might analyze: Billing patterns over time; Relationships between diagnoses and procedures; Provider behavior compared to peers; and Patient visit frequencies and patterns. The model can be trained to output a fraud risk score for each claim or provider, flagging high-risk cases for further investigation.

13.4 API Architecture and Data Flow for AI Integration with EHR and RCM Systems

Integrating AI systems with existing EHR and RCM systems requires a robust, secure, and scalable API architecture. This section outlines the key components of such an architecture and explains the data flow between AI and legacy systems. The API architecture for integrating AI systems with EHR and RCM systems would follow a RESTful design pattern, utilizing HTTPS for secure communication (Kotstein & Bogner, 2021). The API architecture here can be thought of as building a bridge between two islands. One island represents the existing healthcare systems (like patient records and billing systems), and the other island represents the new AI systems that can make predictions and offer insights. The architecture would typically consist of several key components as follows:

1. *API Gateway*: Single entry point for all API requests (like a "GateKeeper"); Handles authentication and authorization; Manages rate limiting and request throttling; Routes requests to appropriate microservices (Zuo et al., 2020).
2. *Microservices*: Separate services for different functionalities (e.g., patient data, billing, AI predictions) (like "Specialized Lanes"); Allows for independent scaling and deployment; Improves fault isolation and system resilience (Dudjak & Martinović, 2020).
3. *Data Transformation Layer*: Converts data between formats used by legacy systems and AI models (like a "Translator"); Handles data normalization and standardization.
4. *AI Model Serving Layer*: Hosts trained AI models (like the "Brain" of the AI); Processes incoming data and returns predictions.
5. *Message Queue*: Manages asynchronous communication between services and is able to hold on to requests when there is too much traffic (like a "Waiting Area"); Ensures reliable data transfer and processing.
6. *Caching Layer*: Improves performance by storing frequently accessed data (like a "Quick Access Zone"); Reduces load on backend systems.

A simplistic example of the flow of data is presented in Figure 13.2.

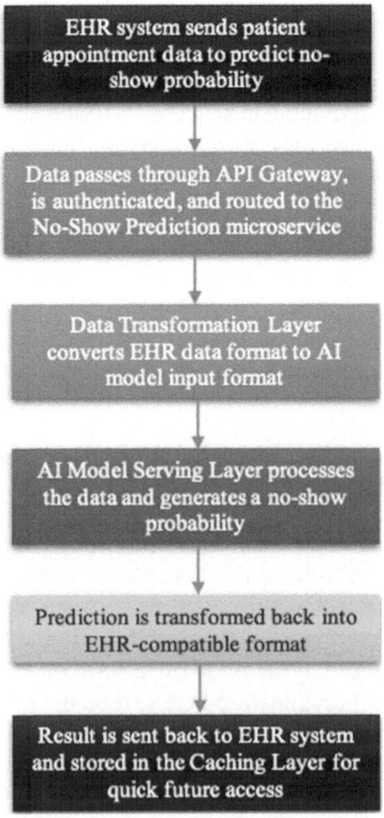

FIGURE 13.2 Visualization of data flow between AI and legacy systems (self-created).

13.5 AI SYSTEM TRAINING AND VALIDATION IN HEALTHCARE RCM

The effectiveness of AI models in healthcare RCM heavily depends on proper data preparation, training, and validation. This section explains key processes and techniques used in developing robust AI models for healthcare financial applications.

13.5.1 Data Preparation

a. Feature Engineering for Healthcare Data: Feature engineering is crucial in healthcare RCM to capture relevant patterns and relationships (Verdonck et al., 2024). Some techniques include:
   - Temporal features: Creating time-based features such as days since last visit.
   - Medical history aggregation: Summarizing patient history into meaningful features (e.g., number of previous no-shows, average length of stay).
   - Billing code grouping: Clustering similar procedure or diagnosis codes to reduce dimensionality.

b. Handling Missing Data and Outliers: Healthcare data often contains missing values and outliers due to various factors. Approaches to handle these include (Emmanuel et al., 2021):
   - Multiple Imputation: Using statistical methods to fill in missing values multiple times, creating several complete datasets.
   - Domain-specific imputation: Using medical knowledge to impute missing values (e.g., assuming a missing test result is negative).
   - Outlier detection: Using techniques like Interquartile Range to identify and handle outliers.

13.5.2 Training Process

For healthcare data, stratified k-fold is preferred to maintain class balance across folds, i.e., ensure the model will work consistently for different groups of patients or different types of medical cases (Prusty et al., 2022).

13.5.3 Model Evaluation Metrics

Area UNDER the ROC Curve (AUC) works well even when classes are imbalanced (fraud is rare compared to legitimate claims), which is often the case in healthcare data. MAE is useful in healthcare AIS, especially for tasks like predicting costs or revenues since it can indicate, on average, how many dollars off the predictions are and is easy to interpret (Naser & Alavi, 2023). The F1 score is also useful in healthcare AIS, especially for tasks like predicting claim denials. It provides a single score that balances two important factors: Precision (*How many of the claims the model predicted would be denied were actually denied?*) and Recall (*Out of all the claims that were actually denied, how many did the model correctly predict?*). This metric is valuable in healthcare because it helps one understand how well the model is performing when both false positives and false negatives are important to avoid. In the case of claim denials, the goal is to accurately predict denials to address issues proactively and not unnecessarily flag claims that won't be denied.

13.6 CHALLENGES IN USING GENERATIVE AI SYSTEMS IN HEALTHCARE

Smaller healthcare organizations may struggle to adopt AI technologies, and this may widen the technology gap between well-funded and under-resourced healthcare providers. Data quality and heterogeneity can also pose challenges for AI models, requiring careful data preparation and standardization (Albahri et al., 2023). There are several challenges to note here – inconsistent data formats across different healthcare systems, missing or incomplete data in patient records, errors in data entry due to manual processes, lack of standardization in medical coding and terminology, and bias in historical data that can be perpetuated or amplified by AI models. AI models trained on poor-quality data may produce inaccurate or unreliable results. Heterogeneous data can also lead to difficulties in integrating information from multiple sources. Biased data can result in discriminatory outcomes, potentially exacerbating healthcare disparities.

The complexity of integrating AI into existing EHR and RCM systems and the potential for errors in AI-generated outputs also require careful consideration. There are several challenges to note here – incompatibility between legacy systems and modern AI technologies; deficient data flow between AI and existing systems; maintenance of system performance during integration and potential disruptions; and staff training to effectively use integrated AI tools. Staff may be resistant to change if they are accustomed to existing workflows or if they are concerned about job displacement due to AI automation.

There are also significant issues in ensuring the accuracy and reliability of AI models in healthcare settings. For example, rare medical conditions or unusual financial scenarios are not well-represented in training data. AI models also may not generalize well across different patient populations. It might also be challenging to maintain model performance over time as healthcare practices evolve. Maintaining human oversight through regular audits and reviews can help mitigate these risks. Providing education and training to healthcare staff about responsible use and reliance on AI systems is also a good strategy.

13.7 COMPARISON OF AI-DRIVEN SOLUTIONS WITH TRADITIONAL METHODS IN HEALTHCARE RCM

AI-driven solutions have the following benefits – increased efficiency and speed in processing, higher accuracy in routine tasks, ability to handle large volumes of data, real-time analysis and decision-making, and adaptability to changing patterns and regulations. However, they do have their limitations – high initial implementation costs, dependence on quality and quantity of training data, the potential for biases if not properly managed, challenges in handling very unusual or complex cases, and the need for ongoing monitoring and adjustment (Ahmed et al., 2023).

In contrast, traditional methods still have some benefits – better handling of exceptional cases, more personal touch in patient interactions, easier to understand and explain processes, less dependence on technology infrastructure, and preference by some patients and staff that are resistant to change. However, they do have significant limitations – slower processing times, prone to human error, limited ability to handle large volumes, less adaptable to changes, and inconsistent application of rules and policies. The ideal approach for many healthcare organizations may be a hybrid model that uses AI for routine tasks and data analysis while retaining human oversight for complex decision-making and patient interactions.

13.8 PRIVACY AND SECURITY CONSIDERATIONS IN AI IMPLEMENTATION FOR HEALTHCARE RCM

AI systems require access to large volumes of patient and financial data, increasing the risk of unauthorized access or breaches. Also, transferring data between systems (e.g., from EHR to AI platforms) creates potential vulnerabilities. Moreover, the use of patient data to train AI models raises questions about data ownership and consent (Marks and Haupt, 2023). The "black box" nature of some AI algorithms can also make it difficult to audit for privacy compliance. Lastly, the integration with external services may involve sharing data with third parties, complicating governance. Privacy and security concerns must be addressed to ensure compliance with regulations like the Health Insurance Portability and Accountability Act (HIPAA). In addition to implementing all the traditional safeguards for HIPAA data, the following two measures should be adopted.

1. *Secure Model Training*: Use federated learning methods to train AI models without centralizing sensitive data.
2. *Explainable AI*: Prioritize the use of interpretable AI models in healthcare applications, facilitating compliance audits.

To ensure comprehensive HIPAA Security Rule compliance, organizations should conduct regular risk analysis of AI systems and infrastructure. To ensure comprehensive HIPAA Breach Notification Rule compliance, they need to establish protocols for identifying and reporting AI-related data breaches.

13.9 CONCLUSION

Generative AI is already changing healthcare AIS, particularly in the domain of RCM. By collaborating with EHR and RCM vendors, allocating resources, and ensuring human oversight, healthcare organizations can successfully use the power of generative AI to strengthen their financial stability and deliver better patient outcomes. As the field of AI in healthcare RCM continues to evolve, several promising areas for future research emerge. Future work should focus on developing more sophisticated NLP models capable of accurately interpreting complex medical narratives, extracting billable items from unstructured clinical notes, and generating compliant medical coding suggestions in real-time. I propose two important future research questions that remain unexplored:

1. How can reinforcement learning (model learns to make decisions by taking actions in an environment where feedback is in the form of rewards or penalties) be applied to balance revenue optimization with patient affordability in healthcare pricing?
2. How can AI models effectively incorporate both clinical and financial data for more accurate revenue predictions?

There needs to be investigations into the synergies between blockchain technology and AI for enhancing security and transparency in healthcare RCM. Blockchain-based systems can help with the secure sharing of AI models and healthcare data (Desai, 2023a, 2023b). Blockchain can also be leveraged to create an immutable audit trail of AI decisions in healthcare RCM.

NOTE

1 The most commonly used procedure coding systems in the United States are: (i) *Current Procedural Terminology (CPT) Codes* that are developed and maintained by the American Medical Association (AMA). These five-digit codes are divided into three categories: Category I (codes for commonly performed procedures and services), Category II (supplementary tracking codes for performance measurement), and Category III (temporary codes for emerging technologies, services, and procedures); (ii) *Healthcare Common Procedure Coding System (HCPCS) Codes* that are published by Centers for Medicare & Medicaid Services (CMS). These codes are divided into two levels: Level I (CPT codes) and Level II (alphanumeric codes used to identify products, supplies, and services not included in the CPT codes, such as ambulance services, durable medical equipment, and prosthetics); (iii) *International Classification of Diseases, 10th Revision, Procedure Coding System (ICD-10-PCS) Codes* that are more detailed and specific than CPT codes and used in hospital inpatient settings to report procedures performed.

REFERENCES

Ahmed, M. I., Spooner, B., Isherwood, J., Lane, M., Orrock, E., & Dennison, A. (2023). A systematic review of the barriers to the implementation of artificial intelligence in healthcare. *Cureus*, *15*(10). https://doi.org/10.7759%2Fcureus.46454

Albahri, A. S., Duhaim, A. M., Fadhel, M. A., Alnoor, A., Baqer, N. S., Alzubaidi, L., … & Deveci, M. (2023). A systematic review of trustworthy and explainable artificial intelligence in healthcare: Assessment of quality, bias risk, and data fusion. *Information Fusion*, *96*, 156–191. https://doi.org/10.1016/j.inffus.2023.03.008

American Hospital Association (2023). The Financial Stability of America's Hospitals and Health Systems Is at Risk as the Costs of Caring Continue to Rise. Retrieved from https://www.aha.org/system/files/media/file/2023/04/Cost-of-Caring-2023-The-Financial-Stability-of-Americas-Hospitals-and-Health-Systems-Is-at-Risk.pdf

Atluri, H., & Thummisetti, B. S. P. (2023). Optimizing Revenue Cycle Management in Healthcare: A Comprehensive Analysis of the Charge Navigator System. *International Numeric Journal of Machine Learning and Robots*, *7*(7), 1–13.

Bentéjac, C., Csörgő, A., & Martínez-Muñoz, G. (2021). A comparative analysis of gradient boosting algorithms. *Artificial Intelligence Review*, *54*, 1937–1967. https://doi.org/10.1007/s10462-020-09896-5

Chandawarkar, R., Nadkarni, P., Barmash, E., Thomas, S., Capek, A., Casey, K., & Carradero, F. (2024). Revenue Cycle Management: The Art and the Science. *Plastic and Reconstructive Surgery–Global Open*, *12*(7), e5756. https://doi.org/10.1097/GOX.0000000000005756

Derricks, J. (2021). Overview of the claims submission, medical billing, and revenue cycle management processes. *The Medical-Legal Aspects of Acute Care Medicine: A Resource for Clinicians, Administrators, and Risk Managers*, 251–276. https://doi.org/10.1007/978-3-030-68570-6_11

Desai, H. (2022). Are firms biasing stakeholder expectations by attributing prior poor performance to COVID-19? *IIM Kozhikode Society & Management Review*, *11*(2), pp. 171–182. https://doi.org/10.1177/22779752211061207

Desai, H. (2023a). Infusing Blockchain in accounting curricula and practice: expectations, challenges, and strategies. *The International Journal of Digital Accounting Research*, *23*, 97–135. https://doi.org/10.4192/1577-8517-v23_5

Desai, H. (2023b). An Auditor's Perspective on Smart Contracts and DAOs. *The CPA Journal*, *93*(7/8), 60–63 Publisher: New York State Society of CPAs. https://doi.org/10.13140/RG.2.2.18319.56481

Dudjak, M., & Martinović, G. (2020). An API-first methodology for designing a microservice-based Backend as a Service platform. *Information Technology and Control*, *49*(2), 206–223. https://doi.org/10.5755/j01.itc.49.2.23757

Emmanuel, T., Maupong, T., Mpoeleng, D., Semong, T., Mphago, B., & Tabona, O. (2021). A survey on missing data in machine learning. *Journal of Big data*, *8*, 1–37. https://doi.org/10.1186/s40537-021-00516-9

Guo, J., Yun, S., Meng, Y., He, N., Ye, D., Zhao, Z., ... & Yang, L. (2023). Prediction of heating and cooling loads based on light gradient boosting machine algorithms. *Building and Environment*, *236*, 110252. https://doi.org/10.1016/j.buildenv.2023.110252

Kotstein, S., & Bogner, J. (2021). Which restful api design rules are important and how do they improve software quality? a delphi study with industry experts. In *Service-Oriented Computing: 15th Symposium and Summer School, SummerSOC 2021, Virtual Event, September 13–17, 2021, Proceedings 15* (pp. 154–173). Springer International Publishing. https://doi.org/10.1007/978-3-030-87568-8_10

Mafarja, M., Thaher, T., Al-Betar, M. A., Too, J., Awadallah, M. A., Abu Doush, I., & Turabieh, H. (2023). Classification framework for faulty-software using enhanced exploratory whale optimizer-based feature selection scheme and random forest ensemble learning. *Applied Intelligence*, *53*(15), 18715–18757. https://doi.org/10.1007/s10489-022-04427-x

Marks, M., & Haupt, C. E. (2023). AI chatbots, health privacy, and challenges to HIPAA compliance. *JAMA*. https://doi.org/10.1001/jama.2023.9458

Naser, M. Z., & Alavi, A. H. (2023). Error metrics and performance fitness indicators for artificial intelligence and machine learning in engineering and sciences. *Architecture, Structures and Construction*, *3*(4), 499–517. https://doi.org/10.1007/s44150-021-00015-8

Parmar, A., Katariya, R., & Patel, V. (2019). A review on random forest: An ensemble classifier. In *International conference on intelligent data communication technologies and internet of things (ICICI) 2018* (pp. 758–763). Springer International Publishing. https://doi.org/10.1007/978-3-030-03146-6_86

Pazoki, M., & Samarghandi, H. (2021). Regulating patient care in walk-in clinics. *Omega*, 99, 102200. https://doi.org/10.1016/j.omega.2020.102200

Prusty, S., Patnaik, S., & Dash, S. K. (2022). SKCV: Stratified K-fold cross-validation on ML classifiers for predicting cervical cancer. *Frontiers in Nanotechnology*, *4*, 972421. https://doi.org/10.3389/fnano.2022.972421

Sharifani, K., & Amini, M. (2023). Machine learning and deep learning: A review of methods and applications. *World Information Technology and Engineering Journal*, *10*(07), 3897–3904.

Taye, M. M. (2023). Understanding of machine learning with deep learning: architectures, workflow, applications and future directions. *Computers*, *12*(5), 91. https://doi.org/10.3390/computers12050091

Verdonck, T., Baesens, B., Óskarsdóttir, M., & Vanden Broucke, S. (2024). Special issue on feature engineering editorial. *Machine learning*, *113*(7), 3917–3928. https://doi.org/10.1007/s10994-021-06042-2

Zuo, X., Su, Y., Wang, Q., & Xie, Y. (2020). An API gateway design strategy optimized for persistence and coupling. *Advances in Engineering Software*, *148*, 102878. https://doi.org/10.1016/j.advengsoft.2020.102878

14 Canadian Rural Medicare 2047

Envisioning Equal Access Through Digitalization

Lionel Huntley Henderson and John Wilson

14.1 INTRODUCTION

Rural communities have the greatest disadvantage in accessing healthcare and, in the context of increasing global urbanization trends, are at risk of becoming a lost voice in the relevant discourse. Consequently, rural communities would experience the greatest potential benefits of digital innovations, including those in developed nations whose systems may be viewed by some as an exemplary model of healthcare services. This chapter plans to correct such views and inform readers of the consequences of an absence to clearly articulate, on the part of Canada Health Infoway, a federal agency responsible for the utilization of Electronic Health Records (EHR), of a national strategy to expand the use of such files, including in rural communities. Artificial Intelligence (AI) can significantly influence EHR solutions to provide equal access in healthcare to rural Canadian communities, as demonstrated by the findings in this chapter. Methodologically, a modified Nominal Group Technique (NGT) was used with data collected from physicians, nurses, administrators and patients in New Brunswick, Canada, and formed the basis to understand priorities to explore solutions to equal healthcare access and outcomes in 2047. In addressing the issue, it also contributes to the evidence and literature relating to healthcare in developed countries. The core contributions of the chapter are now presented.

- Highlighting the need for a national strategy for the utilization of EHR that considers effective expansion to rural communities viz. digital accessibility.
- Updating the use of consensus for provincial research priorities in healthcare to support national policy for equal access in rural communities with the application of a modified NGT.
- Framing the successful integration of AI solutions in rural Canadian healthcare based on lagging (i.e., technical) and leading (user-related) indicators to address digital accessibility.

DOI: 10.1201/9781003503385-14

14.2 CANADIAN HEALTHCARE

Canada is one of the world's most developed economies and largest nations. The nature of Canada's population distribution, when combined with the current and projected demographics of the country, presents several challenges, not least in relation to healthcare. Canada's healthcare system was introduced in 1947 in the province of Saskatchewan implementing universal hospital healthcare. It developed into the Medical Care (Medicare) Act in 1966, by which national healthcare for all citizens is offered (Quinlan et al., 2008). Medicare is defined as Canada's publicly funded health care system that involves federal and provincial-level involvement. At the provincial, or territorial, level, health insurance plans (and their management) offer free health care services to residents (Government of Canada website, 2016). The federal level is responsible for national health standards and funding to provinces and their health care and insurance (Government of Canada website 2016). However, since the 1966 Medicare Act, significant disparities have developed, leading to rural communities being disadvantaged, despite the subsequent development of the Canada Health Act (CHA) in 1984 that defines *"reasonable access"* to health services (Minister of Justice, 2011). This underlying disadvantage is exacerbated by the lack of a national periodic process to measure disparities in healthcare access, provision and outcomes, particularly relating to independent provincial-level government organizations (Mossialos et al., 2017). The significance and implications of the disparities are potentially increased by the fact that Canada Health Infoway lacks a national strategy relating to its key area of responsibility, i.e. the management of patients' EHR (Mossialos et al., 2017).

This research has one aim. Based on a timescale of 2047 (the centennial mark of Canada's healthcare system), it explores possible solutions to the prevalent disparities in healthcare access and provision, which particularly disadvantage rural communities. In doing so, the appropriate strategy for EHR is considered, particularly the opportunities afforded by AI.

Statistics Canada (2015) forecasts of age and sex are published over low, medium and high population growth scenarios with the dependency ratio (a ratio that observes the number of dependents aged 0 to 14 and over the age of 65). Table 14.1 outlines the two closest years of published data (2021–2046) that align with the present and foresight of this research. A 10% growth in dependents is present in all scenarios,

TABLE 14.1
Forecast dependency ratios in Canada for low, medium and high population growth scenarios for Canada for 2021 and 2046 (Statistics Canada, 2015)

Scenario	Low		Medium		High	
Age/Year	**2021**	**2046**	**2021**	**2046**	**2021**	**2046**
0 – 14	23.9	23.0	26.0	25.7	28.0	28.3
65 +	28.6	42.4	28.5	40.4	28.4	38.4
Total	52.5	65.4	54.5	66.1	56.4	66.8

TABLE 14.2
Forecast dependency ratios in New Brunswick for low, medium and high population growth scenarios for New Brunswick from 2021 to 2036 (Statistics Canada, 2015)

Scenario	Low		Medium		High	
Age/Year	**2021**	**2036**	**2021**	**2036**	**2021**	**2036**
0 – 14	20.8	20.4	22.3	22.5	24.7	25.4
65 +	35.6	51.5	36.7	54.1	36.0	50.7
Total	56.4	71.9	58.9	76.6	60.7	76.1

with a greater number of seniors aged 65 or over, suggesting further advancements in healthcare to support the elderly. For the first time in its history, Canada is experiencing (from 2015 to 2021) more citizens over the age of 65 than those who are under 14 years of age. The trend is particularly acute in Atlantic Canada, where the province of New Brunswick is located, and, albeit on different end dates (2046 and 2036) has forecasted dependency ratios that are approximately 10% higher than the national average (see Tables 14.1 and 14.2). The year 2036 is the furthest date published by Statistics Canada (2015) for the province (see web-link for further detail), and it seems reasonable to assume the approximate 10% differential ratio will increase by 2046. The lack of published data toward this timescale, coupled with the significantly aging population, demonstrates the importance of conducting futures research in Canada and specifically into the healthcare systems of provinces such as New Brunswick. Senior citizens comprise 20.8% of the population of New Brunswick, the greatest proportion in Canada compared to a 17.2% national average (Statistics Canada, 2018). Further evidence from the media highlighting hospital closures and discontinuation of certain health services (see CBC News, 2019) suggests the need for intervention, perhaps by means such as digitalization and AI.

It is perhaps significant that the CHA, when amended in December 2017, states that "Canadians can achieve further improvements in their well-being through combining individual lifestyles that emphasize fitness, prevention of disease and health promotion with collective action against the social, environmental and occupational causes of disease" and does not explicitly identify digital accessibility, technological literacy or access, specifically, digitalization or AI (Minister of Justice, 2011). In contrast, Sreelakshmi and Anoop's (2023) literature review notes Canada as one of the nations to publish research articles related to big data and cognitive computing for digital health – and suggests a gap in research and how the CHA may be subsequently updated. Literature related to digitalization and AI in healthcare is now considered.

14.3 DIGITALIZATION IN HEALTHCARE

Being a relatively disadvantaged province, of which over a third is populated in rural communities; while leading provincial ranks of aging and low-income status families, digitalization reforms with AI, can plausibly contribute to improve New

Brunswick's healthcare access and outcomes. Guo and Li (2018) have shown AI offers consistency and can equalize resources in medical services e.g. diagnose and treat diseases such as cancer and tuberculosis, which is particularly helpful in circumstances where the number of medical professionals (viz. physicians and nurses) in rural communities is inadequate and falling. Orejana et al.'s (2015) research found that the use of robots reduced primary care visits and offered elderly patients in rural communities an increased quality of life (one example was keeping patients' company and offering them stimulation). EHR are one avenue to reduce inequalities in access by means of data. Publications on their website (see Canada Health Infoway's (2023a) Annual Report 2022–2023 and Canada Health Infoway's (2023b) 2022–2023 Summary Corporate Plan) demonstrate attempts of EHR expansion yet fail to succinctly articulate a plan to penetrate all urban and rural communities. Further concerns arise given the failure of previous attempts to expand EHRs in other Western nations (e.g. France, Germany, Spain, UK) which brings into question the appropriate level (national/provincial/county) of strategy for procuring EHR (Ben-Assuli, 2015). As such, alternative research methods such as futures studies would allow an exploration of ideas to prevent further failure and allow relevant stakeholders to imagine how technology can allow equal access to healthcare across Canada.

14.4 THE NOMINAL GROUP TECHNIQUE (NGT)

The NGT approach originated from Ven and Delbecq's (1972) article "The Nominal Group as a Research Instrument for the Exploratory Health Studies". The NGT approach is used to explore ideas in relation to a question or problem (McMillan et al., 2016) and thus is a complementary methodology to envision plausible solutions to equal access to healthcare in rural communities. Four steps were undertaken by focus groups, i.e. silent idea generation, round robin, idea confirmation and confidential ranking. In the first step, the participants answered the following question, based on Amara and Lapinski's (1983) seven questions approach, i.e., *In the best possible world, what would equal healthcare access and outcomes, viz. digitalization, look like in rural communities in 2047?* Data was collected in New Brunswick, Canada, with 37% of residents, one of the highest of all Canadian provinces, living in rural communities (see Statistics Canada, 2021). The scope of the sample was restricted to the province of New Brunswick, to align the current provincial oversight of disparities and given the indicators of an aging, rural and impoverished communities prevalent in the province that are linked to declining health outcomes. This study had three nominal groups sampling a similar number of physicians to Vella et al.'s (2000) NGT study.: group 1 with ten participants (six physicians, two nurses, one patient and one healthcare administrator); group 2 with four participants (four physicians); group 3 with a physician and a dentist. The physicians had a significant portion of patients from rural communities in their medical practice.

14.5 ANALYSIS

Following the confidential ranking, the themes were analyzed by means of multiple group analysis utilizing the top five themes with a priori (i.e. a pre-classified code,

TABLE 14.3
Higher and sub-order themes prioritized based on marks to rural healthcare outcomes

Higher-Order	Marks	Sub-Order
Video and Telemedicine Advancements	39	• Specialist Access • Patient Interaction • Eliminate Transportation • Home Consultations
Education	35	• Patient Education • Provider Education
Healthcare Staffing Changes	32	• Human Involvement • Nurse Practitioner
Electronic Health Records	25	• Improved Efficiencies • Comprehensive Records • Accessible Nationwide
Patient Monitoring Devices	24	• Limitations • Patient Empowerment
Local Healthcare	15	• Equipment • Decentralization
Privatization	5	• Contradictory Outcomes

one of which was word repetition) basis of coding. The primary coding framework involved "lumping" to complete higher-order themes, with a corresponding accumulated mark (derived from the ranking) from their derived themes and a secondary coding framework involved "splitting" the data for sub-order themes, which then integrated the nine pages of raw data containing the participants' justifications for the rankings. In ascending order of ranked importance, the top five themes to address the research question (see Section 14.4 include patient monitoring devices, EHR, healthcare staffing changes, education and video and telemedicine advancements. See Table 14.3 for the higher-order themes, marks and sub-order themes presented in ascending order of consensus (for higher-order themes based on accumulated marks and for sub-themes a percentage of coded coverage).

14.6 DISCUSSION

Based on the findings, the application of AI in providing equal access to healthcare is now discussed in ascending order of importance. First patient monitoring devices, their AI algorithms should facilitate empowerment and existing limitations to healthcare access. Digital accessibility is the inclusive practice of removing barriers and centers "*on access to technology products, resources, and services across hardware and software*" (Kulkarni, 2019, p. 91), and is underpinned by web accessibility, which "*implies making the perception, comprehension, navigation of, and contributions to the Web easier for persons with disabilities or for those whose abilities may change given the process of bodily ageing*" (Kulkarni, 2019, p. 91). In patient's utilizing such devices, AI applications should consider digital accessibility to be user-friendly for patients who have limited or no experience with modern-day technology. Bai et al.'s (2024) research found that anthropomorphism is linked to the warmth perception that can enhance the positive impact of competence perception (supporting the perception concept of web accessibility) with integrating AI in patient monitoring devices. Separately, anthropomorphism is separately discussed in Omrani et al. (2022) to facilitate initial trust formation, which is relevant, as their data surveyed from more than 30,000 individuals across the EU28 suggests that concerns related to AI are linked to AI trust (supporting the perception and contributions concept of digital accessibility).

Second EHR was suggested to be a nationwide and comprehensive record that can achieve greater efficiencies in health services. Consistency in the management terms (i.e., privacy, confidentiality and security) is recommended by Nowrozy et al.'s (2024) research before implementing EHR expansion and use solutions – i.e., access control, blockchain, cloud-based, and cryptography. Separately, Tertulino et al.'s (2024) systematic review of privacy related to EHR's found a growing interest in privacy research. Their (Tertulino et al.'s 2024) review also observed the lack of a systematic approach between EHR solutions and existing laws and policies that would lead to better strategies to certified processes for patients' digital files. This would require provincial and federal representatives to jointly work on a solution for the Canadian healthcare context – henceforth, and in addition to the raw data findings, it suggests the need for a national strategy for EHR expansion (including in rural communities). AI applications to EHR should consider these aspects.

Third healthcare staffing involvement, which focused on the human involvement and shift to more nurse practitioners. The findings of new healthcare roles as a solution suggest testing all AI applications and EHR systems to Khashan et al.'s (2024) extended Technological Acceptance and Readiness (TRAM) model to help physicians in rural communities integrate EHR and support the use of patient monitoring devices. Khashan et al.'s (2024) model is also pertinent to tackle digital accessibility that healthcare staff themselves may be experiencing.

Fourth was both patient and provider education. The implication being for the end users (both doctors, nurses and patients) was similarly found in Govindarajan et al.'s (2023) research that suggested the need to direct more attention to the end users to support AI's technical components, and specifically their development. Considering the earlier mentioned indicators of poor health outcomes prevalent in New Brunswick – i.e., an aging, rural and impoverished population, education for all end users (doctors, nurses, administrators and patients) is imperative to integrate AI solutions.

Fifth, and most important, video and telemedicine advancements, will allow specialist access, facilitate patient interaction, and eliminate patient transportation constraints while facilitating home care. In consideration of the integration of AI with telemedicine advancements, the use of human-like interactions – i.e., more avatars, less chat boxes, were suggested by Sestino and D'Angelo (2023) for a better patient experience.

14.7 RECOMMENDATION

To address the challenges of rural healthcare in Canada, digital accessibility, and build on Govindarajan et al.'s (2023) research, it is recommended based on the findings to frame the themes toward the future of equal access to healthcare as leading indicators related to the end users (i.e., staffing changes, education, telemedicine advancements – user aspects), that, if addressed, would subsequently allow the lagging indicators of technical innovation related to hardware (patient monitoring devices, telemedicine advancements – technical aspects) and software (EHR) to enable equal access to healthcare for rural Canadians. Separately, the findings suggest that Canada Health Infoway should adopt a national-level strategy to expand the use of EHR with consideration of the rural community context. Singh et al.'s (2024) paper suggests a few strategies for the smooth adaptation of AI services in healthcare that relate to their ease of use, automation efficacy, diagnostic accuracy, and cost efficiency. This chapter puts forward the driver of digital accessibility to Singh et al.'s (2024) strategies to support the rural context.

14.8 LIMITATIONS

This research is based on an NGT approach but was modified to enable mixed groups of physicians, nurses, administrators and patients consider futures for Canadian rural Medicare in 2047. The modification was not without limitations. An asynchronous approach to data collection was integrated with the nominal groups by relying on phone and/or email communication, instead of offline focus groups, as conducted in Shipman et al.'s (2008) study, which also relied heavily on the participation of physicians.

14.9 FUTURE WORK

Research related to expanding the use of EHR, will be of interest to The Public Health Agency of Canada and Canada Health Infoway respectively. A broader study across Atlantic Canada – i.e., the provinces of New Brunswick, Nova Scotia, Prince Edward Island, and Newfoundland – is recommended. The east coast provinces of Canada have similar demographics and regional culture, with many local medical practitioners knowing each other across provincial borderlines. The chance to influence practical research that can identify how AI may most effectively be implemented to help the region, which is expected to collaborate in terms of resource sharing in the future due to budget cutbacks, is of interest. Another consensus technique suggested would be the Delphi Technique to survey across a bigger and geographically spread-out sample of participants.

14.10 CONCLUSION

Canada is globally recognized for its healthcare system, and Medicare is part of Canadians' national identity and culture. As most healthcare treatments and related expenditures occur in the later years of a patient's life, the context of New Brunswick's aging and rural communities has provided evidence of the major themes of what is needed to prioritize to ensure equal healthcare access to all citizens in the future. It is up to not only academics but also practitioners to jointly work and develop these themes to ensure a higher quality of life for Canadians with the assistance of AI.

REFERENCES

Amara, R. & Lapinski. A. J. (1983). *Business Planning for an Uncertain Future: Scenarios and Strategies* (Vol. 228). New York: Pergamon Press.

Bai, S., Yu, D., Han, C., Yang, M., Gupta, B. B., Arya, V., Panigrahi, P.K., Tang, R., He, H., & Zhao, J. (2024). Warmth trumps competence? Uncovering the influence of multimodal AI anthropomorphic interaction experience on intelligent service evaluation: Insights from the high-evoked automated social presence. *Technological Forecasting and Social Change*, 204, 123395. https://doi.org/10.1016/j.techfore.2024.123395

Ben-Assuli, O. (2015). Electronic health records, adoption, quality of care, legal and privacy issues and their implementation in emergency departments. *Health policy*, 119(3), 287–297. https://doi.org/10.1016/j.healthpol.2014.11.014

CBC News (November 26th, 2019). Campbellton hospital takes 'extreme' steps after running out of beds. Retrieved from: https://www.cbc.ca/news/canada/new-brunswick/campbellton-regional-hospital-1.5367670

Canada Health Infoway (2023a). *Annual Report 2022-2023*. Retrieved from: https://www.infoway-inforoute.ca/en/component/edocman/6452-annual-report-2022-2023/view-document?Itemid=103

Canada Health Infoway (2023b). *Summary Corporate Plan 2022-2023*. Retrieved from: https://www.infoway-inforoute.ca/en/component/edocman/6354-summary-corporate-plan-2022-2023/view-document?Itemid=103

Government of Canada website (2016). Canada's health care system. Retrieved from: https://www.canada.ca/en/health-canada/services/canada-health-care-system.html

Govindarajan, U. H., Singh, D. K., & Gohel, H. A. (2023). Forecasting cyber security threats landscape and associated technical trends in telehealth using bidirectional encoder representations from Transformers (Bert). *Computers & Security*, 103404. https://doi.org/10.1016/j.cose.2023.103404

Guo, J., & Li, B. (2018). The application of medical artificial intelligence technology in rural areas of developing countries. *Health equity*, 2(1), 174–181. https://doi.org/10.1089/heq.2018.0037

Khashan, M. A., Alasker, T. H., Ghonim, M. A., & Elsotouhy, M. M. (2024). Understanding physicians' adoption intentions to use Electronic Health Record (EHR) systems in developing countries: an extended TRAM approach. *Marketing Intelligence & Planning*. https://doi.org/10.1108/MIP-05-2023-0225

Kulkarni, M. (2019). Digital accessibility: Challenges and opportunities. *IIMB Management Review*, 31(1), 91–98. https://doi.org/10.1016/j.iimb.2018.05.009

McMillan, S. S., King, M., & Tully, M. P. (2016). How to use the nominal group and Delphi techniques. *International journal of clinical pharmacy*, 38(3), 655–662. doi.org/10.1007/s11096-016-0257-x

Minister of Justice. Canada Health Act. (July 18, 2011). Retrieved from: http://laws-lois.justice.gc.ca/eng/acts/C-6/

Mossialos, E., Djordjevic, A., Osborn, R., & Sarnak, D. (2017). International profiles of health care systems: *Australia, Canada, China, Denmark, England, France, Germany, India, Israel, Italy, Japan, the Netherlands, New Zealand, Norway, Singapore, Sweden, Switzerland, Taiwan, and the United States*. Retrieved on January 29 2020 from: https://www.commonwealthfund.org/sites/default/files/documents/___media_files_publications_fund_report_2017_may_mossialos_intl_profiles_v5.pdf

Nowrozy, R., Ahmed, K., Kayes, A. S. M., Wang, H., & McIntosh, T. R. (2024). Privacy preservation of electronic health records in the modern era: A systematic survey. *ACM Computing Surveys*, 56(8), 1–37. https://doi.org/10.1145/3653297

Omrani, N., Rivieccio, G., Fiore, U., Schiavone, F., & Agreda, S. G. (2022). To trust or not to trust? An assessment of trust in AI-based systems: Concerns, ethics and contexts. *Technological Forecasting and Social Change*, 181, 121763. https://doi.org/10.1016/j.techfore.2022.121763

Orejana, J. R., MacDonald, B. A., Ahn, H. S., Peri, K., & Broadbent, E. (2015, October). Healthcare robots in homes of rural older adults. In *International Conference on Social Robotics* (pp. 512–521). Springer, Cham. doi.org/10.1007/978-3-319-25554-5_51

Quinlan, D., Mahoney, R., Chang, R., & Morris, G. (2008). *The Canadian Challenge*. Oxford University Press.

Sestino, A., & D'Angelo, A. (2023). My doctor is an avatar! The effect of anthropomorphism and emotional receptivity on individuals' intention to use digital-based healthcare services. *Technological Forecasting and Social Change*, 191, 122505. https://doi.org/10.1016/j.techfore.2023.122505

Shipman, C., Gysels, M., White, P., Worth, A., Murray, S. A., Barclay, S., Forrest, S., Shepherd, J., Dale, J., Dewar, S., Peters, M., White, S., Richardson, A., Lorenz, K., Koffman, J., Higginson, I.J. (2008). Improving generalist end of life care: national consultation with practitioners, commissioners, academics, and service user groups. *Bmj*, *337*, a1720. https://doi.org/10.1136/bmj.a1720

Singh, N., Jain, M., Kamal, M. M., Bodhi, R., & Gupta, B. (2024). Technological paradoxes and artificial intelligence implementation in healthcare. An application of paradox theory. *Technological Forecasting and Social Change*, 198, 122967. https://doi.org/10.1016/j.techfore.2023.122967

Sreelakshmi, S., & Anoop, V. S. (2023). Cognitive computing and big data for digital health: Past, present, and the future. In *Era of Artificial Intelligence* (pp. 55–66). Chapman and Hall/CRC. https://doi.org/10.1201/9781003300472

Statistics Canada (2021). Canada's rural population since 1851. Retrieved from: https://www12.statcan.gc.ca/census-recensement/2021/as-sa/fogs-spg/Page.cfm?Lang=E&Dguid=2021A000213&topic=1

Statistics Canada (2015). Population Projections for Canada, Provinces and Territories. Retrieved from: https://www150.statcan.gc.ca/n1/pub/91-520-x/2010001/tablesectlist-listetableauxsect-eng.htm

Statistics Canada (2018). Canada's population estimates: Age and sex, July 1, 2018. Retrieved from: https://www150.statcan.gc.ca/n1/en/daily-quotidien/190125/dq190125a-eng.pdf?st=OdEKiTe2

Tertulino, R., Antunes, N., & Morais, H. (2024). Privacy in electronic health records: a systematic mapping study. *Journal of Public Health*, 32(3), 435–454. https://doi.org/10.1007/s10389-022-01795-z

Van de Ven, A. H., & Delbecq, A. L. (1972). The nominal group as a research instrument for exploratory health studies. *American Journal of Public Health*, 62(3), 337–342. Retrieved from: https://ajph.aphapublications.org/doi/pdf/10.2105/AJPH.62.3.337

Vella, K., Goldfrad, C., Rowan, K., Bion, J., & Black, N. (2000). Use of consensus development to establish national research priorities in critical care. *BMJ*, 320(7240), 976–980. https://doi.org/10.1136/bmj.320.7240.976

15 Revolutionizing Patient Access Through AI in Healthcare

Herat Joshi, Jahanvi Bansal and Parag Shukla

15.1 INTRODUCTION

AI is rapidly transforming numerous sectors, such as healthcare, banking, education, manufacturing, and transportation. The integration of AI in numerous domains has progressed beyond our initial projections, as the theoretically futuristic approach is already a reality (Alowais et al., 2023). A major development in the medical field is AI-driven healthcare. AI is significantly transforming healthcare, from illness diagnosis to medicine development. By 2030, it is anticipated that the global market for AI in healthcare would have grown from 11 billion dollars in 2021 to 188 billion dollars (Bohr & Memarzadeh, 2020). Notably, the current surge in AI is not only a fad but a necessity in light of the urgent need for a healthcare ecosystem that is more effective and efficient. The global healthcare business, valued at $10 trillion, faces significant challenges as a result of increased out-of-pocket expenses, the increasing incidence of illness, and deteriorating health (Khan, 2024). Patient care and access to healthcare services are challenged by these issues.

Through a comprehensive review of the current landscape of AI in healthcare and clinical services, this chapter aims to shed light on its role as a pivotal tool for enhancing healthcare accessibility and effectiveness. However, as it continues to evolve, its ethical and legal implications remain in a state of paradox. Nevertheless, researchers are increasingly dedicated to exploring opportunities to develop intelligent systems for the betterment of humanity (Poalelungi et al., 2023). Concurrent study to assess the benefits and drawbacks of this kind of system is therefore becoming more and more necessary. In light of this, the comprehensive evaluation of this work seeks to accomplish the following objectives:

- To examine the myriads of obstacles preventing patients from receiving necessary medical services.
- To explore the revolutionary potential of AI in removing these obstacles and promoting healthcare delivery systems that are more effective, individualized, affordable, and inclusive.

 DOI: 10.1201/9781003503385-15

Additionally, this paper will cover case studies of patient access in healthcare provision, AI technologies for patient access, challenges in AI applications in the healthcare industry, real-world examples and case studies of patient access in healthcare provision, and the future of AI applications.

15.2 LITERATURE REVIEW

15.2.1 AI Technologies for Patient Access

For patient access, AI technologies inclusive of machine learning (ML), natural language processing (NLP), neural networks, deep learning, and machine vision/computer vision (MV/CV) are applied (Javanmard, 2024). The greater part of medical data entails images and records from electromagnetic radiation (X-ray), magnetic resonance imaging (MRI), and computed tomography (CT) machines. Healthcare systems generate a lot of data each year, necessitating AI solutions as a remedy in the event of processing large amounts of information. In this regard, the integration of AI into health systems allows for proper data processing, speeds up the diagnosis process, cuts down on costs, and leads to ample patient access to healthcare services. Some of the applicable AI tools for processing healthcare data include.

15.2.1.1 Machine Learning (ML)

The ML algorithm allows computers to function just like human beings by determining ample insights, classifying patient data, and making ample predictions, respectively. ML algorithms also entail deep learning, an aspect that enables the development of accurate results in data clustering and predictive endeavors. Deep learning allows for rapid and easy execution of complex and advanced tasks (Saravanan & Sujatha, 2018). Supervised learning integrates labeled and structured datasets in the event of uncovering documents. Semi-supervised learning integrates both unlabeled data and labeled data in training models. Finally, unsupervised learning makes use of raw or unstructured data in the form of images and text in automated processes that determine hidden patterns in data. Neural networks in ML algorithms function by recognizing patterns in the event of clustering or classifying data, respectively. Neural networks detect deviations in a given data set, an aspect that provides for accurate diagnosis mechanisms for health practitioners in aspects such as determining the development of tumors in patients. Table 15.1 outlines the different types of ML facets, including semi-supervised learning, unsupervised learning, and supervised learning, along with their functions.

TABLE 15.1
Machine Learning (ML) Facets

Type	Function
1. Semi-supervised learning	Labeled and unlabeled data
2. Unsupervised learning	Unstructured data
3. Supervised learning	Structured and Labeled datasets

15.2.1.2 Natural Language Processing (NLP)

NLP algorithms are AI tools that present hidden or irregular data from human-developed articles and records entailing medical information. NLP entails two main facets: unstructured data processing and speech recognition capabilities. Speech recognition eradicates the need for manual data input by health practitioners, while unstructured data processing allows for better interpretations through data classifications, summaries, and the extraction of insights (Kinsley & Kukiela, 2020). The NLP algorithms function by retrieving information from medical documents, followed by ample processing measures through its five facets that lead to ample classification and grouping of data. The latter makes it easier to harness information pertaining to historical records of patients and empowers health practitioners by saving time and costs, respectively.

Apparently, ML algorithms simplify data processing for the patient registration process, encompassing the pre-arrival, arrival, and identification stages, increasing productivity and lowering errors. The use of NLP technologies is essential for scheduling and appointment management because they allow for automated, intelligent systems to understand and respond to patients' natural language inputs, resulting in more seamless interactions. ML and deep learning are used to analyze large datasets and find patterns that help patients adapt their financial solutions and quickly verify insurance benefits (Siwicki, 2023). These applications include financial counseling and support, eligibility verification, and benefit verification. Table 15.2 lists various AI tools used in healthcare provision, such as ML and NLP, and their corresponding functions in data prediction and processing.

15.2.2 Enhancing Patient Access through AI

Medical practices empowered by AI involve three basic considerations: administrative, pharmacological, and clinical components, where the latter functions by automating, fostering, or enhancing these aspects. For example, AI applications from a clinical perspective led to improved patient access experiences by developing better treatment notions with a focus on quality provision, improving accuracy levels, and integrating speed-based notions in processes such as diagnosis (Petersson et al., 2022). AI applications in the pharmaceutical field entail empowerment in the compilation of reports or the enhancement of research processes that lead to the development of new drugs. Applications of AI in the administrative facet involve the automation of the revenue cycle, with ample management of bureaucratic endeavors that follow on automation in data processing methods. Practical enhancements to patient access may include.

TABLE 15.2
AI Tools in Healthcare Provision

AI Tool	Functions
1. Machine Learning (ML)	• Data Prediction • Data Clustering
2. Natural Language Processing (NLP)	• Simplify data processing

1. *Medical data and record management*: In the context of history and medical records, AI involves aspects of data analysis. The endeavor mainly focuses on the management of data as a field of digital automation through data collection. Storage, reformatting, and tracing for faster and more consistent access to data are additional features from AI in healthcare provision. (Petersson et al., 2022).
2. *Repetitiveness*: The use of robots in AI is a recent development that allows for the processing of various data-based aspects through an integral analysis of tests, CT scans, X-rays, and data entry endeavors at large. Huge amounts of data are a common endeavor for healthcare providers in fields such as radiology and cardiology, which calls for the use of robots as a way of simplifying complex data and saving time.
3. *Consultations and Treatment*: A digital approach that empowers patient healthcare experiences in a digital world involves the use of applications that cater to the consolation needs of a patient. The application combines medical knowledge with patient medical information, allowing users to feed their symptoms into an app for comparison against databases. Consequently, on processing the information, the applications consequently provide recommendations and offer a suitable course of action for the patient. Furthermore, systems involving AI allow for the analysis of reports and notes containing patient information and may extend to clinical experiences and external research in a bid to select the correct and customized treatment methods (Bonaccorso et al., 2018).
4. *Virtual Services*: "Molly," a recent technological development, emerges as a program that allows patients to monitor their health conditions. These integral processes involve empowering treatment follow-ups that emerge between patient-doctor interactions. Notably, the programs integrate ML into enhancing patient experiences (Chen & Decary, 2019).
5. *Drug Development*: Pharmaceuticals undergo eminent clinical trials, especially in the development of drugs, a process that takes ample time and costs, respectively. AI emerges as a cheap and faster remedy that counters time wastage and unprecedented costs, respectively. AI-powered programs integrated with medicine scanning capabilities and other related endeavors promote a more informed approach to drugs and their viability (Siwicki, 2023).
6. *AI in Drug Development Using Python*: The drug development process has been revolutionized by AI, particularly through the use of Python. A pharmaceutical company commenced using the Python libraries SciPy and NumPy to speed up the process of drug discovery. When studying drug effectiveness and safety, these libraries and massive data sets have made ML algorithms very effective. A study clearly showed how these computational techniques might be used to find prospective drug candidates that had a high rate of success in clinical trials (Joshi, 2024). This contrasts with the conventional approaches to drug development, which consume a lot more time and money and provide results that, in practice, are often ineffective.
7. *Precision in Medicines*: The connections between diseases and genetic mutations are based on information we have gleaned from DNA. With the

advent of AI, technologies that support body scans now allow health practitioners to identify culpable agents in a disease's constellation of symptoms. These health practitioners can now make predictions about what kind of health-related problem is affecting a person based on where mutations present themselves on the DNA strand. AI has substantially moved the needle forward with precision medicine, especially when applying AI through Java-based frameworks. For instance, Weka, a Java-based data mining tool, has found application in precision medicine by facilitating predictive modeling and performing data analysis (Kumar et al. 2021). Python programming has found widespread use in precision medicine. For example, its scikit-learn, TensorFlow, and Pandas libraries are widely used in ML and AI fields. One such scenario in which a research team created a Python ML model that, when combined with the patient's genetic and clinical data, predicts the patient's response to cancer therapy (Zhang et al., 2022).

8. *Monitoring Health Status*: Monitoring of activity levels as well as heart rates includes Garmin, Apple, and FitBit. Eminent applications send alerts to doctors and provide information about a patient's habits and needs.
9. *Detection mechanisms*: Apparently, various AI developments in the healthcare perspective today are known to outperform health practitioners, such as doctors, in the context of accuracy, especially in the diagnosis of cancer patients. (Kinsley & Kukiela, 2020).
10. *Analyzing Healthcare Systems*: The application of AI technologies for consequent workflows remains dynamic and unique for each facet and may entail:
    a. Pre-authorization: use of ML to review patient data against insurance policies to get instant approvals.
    b. Healthcare Navigation: Medical systems are large and complex, but leveraging NLP and Neural Network, we can provide digital navigation, personalized advice, and support.
    c. Language Barrier: Use of NLP enables real-time translation services to ensure patients understand complex medical terms in their native language.
    d. Telehealth Services: Deep Learning and MV/CV for remote diagnostics and patient monitoring with brining specialist care to patient's remote location.
    e. Patient Portal: Use a combination of all AI technologies to offer the most interactive way to manage patient health information access and use of ML algorithms to analyze patient health information to provide education for self-management of acute cases.
    f. Outreach Services: Use of ML and NLP to identify population health trends and community in need of specific health intervention. Specifically for rural populations to allocate right health care resources and services use of these technologies are important.
    g. Patient Portal: Use a combination of all AI technologies to offer most interactive way to manage patient health information access and use of ML algorithms to analyze patient health information to provide education for self-management of acute cases.

15.2.3 Real-world Examples and Case Studies of Patient Access

The chapter will focus on effective AI applications in healthcare access and explain the main lessons and best practices learned from these encounters. It will explore the best practices and lessons discovered, providing insights into the revolutionary potential of AI in transforming the provision of medical care.

15.2.3.1 Pre-authorization

In the healthcare industry, prior authorization is a mechanism used by payers or insurance companies to decide whether to pay for a recommended treatment, surgery, or drug. The healthcare professional must first obtain approval from the patient's health insurance company's approval before a patient can receive specific services or prescriptions. The healthcare provider is subsequently informed by the insurance company of the decision about the patient's benefits plan, whether it is accepted, rejected, or partially accepted. The purpose of prior authorization is to prevent overuse of services and prescriptions that may not be the best course of action, in an effort to control costs. If there is a denial that necessitates an appeal, it may also result in delays in service, more paperwork for medical professionals, and occasionally annoyance for patients. Figure 15.1 demonstrates typical workflow of how information is being transferred from Healthcare EMR system to insurance company data base for submission of prior authorization.

As explained in Figure 15.2, the ML will be used and trained to classify prior authorization applications into accepted, rejected, or partially accepted. By analyzing historical authorization requests, a ML platform can determine the circumstances that are most likely to lead to approval. For instance, a patient needs to have an X-ray, try physical therapy, and take anti-inflammatory medicine before being authorized for an MRI of the knee. The payers can create a system that automatically approves incoming requests that satisfy certain requirements based on these factors, significantly reducing the workload. Those who don't fit the requirements will be marked for manual evaluation (Scott, 2021).

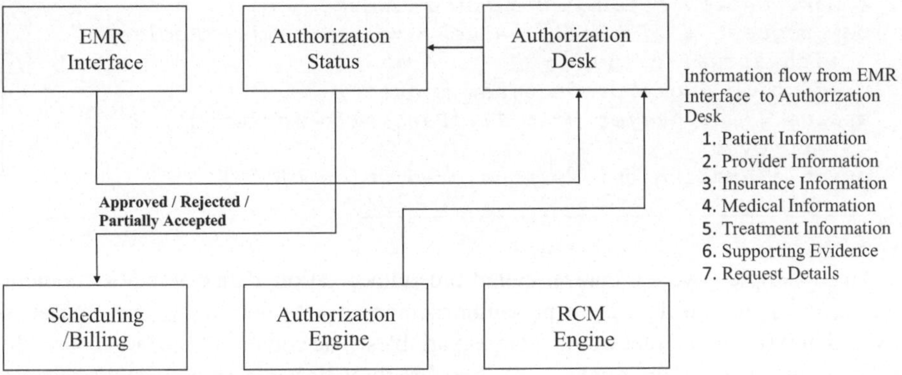

FIGURE 15.1 Typical prior-authorization workflow.

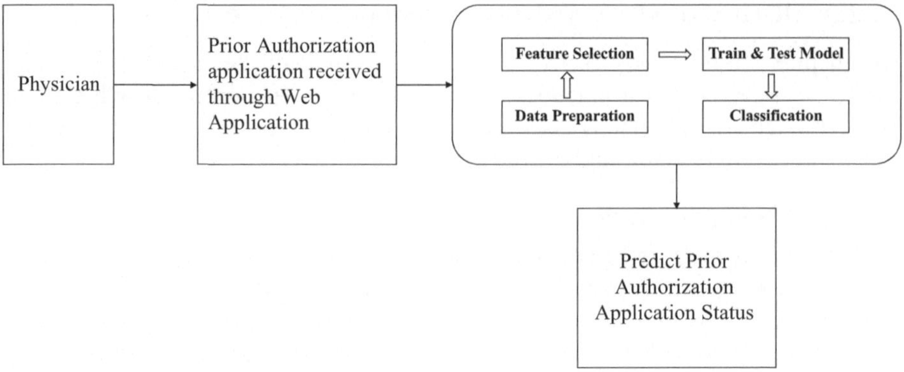

FIGURE 15.2 Use of Machine Learning (ML) classify prior authorization response.

PYTHON IMPLEMENTATION: AUTOMATED PRE-AUTHORIZATION WITH ML

```
import pandas as pd
from sklearn.model_selection import train_test_split
from sklearn.ensemble import RandomForestClassifier
# Load dataset
data = pd.read_csv('pre_authorization_data.csv')
# Preprocess data
X = data.drop('status', axis=1)
y = data['status']
# Split data
X_train, X_test, y_train, y_test = train_test_split(X, y,
  test_size=0.2, random_state=42)
# Train model
clf = RandomForestClassifier(n_estimators=100,
  random_state=42)
clf.fit(X_train, y_train)
# Make a prediction for a new request
new_request = [[value1, value2, value3, ...]] # Replace
  with actual values
prediction = clf.predict(new_request)
status = {0: 'Rejected', 1: 'Partially Approved', 2:
  'Approved'}
print(f"Prediction: {status[prediction[0]]}")
```

This example covers a dataset called pre_authorization_data.csv, whose content represents Historical data from pre-authorization request decisions. The dataset is divided into two parts: features and target variables. The content of the target variable indicates the status of the request, and there are three possible outcomes: the request is either approved, denied, or partially approved. To predict the status of new requests, we trained a random forest classifier on this dataset. Using ML to predict decision outcomes on a pre-authorization request could alleviate some of the administrative burden and improve the speed and accuracy of the pre-authorization decision-making process.

15.2.3.2 Healthcare Navigation

The literature highlights the significance of navigational systems in hospitals while looking at the concept of healthcare navigation from many angles. These mechanisms contribute to ensuring that all members of the population, including those with restricted mobility, may use the services provided. This framework makes it possible to comprehend the human and environmental aspects that affect a person's ability to access the healthcare system.

A leading tech company recently launched a revolutionary AI-enabled patient navigation service, representing a huge leap forward in the digital health arena. Dubbed the "digital front door," this service stitches together data from different health systems and puts it all in one place, making it that much easier for patients to find their way to the services they're after (Fox, 2023). An AI-powered patient direction service, as shown in Figure 15.3, pulls data from multiple health systems to help direct patients to the appropriate services. The service uses NLP and neural networks to accomplish this task.

NPL can process and evaluate free text, predict text outcomes, and create diagnostic models (Locke et al., 2021). By providing real-time translation services for patients, NLP has the potential to revolutionize healthcare as mentioned in Figure 15.3. But for NLP applications in languages other than English to be successful, gold-standard clinical corpora in those languages must be created (AlShuweihi et al., 2020).

PYTHON IMPLEMENTATION: AI FOR HEALTHCARE NAVIGATION

```
import nltk from import nltk.chat.util Define
   conversation pairings in Chat, Reflections.
pairs = [['I need to find a cardiologist.', ['You
   can find a cardiologist at our main campus on the
   second floor.']], ['Where is the pharmacy?', ['The
   pharmacy is located on the ground floor, near the main
   entrance.']], ['How do I schedule an appointment?',
   ['You can schedule an appointment by calling our main
   line at (555) 123-4567 or visiting our website.']],
   ['(.*)', ['I apologize; I do not comprehend. For
   further assistance, please contact our support
   desk.']]]
# Launch the chatbot chatbot.converse() chatbot =
   Chat(pairs, reflections)
```

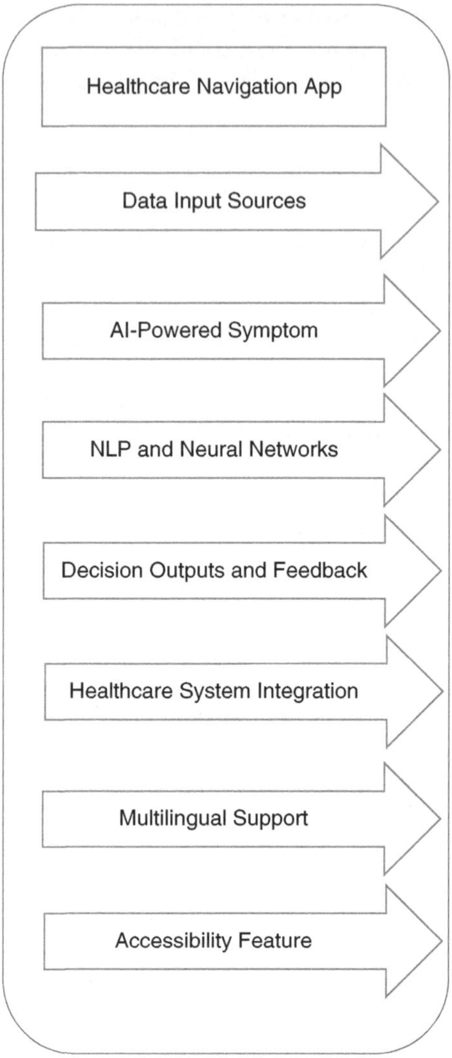

FIGURE 15.3 Use of NLP and Neural Network for healthcare navigation.

Here we have a straightforward instance of a chatbot created with Python. This one assists patients with wayfinding in a healthcare facility and gives them information that helps them get to the right place within the facility. The chatbot has a very simple structure. It uses conversation pairs and has rendered the conversation in the form of a tree. The assistant won't let you get "lost," which is a good feature for AI when you're talking about healthcare or any kind of critical situation.

15.2.3.3 Telehealth Services

The increased use of telehealth for remote diagnostics and patient monitoring is now much more effective, thanks to deep learning and the telehealth/machine vision revolution. These technologies are combined with other vital components of the telehealth system to improve the kinds of health services that patients receive from a distance. This capability is necessary and useful when healthcare situations don't allow the luxury of being right there at hand. Relative to remote health monitoring, deep learning on the Internet of Things (IoT) has garnered a lot of attention lately. IoT-based devices are capable of collecting and analyzing a wide range of physiological data, including body temperatures, heart rates, blood oxygen levels, and electrocardiogram (ECG) signals (Bhatt & Chakraborty, 2023). They can likewise provide immediate feedback to medical professionals, enabling them to react suitably and within the necessary time constraints (Islam et al., 2023). Figure 15.4 illustrates how computer vision and patient learning are utilized in telemedicine to facilitate remote diagnosis and patient monitorin. To provide specialized treatment remotely, telemedicine requires clinical data. This may include everything from body temperature to medical imaging.

15.2.3.4 Python Implementation in Telehealth

Telehealth services have seen significant transformations as a result of the integration of AI, especially Python. The development of a remote diagnostic tool using Python's TensorFlow and Keras modules is one noteworthy application. This device provides real-time diagnostic feedback to healthcare professionals by evaluating physiological data, such as body temperature and electrocardiogram (ECG) signals (Petmezas et al. 2022). An additional example might be the real-time video analysis performed with Python's OpenCV library during telemedicine consultations. By providing additional data points, video feeds allow for the remote diagnosis of patient vitals, including heart rate and respiratory rate.

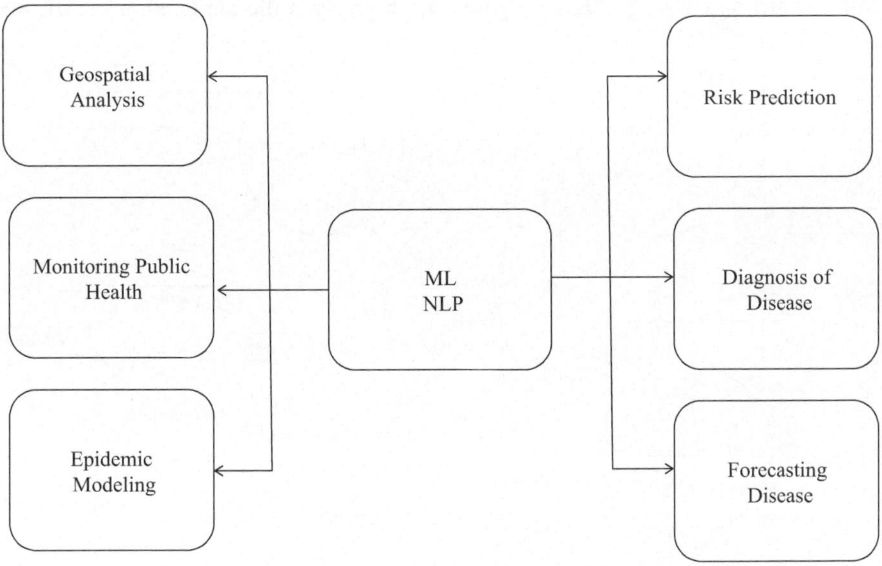

FIGURE 15.4 Taxonomy of Machine Learning (ML) and computer vision for telemedicine.

15.2.3.5 Patient Portal

Increased patient involvement and a higher chance of chronic illness self-management may result from better usage of patient portals (Balsdon, 2021). Patients should be able to access the most current studies via their portals. Using AI to auto-summarize dense biomedical literature, it was discovered that their system's ability to make the material readable for non-specialist users was its greatest advantage. Since the portal is now a means of direct contact between physicians and patients, people need to have access to the same kinds of summaries that their doctors do. One important area of potential and responsibility for AI is writing these summaries.

Enhancing Patient Portals with Python: Patient portal functionality has changed due to AI. One notable example is the creation of NLP models that classify and prioritize patient communications using Python's Natural Language Toolkit (NLTK) and the SpaCy libraries. These NLP models enable a healthcare professional to expedite patient inquiry response times. Messages deemed urgent are automatically sent to the front of the line, allowing pertinent information to reach the patient as soon as possible. By prioritizing the activities that are most important to them, this approach not only improves patient satisfaction but also aids healthcare professionals in their day-to-day jobs. At this stage, an entirely new division of labor may be established. Another study demonstrated how sentiment analysis, which was also carried out with the use of some of Python's textual libraries, could be utilized to learn more about patients' overall portal experiences (Carini et al., 2021).

15.2.3.6 Outreach Services

Finding trends in the health of large populations using ML and NLP is a relatively new field. This field of study often examines rural populations and the particular health issues they face, and it typically seeks solutions to help these communities' health (Ward and Young, 2020). Figure 15.5 highlights the application of ML and

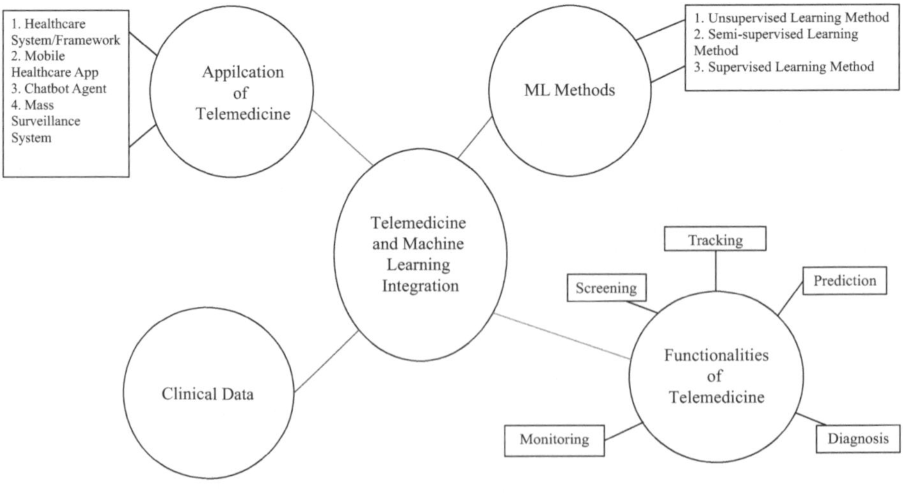

FIGURE 15.5 Utilizing ML and NLP for identifying health trends and allocating resources in rural areas.

NLP to identify health trends and allocate healthcare resources effectively in rural areas. AI has the potential to greatly improve healthcare services and the efficacy of public health programs, particularly with regard to patient access and outreach activities. AI has historically been employed in the provision of healthcare, primarily for administrative and medical purposes. However, applying AI to public health represents a significant step forward in addressing the real-world problems that public health practitioners and agencies face on a daily basis. AI is quite new in public health, but its potential is astounding, and we want to make sure that the pathway to use is clear.

15.2.3.7 ML and NLP for Rural Health

Using the Python scikit-learn and Pandas libraries, researchers developed ML models that look at health trends in rural regions. An AI-driven outreach program developed using Python's PyTorch library was used to identify high-risk individuals for diabetes living in remote locations. The program provided personalized health recommendations over the course of two years, which led to a 20% reduction in new diabetes cases (Tafti et al., 2019).

15.2.4 Challenges in AI Applications in the Healthcare Industry

The chapter goes into the ethical, regulatory, and privacy implications of AI making its way into healthcare. What is more, just these sorts of issues have generated some pretty good controversy in areas like self-driving cars and facial recognition software, not to mention those nascent careers in bioethics that have sprung up in response to too many ethical dilemmas. But this is the critical need to balance technological advancements with ethical considerations to ensure the future "equitable and responsible delivery of healthcare that is both accessible and effective." The healthcare system is seeing a lot of influence from AI and technological advancements. The infusion of technology has, without a doubt, improved the system's current circumstances. We're seeing a lot of great things: improved patient outcomes, more sense made of system processes, and better mechanisms for making diagnoses. Moreover, ML algorithms are the force behind ample detection of frauds, enhanced billing systems, the accordance of medical decision support mechanisms, and the development of ample imaging notions in healthcare systems (Velichko, 2021). Despite its eminent merits, some challenges involving the integration of AI in healthcare systems remain eminently present and emerge as a setback altogether.

1. *Data Quality Challenges*: The relationship between healthcare and AI focuses on large data processing and management. The phenomenon remains prone to inaccuracies, inconsistencies, and incomplete aspects of the final results. Apparently, inconsistent data sets include errors, which lead to mistakes in patient outcomes and perpetuate disparities in healthcare. Inconsistent data hinders extensive data exchange and comparison for healthcare providers, limiting the insights emerging from eminent data analysis endeavors (Petersson et al., 2022). Normalization is a determinant facet in the application of AI in healthcare. The lack of normalization leads

to compromised AI models with errors in eminent predictions. Healthcare data remains huge and vast with immense patient data, an aspect that poses AI algorithms as facets that require ample data quality and accuracy for their effectiveness. Apparently, heterogeneous and complex data from healthcare systems normally finds storage in most systems, an aspect that hinders the aggregation of data, an aspect that involves the storage of data in different formats and systems, respectively. These notions play a role in undermining data quality and processing, respectively (Aggarwal, 2018). Eminent data quality challenges call for the development of data strategies, especially by using similar or common data models, ample data formats, and setting vocabulary standards. Mitigating data quality challenges leads to ample data exchange endeavors between systems and improves the quality of data altogether.

2. *Interoperability Challenges*: Interoperability challenges emerge in the context of integrating diverse sources of data in the integration of AI in healthcare systems. Interoperability challenges relate to the lack of application programming interfaces (APIs) in healthcare applications. API's function is as a set of standards for protocols, an aspect that influences the integration and retrieval of data, especially for data retrieved from several sources (Pournik et al., 2023). In a bid to counter interoperability challenges, the main mitigation factors include the use of frameworks and standards as major determinants in developing data strategies.
3. *Security Challenges*: Healthcare organizations expand spontaneously, serving many patients at once, an aspect that calls for consideration of regulatory, ethical, and security measures. Ample expansions imply that a consistent increase in patient data remains important for an organization. Apparently, security challenges arise in the context of data misuse, breaches, and access by unauthorized entities. The main idea behind countering security challenges entails securing workloads with ample protective measures on sensitive data, an aspect that relates to the Zero Trust security measure. Protected health information (PHI) fosters security and privacy measures that are compliant with legal requirements.
4. *Infrastructural Challenges*: The use of AI in healthcare practices calls for the standardization of infrastructure through the use of eminent tools. For instance, integrating the graphical processing unit (GPU) in AI models may pose ample impacts, but ample setbacks include the fact that GPUs remain inaccessible and costly to implement. Inaccessibility of the latter may hinder the proper implementation of AI models and schemes. Solutions to the setback include the integration of standard and strategized planning notions, with consequent considerations for scalable infrastructural alternatives as a whole.
5. *High Purchasing Costs and Skill Gaps*: Successful AI implementation necessitates an equally trained and informed workforce for the use of AI-based applications. Nonetheless, a skill gap involving the lack of ample know-how in various AI facets undermines the successful implementation of AI in the healthcare industry. Each AI-based initiative sets in with its

own requirements in terms of engineering, data science, and healthcare, an aspect that leaves organizations with a shortage of skilled manpower for the successful integration of AI with respect to healthcare provision; the latter calls for ample investments in education in a bid to counter eminent skill gaps that undermine ample harnessing opportunities in AI-based provisions.

6. *Ethical Implications and Potential Risks*: While there are several benefits to incorporating AI into the healthcare system, there are also considerable dangers and ethical considerations. Concerns about privacy and secrecy, prejudice and injustice, the often-deadly superhuman abilities of AI, and accountability ambiguity are a few of them. These are not little problems. We must pay attention to these fundamental ethical principles and implement regulations that place appropriate restrictions on AI operations in the healthcare industry if we want AI to function at a rate that is consistent with them. We also need to think carefully about what is best for the people who are being treated by our medical system (Tim et al., 2023).
7. *Integrity and Accountability*: AI systems in the critical care unit may use opaque or even hidden decision-making procedures. The seeming opacity presents us with a challenge to employ the AI system responsibly in the text. Conversely, in a high-stakes, trust-based environment such as the ICU, it is no less reckless to feed the AI system healthcare data if we just act as if we know what's happening inside.
8. *Regulatory and Legal Challenges*: One major obstacle to the use of AI in healthcare is the intricate network of rules and laws. The complex, tangled, and sometimes conflicting rules that govern the healthcare sector must be adhered to by the AI technologies that analyze patient data and offer treatment recommendations. As a result, many were written with only the most rudimentary concept of computer security in mind.
9. *Ethical Use of AI*: In healthcare, AI's ethical application must achieve two goals: augmenting rather than diminishing human inputs and enhancing rather than diminishing human outputs. The human inputs we must look to AI to augment include the essential clinical judgments that healthcare professionals make every day. These decisions cannot and must not be rendered by AI, for doing so would remove an irreplaceable human element from the quality of care provided to patients. Indeed, would we even give our informed consent to having a computer "decide" our fate in a manner akin to the way it now "decides" issues of security clearance, creditworthiness, or sentencing in a court of law?

15.2.5 Future of AI Application in Healthcare Provision

Regulation with respect to the Food and Drug Administration (FDA) entails any potential and present applications of AI in the development of medicinal drugs. Nonetheless, healthcare providers need to consider data quality and standard model developments in drug developmental endeavors. Future plans encompassing the integration of AI in healthcare systems consider the amendment of current regulations for the utmost harnessing of the potentials posed by AI at large. For instance, AI integration in current frameworks serves as an eminent and reliable way of attaining ample accuracy and efficacy standards in the healthcare industry. The latter entails regular AI updates and control measures, respectively. Current problems and challenges in the healthcare industry, such as inefficiencies in diagnosis, call for a future that involves AI integration, such as image reconstruction in related medical treatments and diagnosis, for ample accuracy, effectiveness, and accessibility. Another consideration involves using AI in administrative schedules by integrating AI-based assistance in applicable areas.

Apparently, technologies associated with AI include NLP, ML, and deep learning. The latter are causative agents in the current technological experience eminent in healthcare centers and serve to increase accuracy levels by eradicating errors, saving lives, and enhancing patient access to healthcare provisions. In this regard, expansions in AI's influence and scope bear immense potential in the healthcare sector as a source of optimization and a determinant factor in the realization of patient outcomes (Siwicki, 2023). The application of AI in healthcare practices in the near future takes on several forms that include the development of patient trust, the realization of cost-effective incorporation, robotic-aided surgery endeavors, reliable disease detection mechanisms, and improved diagnosis methods amalgamated with easy and fast access to data.

15.2.6 Stakeholder Perspectives on the Impact of AI on Patient Access

AI technologies have significantly improved patient access to healthcare services, but the impact varies across different stakeholder groups. While patients benefit from quicker diagnosis and treatment, healthcare providers and policymakers face challenges related to ethical concerns and resource allocation. Table 15.3 summarizes the perspectives of different stakeholder groups, including patients, healthcare providers, and policymakers, on the benefits and challenges of AI in patient access.

15.2.7 Real-World Examples and Case Studies of Patient Access in the provided document

An in-depth exploration of relevant cases would vastly enhance comprehension of the manifold applications and implications of AI technologies in the healthcare domain. A nuanced examination of particularly illustrative real-world examples has the potential to offer profound insights for all stakeholders invested in optimizing both the advantages and addressing the shortcomings of these nascent yet rapidly advancing tools.

15.2.7.1 Prior Authorization Streamlining Case Study

One illustrative example concerns a large integrated healthcare network seeking to reduce inefficiencies in prior authorization with AI (Khan, 2024). After analyzing over five years of de-identified insurance approval records totaling 200,000 entries, researchers trained several ML classification models. As a baseline, traditional non-AI processes averaged 30 days to resolution with 85% accuracy. The AI system was able to automatically adjudicate 45% of common authorization types in just 3 days on

TABLE 15.3
Stakeholder Perspectives on the Impact of AI on Patient Access

Stakeholder Group	Perspectives on Benefits of AI	Perspectives on Challenges of AI
Patients	Increased access to specialists in remote areas via telehealth Enhanced personalization of care through predictive analytics and precision medicine Empowerment through access to one's own health records	Privacy and security of personal health information Lack of understanding of how AI systems reach decisions Potential for bias and unfair treatment based on algorithmic decisions
Healthcare Providers	Administrative efficiencies reducing clerical burdens Diagnostic support enhancing accuracy and consistency Population health management insights improving care delivery Filling gaps in areas with physician shortages	Malpractice liability if AI recommendations lead to poor outcomes Disruption of clinical workflows and traditional decision-making models Requirements for extensive staff training and IT infrastructure upgrades
Policymakers	Containment of rising healthcare costs through optimized resource allocation and preventative care Avenues for greater equity in access through telehealth and mobile apps Economic growth potential of AI sector development	Ensuring responsible governance and regulation of AI to prevent harms Mitigating consequences of job losses from AI automation on healthcare workforce Difficulty in assessing long-term impacts and benefits of new technologies

average. This resulted in a 60% decrease in average turnaround times for these standard requests. With 98% accuracy on par with manual review, the AI realized notable productivity benefits. A more thorough analysis uncovered possible biases and found that specific patient populations were denied AI decisions at an initial rate 10-15% higher than their peers (Jones et al., 2023). These biases expose a risk that, if left unaddressed, could lead to a systematic denial of access to vulnerable communities. In response, the researchers built new models and used the old decision-making parameters to make the new AIs "equal opportunity" AI. They did this by adding some socio-economic variables, a bit of demographic data, and some clinical variables, which are not part of the decision-making process for "medical necessity" to the old parameter set. Then they retrained the decision-making algorithm using the new parameter set.

As healthcare and social dynamics are always changing, experts emphasized the necessity for continual oversight, even as they initially reduced prejudice (Chen & Decary, 2019). In order to tackle this issue, networks implemented quarterly performance audits and created avenues for stakeholders to provide input that might impact further algorithmic improvements. The AI implementation illustrated how, with careful examination, such technologies may help remove rather than exacerbate obstacles to care by maintaining accountability even as procedures become faster and more scalable. Continued monitoring is essential to guarantee fair, compassionate, and just application over the long run.

15.2.7.2 Remote Telehealth Case Study

Another instructive case involved a pilot program offering AI-powered telehealth services for patients in remote, underserved regions across three Midwestern states (Gedefaw et al., 2023). Researchers partnered with community health centers to deploy videoconferencing devices integrated with a deep learning-based diagnosis support tool. For one year, four primary care clinics participated, enrolling 500 patients living 50+ miles from specialty care. The AI classifier was trained on millions of anonymous electronic health records to help clinicians by offering differential diagnoses and tied medical literature. Evaluations found no statistical difference in health outcomes compared with in-person appointments, and specialists reported average 10-minute savings in call times aided by AI prompting. Qualitative surveys with patients highlighted relief from travel burdens and improved ability to receive preventive screenings and ongoing management for chronic needs like diabetes and hypertension (Stone, 2019). Communities experienced fewer emergent transports. However, providers noted the need for full-time IT staff at clinics to address technological barriers caused by poor rural connectivity and end-user digital literacy challenges among some older patients.

15.2.7.3 Drug Discovery Case Study

It was investigated in a big study how AI may help to streamline pharmaceutical R&D pipelines. NLP models trained on more than 50 million biomedical abstracts and drug trial data were used by researchers at a top five global innovator to identify novel candidate molecular targets. They said that AI screening capabilities were equivalent to 200 scientists examining 200 papers each day without fatigability. Four years ahead of schedule for typical literature reviews, AI found eight targets in less than a year, which were then verified by in vitro testing. The estimated savings from an accelerated time to market exceeded $50 million for each innovative therapy that became successful.

At the same time, observers stressed the necessity to safeguard AI against misuse that might endanger certain communities. For example, privacy protection is paramount since reidentification of individuals in biomedical data may result in legal consequences, and erosion of public trust in data is essential for the growth of data sharing. Algorithms must also be checked for any social biases that might damage study goals, such as amplifying diseases that mostly affect affluent demographics (Al Kuwaiti et al., 2023). Leaders in the area of AI have accurately identified the need for enhancing model explainability using techniques like attribution mapping, given the black-box nature of AI, to ensure that reasoning conforms to scientific criteria of impartiality, generalizability, and safety.

15.3 DISCUSSION AND CONCLUSIONS

Patient engagement and access to healthcare have long been unresolved issues, leading to ineffective outcomes. AI is gaining dynamic popularity in the healthcare sector due to various reasons, including the provision of easy and reliable access to complex data. AI applications gather, analyze, and store health records effectively in digital form and are the main factors behind the speedy exertion of processes in health-based organizations.

The application of IoT-enabled technology puts caregivers at ease and ensures better participation (Bhatt & Chakraborty, 2023). Notably, AI integration in health centers leads to efficient diagnosis efforts that allow for timely and early detection of diseases. AI algorithms can be used to identify the early spread of any dangerous or contagious diseases so that preventive action can be taken. However, for AI to gain public acceptance in healthcare, it is crucial to increase awareness and build trust. It is important to highlight that AI will not replace medical practitioners or doctors; rather, it should be seen as a tool to enhance their efficiency (Jiang et al., 2021). AI should be considered a means of improving medical efficacy rather than an intimidating threat to human existence or professions. The era of AI has begun, and the healthcare sector will not be immune to its disruptive influence. Different players—legislators, AI researchers, and those in the medical domain, among others—will need to come together to foster the necessary trust that will make healthcare AI's next frontier (Pongtriang et al., 2023). Nonetheless, employing AI in health care could create ethical problems associated with accountability, confidentiality, precision, and permission. To achieve the AI-driven healthcare vision, a concentrated and extensive effort is required to ensure that healthcare professionals at all levels understand the implications of AI and are skilled at implementing it. While the upskilling of our workforce is vital, it is equally necessary to put in place robust guidelines for the ethical processing of patient data and to construct sufficient infrastructure to support real-time decision-making for AI in health care to be effective and sustainable.

In summary, this chapter has provided a comprehensive dissection of the groundbreaking impacts of AI on patients' access to medical care. It has augmented the burgeoning body of work about AI in healthcare by scrutinizing contemporary access challenges in detail, along with real-world examples and layered solutions. It has also proposed some future scenarios to highlight how serious this moment is and how much access could be enhanced if we win the next series of decisions about AI's role in these spaces.

REFERENCES

Aggarwal, C. C. (2018). *Neural networks and deep learning*. Springer International Publishing. https://doi.org/10.1007/978-3-319-94463-0

Al Kuwaiti, A., Nazer, K., Al-Reedy, A., Al-Shehri, S., AlMuhanna, A., Subbarayalu, A. V., Al Muhanna, D., & AlMuhanna, F. A. (2023). A review of the role of artificial intelligence in healthcare. *Journal of Personalized Medicine*, *13*(6), 951. https://doi.org/10.3390/jpm13060951

Alowais, S. A., Alghamdi, S. S., Alsuhebany, N., Alqahtani, T., Alshaya, A. I., Almohareb, S. N., & Albekairy, A. M. (2023). Revolutionizing healthcare: The role of artificial intelligence in clinical practice. *BMC Medical Education*, *23*(1), 689. https://doi.org/10.1186/s12909-023-04698-z

AlShuweihi, M., Salloum, S. A., & Shaalan, K. (2020). Biomedical corpora and natural language processing on clinical text in languages other than English: A systematic review. In *Studies in Systems, Decision and Control* (pp. 491–509). Springer International Publishing. https://doi.org/10.1007/978-3-030-47411-9_27

Balsdon, H. (2021). Introducing a digital portal that enables patients to access their health records. *Nursing Management*, *28*(6), 36–42. https://doi.org/10.7748/nm.2021.1994

Bhatt, V., & Chakraborty, S. (2023). Improving service engagement in healthcare through internet of things based healthcare systems. *Journal of Science and Technology Policy Management*, *14*(1), 53–73.

Bohr, A., & Memarzadeh, K. (2020). The rise of artificial intelligence in healthcare applications. In *Artificial Intelligence in Healthcare* (pp. 25–60). Academic Press.

Bonaccorso, G., Fandango, A., & Shanmugamani, R. (2018). *Python Advanced Guide to Artificial Intelligence*. Packt Publishing.

Carini, E., Villani, L., Pezzullo, A. M., Gentili, A., Barbara, A., Ricciardi, W., & Boccia, S. (2021). The impact of digital patient portals on health outcomes, system efficiency, and patient attitudes: Updated systematic literature review. *Journal of Medical Internet Research*, *23*(9), e26189. https://doi.org/10.2196/26189

Chen, M., & Decary, M. (2019). Artificial intelligence in healthcare: An essential guide for health leaders. *Healthcare Management Forum*, *33*(1), 10–18. https://doi.org/10.1177/0840470419873123

Fox, A. (2023, September 5). Orion Health launches new healthcare AI-enabled patient navigation services. *Healthcare IT News*. Retrieved from https://www.healthcareitnews.com/news/orion-health-launches-new-healthcare-ai-enabled-patient-navigation-services

Gedefaw, L., Liu, C. F., Ip, R. K., Tse, H. F., Yeung, M. H., Yip, S. P., & Huang, C. L. (2023). Artificial intelligence-assisted diagnostic cytology and genomic testing for hematologic disorders. *Cells*, *12*(1755), 1755. https://doi.org/10.3390/cells12131755

Islam, Md. R., Kabir, Md. M., Mridha, M. F., Alfarhood, S., Safran, M., & Che, D. (2023). Deep learning-based IoT system for remote monitoring and early detection of health issues in real-time. *Sensors*, *23*(11), 5204. https://doi.org/10.3390/s23115204

Javanmard, S. (2024). Revolutionizing medical practice: The impact of artificial intelligence (AI) on healthcare. *Open Access Journal of Applied Science and Technology*, *2*(1), 01–16.

Jiang, L., Wu, Z., Xu, X., Zhan, Y., Jin, X., Wang, L., & Qiu, Y. (2021). Opportunities and challenges of artificial intelligence in the medical field: Current application, emerging problems, and problem-solving strategies. *Journal of International Medical Research*, *49*(3), 03000605211000157.

Jones, C., Thornton, J., & Wyatt, J. C. (2023). Artificial intelligence and clinical decision support: clinicians' perspectives on trust, trustworthiness, and liability. *Medical law review*, *31*(4), 501–520.

Joshi, H. (2024). Enabling next-gen healthcare: Advanced interoperability and integration with AI, IoMT, and precision medicine. *International Journal of Advanced Research in Science, Engineering and Technology*, *8*(1). https://doi.org/10.17148/iarjset.2021.8116

Khan, F. (2024). Regulating the revolution: A legal roadmap to optimizing AI in healthcare. *Minnesota Journal of Law, Science & Technology*, Spring.

Kinsley, H., & Kukiela, D. (2020). *Neural networks from scratch in Python*. Retrieved from https://nnfs.io

Kumar, S., Nehra, M., Khurana, S., Dilbaghi, N., Kumar, V., Kaushik, A., & Kim, K. H. (2021). Aspects of point-of-care diagnostics for personalized health wellness. *International Nanomedicine*, *16*, 383–402. https://doi.org/10.2147/IJN.S267212

Locke, S., Bashall, A., Al-Adely, S., Moore, J., Wilson, A., & Kitchen, G. B. (2021). Natural language processing in medicine: A review. *Trends in Anaesthesia and Critical Care*, *38*, 4–9. https://doi.org/10.1016/j.tacc.2021.02.007

Petersson, L., Larsson, I., Nygren, J. M., Nilsen, P., Neher, M., Reed, J. E., Tyskbo, D., & Svedberg, P. (2022). Challenges to implementing artificial intelligence in healthcare: A qualitative interview study with healthcare leaders in Sweden. *BMC Health Services Research*, *22*(1). https://doi.org/10.1186/s12913-022-08215-8

Petmezas, G., Stefanopoulos, L., Kilintzis, V., Tzavelis, A., Rogers, J. A., Katsaggelos, A. K., & Maglaveras, N. (2022). State-of-the-art deep learning methods on electrocardiogram data: Systematic review. *JMIR Medical Informatics*, *10*(8), e38454. https://doi.org/10.2196/38454

Poalelungi, D. G., Musat, C. L., Fulga, A., Neagu, M., Neagu, A. I., Piraianu, A. I., & Fulga, I. (2023). Advancing patient care: How artificial intelligence is transforming healthcare. *Journal of Personalized Medicine*, *13*(8), 1214.

Pongtriang, P., Rakhab, A., Bian, J., Guo, Y., & Maitree, K. (2023). Challenges in adopting artificial intelligence to improve healthcare systems and outcomes in Thailand. *Healthcare Informatics Research*, *29*(3), 280–282.

Pournik, O., Mukherjee, T., Ghalichi, L., & Arvanitis, T. N. (2023). How interoperability challenges are addressed in healthcare IoT projects. In *Telehealth Ecosystems in Practice*. IOS Press. https://doi.org/10.3233/TEP-2022-110

Saravanan, R., & Sujatha, P. (2018). A state of art techniques on machine learning algorithms: A perspective of supervised learning approaches in data classification. In *2018 Second International Conference on Intelligent Computing and Control Systems (ICICCS)*. IEEE. https://doi.org/10.1109/iccons.2018.8663155

Scott, M. (2021, December 6). How AI can solve prior authorization. *Insurance Thought Leadership*. Retrieved from https://insurancethoughtleadership.com/life-health/how-ai-can-solve-prior-authorization

Siwicki, B. (2023, August 24). Where generative AI can make headway in healthcare. *Healthcare IT News*. Retrieved from https://healthcareitnews.com/news/where-generative-ai-can-make-headway-healthcare

Stone, J. V. (2019). *Artificial intelligence engines: A tutorial introduction to the mathematics of deep learning*. Sebtel Press.

Tafti, A. P., Fu, S., Khurana, A., Mastorakos, G. M., Poole, K. G., Traub, S. J., Yiannias, J. A., & Liu, H. (2019). Artificial intelligence to organize patient portal messages: A journey from an ensemble deep learning text classification to rule-based named entity recognition. In *2019 IEEE International Conference on Bioinformatics and Biomedicine (BIBM)*. IEEE. https://doi.org/10.1109/bibm47256.2019.8982942

Tim, Y., Chiew, T. K., Lim, H. M., Teo, C. H., & Ng, C. J. (2023). Design process knowledge for crisis-driven information systems solutions: Insights on building digital resilience from an action design research study. *Information Systems Journal*, *33*(6), 1343–1369.

Velichko, Y. (2021, December 2). Types and applications of AI in healthcare. *Postindustria*. Retrieved from https://postindustria.com/types-and-applications-of-ai-in-healthcare

Ward, P. J., & Young, A. M. (2020). Natural language processing and machine learning methods in public health surveillance: A narrative review (Preprint). *JMIR Publications Inc*. https://doi.org/10.2196/preprints.26351

Zhang, C., Liu, X., Jin, S., Chen, Y., & Guo, R. (2022). Ferroptosis in cancer therapy: A novel approach to reversing drug resistance. *Molecular Cancer*, *21*(1). https://doi.org/10.1186/s12943-022-01530-y

16 Transformation of Insurance Sector in the Era of Artificial Intelligence

Suhasini Verma, Jeevesh Sharma, V. S. Anoop and Shweta Goyal

16.1 INTRODUCTION

Technology has revolutionized how businesses are operated in this era. It has influenced businesses globally and has shown a dramatic shift in business models (Cortis et al., 2019). Technology has created a competitive advantage with the emergence of Artificial Intelligence (AI) (Riikkinen et al., 2018), Big Data (Arumugam & Bhargavi, 2019), machine learning (Baudry & Robert, 2019) Blockchain (Brophy, 2019), IoT (Nayak & Bhattacharyya, 2020), etc., and digitalizing the businesses (Agbo et al., 2019; Baecke & Bocca, 2017; Barry & Charpentier, 2020; Brophy, 2019). The business sector is likewise trying to deal with the demanding and evolving client behavior about goods, comfort, services, etc. (Cappiello, 2020). A "one-size-fits-all" strategy is being replaced by "bite-size insurance" and "sachet-model insurance" products in the market (Mokkarala, 2019). With the help of technology, firms are offering innovative products at a minimized cost (Fitzgerald et al., 2014).

Technology has disrupted many businesses, and the insurance business is also impacted by it. The adoption of technology is hastening the transformative change in the insurance industry. The impact of this widespread use of technology in the insurance sector is so vast that the new term "Insurtech" is coined. Insurtech is "an insurance firm, middleman or an expert in the insurance value chain, which makes use of technology to compete or to offer value-added advantages for the insurance sector" (Yan et al., 2018). This emerging phenomenon called Insurtech has the potential to re-establish customer relationships in the insurance sector (Yan et al., 2018). Asymmetric information, adverse selection, and moral hazard are features of the insurance market. Insurtech offers the ability to close this knowledge gap, lowering the likelihood of moral hazards and adverse selection (Malik et al., 2022). The Indian insurance industry is evolving fast with the emergence of Insurtech start-ups (Mokkarala, 2019). The old economy corporations are under competition from Insurtech firms (Saeed et al., 2022).

DOI: 10.1201/9781003503385-16

These changing dynamics are putting pressure on conventional firms. They need to update their business model, product offerings, operations, and customer relationship management to avoid being left behind by new-age insurance companies. In this direction, this study attempts to provide a thorough grasp of Insurtech in the present environment while simultaneously analyzing how Insurtech companies are using AI and other technologies to provide better and new innovative products and streamline their operations, so that conventional companies may use this insight for their betterment and stay ahead in the competition.

The chapter is structured in six sections. Section 16.2 conceptualizes the background of the study by analyzing the technology disruption in the insurance sector. Section 16.2 details the technologies being used in the insurance sector, followed by the impact of AI on the insurance business in Section 16.4. Section 16.5 provides concluding remarks and ends by presenting the recommendations, limitations, and future research of the study in Section 16.6.

16.2 TECHNOLOGY AND INSURANCE SECTOR: INSURTECH

Digital shift refers to the application and integration of information and developing technology to fundamentally change various areas of a firm, including the development of new business models and adjustments to operational procedures and customer service. The advent of new digital technology offers significant and transformative prospects for both the public sector and businesses of all scales. Due to the nature of their dealings with intangibles, financial services are particularly well-suited for digitization to cut down on processing expenses and speed up service delivery. The use of digital technology has had an enormous impact on how services are delivered, how they are used, and ultimately how businesses relate to their customers.

The use of digital technologies has transformed how customers hunt for information, make decisions, purchase goods, and generate new requirements. Most businesses are implementing different technologies as part of their operations' digital transformation; the insurance sector is not an exception. Insurance firms employ technology as a tool to streamline their offerings and improve client satisfaction.

The now unstoppable digitization process is having a significant impact on insurance companies and pressuring drastic shifts in corporate culture, products and services, relationship management, and relations with the sector's various competitors (Albrecher et al., 2019). Its growth is being fueled by the acceleration of digitalization, the emergence of innovators, and applicable technologies like AI, big data, machine learning, and the Internet of Things (Okada, 2018).

Insurance businesses may increase their efficiency through cost reduction and pricing strategies by cutting down on interactions owing to the digitalization of distribution channels (Cappiello, 2020). Numerous innovative technologies can optimize processes across the value chain on both front and back ends. Big data, AI, cognitive computing, predictive modeling, telematics, the IoT, pricing/underwriting, sales and distribution, policy and claims administration, asset and risk management, and more are affecting the insurance value chain. The Insurtech firms concentrate on streamlining the insurance industry's technological environment and enhancing operations (Yan et al., 2018; Yeole & Kalbande, 2016). By using big data, AI/

cognitive computing, predictive models, wearable technologies, telematics, and the Internet of Things (IoT) to create value chains, Insurtech is transforming communications, information exchange, and the insurance business model. Companies have started to innovate using technologies like IoT, blockchain, and AI to reduce the product's complexity.

16.3 TECHNOLOGIES APPLIED IN THE INSURANCE SECTOR

Technological advancements such as AI, IoT, machine learning, cloud computing, telematics, IoT, mobile devices, and predictive modeling have significantly influenced the insurance industry (Cappiello, 2020). As emerging technologies advance and reach a higher level of sophistication, the process of converting information into a digital format will continue to exert a substantial impact on the sequence of activities involved in the insurance industry (Eling & Lehmann, 2018). The application and implementation of such technologies and the resulting data variety have huge potential for the health and health care insurance market. This kind of technology is already being used by insurers from a variety of industries in areas like customer interaction, promotion, and assessment (Spender et al., 2019) (Figure 16.1).

16.3.1 Artificial Intelligence and Insurance

AI refers to the use of computers to simulate human intelligence (Hamet & Tremblay, 2017). AI applications are highly effective in various areas, particularly in marketing

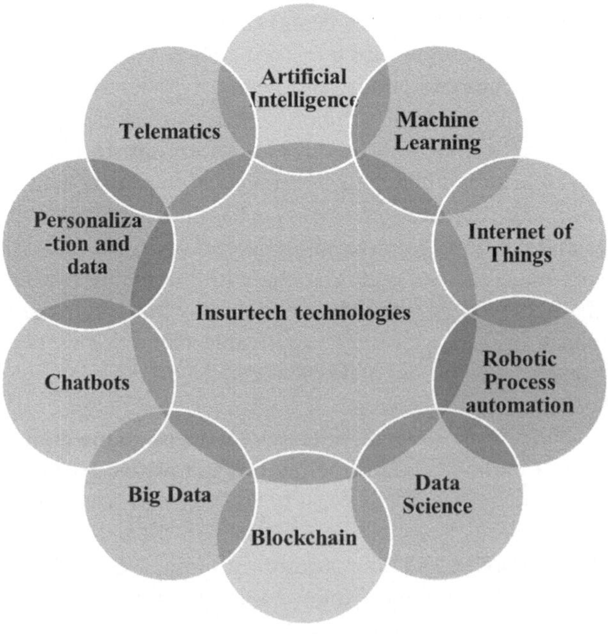

FIGURE 16.1 Technologies applied in insurance sector.

and finance, due to their widespread acceptance and the development of innovative approaches. AI has the potential to improve and evolve daily, based on the judgments made yesterday. The system continuously acquires knowledge from the enormous volume of data that is available to it (Kumar et al., 2019).

Through strengthening risk pooling and risk reduction, mitigation, and prevention, the application of AI in insurance has the potential to produce economic and societal advantages that transcend beyond insurers and their clients (Riikkinen et al., 2018). The move from manual to computerized data processing is only the beginning of the insurance sector's advanced digitalization. Insurance companies must gain the trust of clients by appropriately using modern technologies to promote the use of AI systems and realize these benefits (Stoeckli et al., 2018). By rethinking their conventional roles in the economy, these ecosystems provide insurance firms the chance to not only join new income streams but also incorporate their insurance products into seamless client experiences (Eling & Lehmann, 2018).

Insurers must gain the trust of their clients by carefully using innovative technology to promote the use of AI systems and reap the benefits. AI showed its value in several commercial sectors by quickly building automated, controlled settings that maximize production (Kumar et al., 2019). Additionally, AI can aid insurers in enhancing their position in risk mitigation, prevention, and reduction. The following are the benefits of AI in insurance (Table 16.1).

16.3.2 IoT and Insurance

Big data, IoT, and other technologies triggered the fourth industrial revolution in insurance in the industrialized world. The industry is working to make remote sensing technology more user-friendly to increase customer acceptance. A way to

TABLE 16.1
Advantages of AI in Insurance

Extend the Scope of Risk Pooling	Reduce the Cost of Risk Pooling	Mitigate and Prevent Risks
• By simplifying access to individualized products (such as life insurance for those with pre-existing illnesses), insurance coverage may be extended to new and previously uninsured client segments. • Increased risk insights will increase the number of hazards for which insurance coverage is accessible (e.g., cyber risks).	By automating some operations, doing better risk assessments, and reducing moral hazard and adverse selection, you may provide insurance at a lower cost.	• Yield fresh insights about the risk that may be used to reduce and avoid dangers. • Make early warning systems available so that losses can be reduced.

Source: Keller, 2020.

increase insurance penetration may be found in emerging economies' use of IoT (Saeed et al., 2022). IoT uses the internet to create a worldwide network of connections between billions of people and physical items. Due to factors such as increasing medical expenses, a growing elderly population requiring remote surveillance due to chronic diseases, limited access to medical services, and a need for eHealth in developing countries, the IoT has emerged as an intriguing subject in healthcare systems (Kashani et al., 2021).

A typical IoT ecosystem also includes sensors, sophisticated algorithms, communication interfaces, and cloud interfaces. Patient monitoring, detection, and surveillance are crucial for improving the health insurance system. Medical technology and the available instruments, however, are unable to correctly fulfill the same because of the current state of inadequate healthcare (Kodali et al., 2015). Sensors from various gadgets collect data. It presents a web mobile medical service to track, identify, and predict serious conditions. IoT innovations can raise productivity, corporate profitability overall, and portfolio risk profiles. IoT enables insurers to communicate with customers more effectively by introducing crucial touchpoints during delicate times like purchases and claims. IoT technologies are used in different medical fields, making them convenient for doctors and patients in the current medical environment, such as real-time monitoring, patient information management, and healthcare management. The wireless sensing devices make it easier to check health indicators, including blood glucose levels, heart rate, blood pressure, body temperature, and respiration rate.

16.3.3 Robotic Process Automation, Chatbots and Insurance

The last few years have seen a lot of interest in software robotics. Through instantly automating manual consumer and back-office procedures, Software Robotics claims to be able to increase their speed, cost-effectiveness, consistency, and regulatory compliance. The return on investment for all these advantages often happens in less than a year (Lamberton et al., 2017). RPA may be applied in a wide variety of corporate and industrial organizations. RPA may be used as a platform for many business process automation. Many different industries and business organizations may use RPA. Several business process automations may be supported by RPA as a platform. To assess the market, identify potential consumers, and ascertain their needs, insurance companies are already using RPA. RPA will assist in fusing innovative methods, securing them against updates in the future. RPA's elevated level of automation will make it possible to report and analyze fraud tendencies. After the description of technologies used in the insurance sector, including healthcare, Table 16.2 summarizes each technology applied in Insurtech.

16.3.4 Machine Learning in Insurance

A fundamental component of contemporary financial systems, the insurance sector is progressively leveraging machine learning (ML) to optimize its operations. ML is a distinct branch of AI that encompasses methods that allow computers to acquire knowledge from data and enhance their performance without the need for explicit programming. ML applications in the insurance industry encompass a wide range

TABLE 16.2
Technology Adoption in Insurance Sector

Sl. No.	Technologies	Description	References
1.	Artificial Intelligence	It can help gather data, classify information, improve risk assessments, and enhance customer interactions.	Johnson et al., 2021
2.	Machine Learning	Beneficial for building chatbots, finding trends, detecting fraud, and categorizing substantial amounts of data.	Paruchuri, 2020; Baudry & Robert, 2019;
3.	Internet of Things	IoT solutions enable continuous data collection and sharing across networks, accelerating and optimizing the claims process, reducing data duplications, and essentially eliminating consumer annoyance.	Kashani et al., 2021; Kodali et al., 2015; Darshan & Anandakumar, 2015;
4.	Robotic Process Automation	It is a collection of tools that helps organizations run more quickly by giving monotonous, repetitive, iterative jobs to bots and creating possibilities for effectively using human labor.	Bhatnagar, 2019; Lamberton et al., 2017;
5.	Big Data	The healthcare industry uses the term "big data" to describe the vast quantities of information generated via the use of digital technologies for collecting patient records and monitoring hospital performance.	Berthele, 2018; Kenyon & Eloff, 2017; keller et al., 2018; Hussain & Prieto, 2016
8.	Personalization and Data	Insurance firms integrate information gathered from gadgets and cell phones to determine the requirements and preferences of their clients and design plans that are suitable for those demands. A more positive customer experience and precise risk evaluations are made possible by using data to target individuals.	Barry & Charpentier, 2020; Xu & Dukes, 2022
9.	Telematics	Telematics is a tool that auto insurance firms use to get real-time data on the policyholder and driver. Observing driver behavior, vehicle condition, and mileage are a few of the frequent use cases. Usage-based insurance (UBI), pay-as-you-drive (PAYD), and pay-how-you-drive (PHYD) are a few insurance forms that lead to telematics.	Baecke & Bocca, 2017; Eling & Kraft, 2020; Constantinescu et al., 2018; Guillen et al., 2019
10.	Chatbots	The bots would be capable of answering consumer questions without the need for human interaction, saving insurance firms a great deal of time and money. Additionally, it enables 24-hour assistance and smooth consumer engagement.	Riikkinen et al., 2018

Source: Author's Compilation.

of tasks such as underwriting, risk assessment, fraud detection, and customer support. These applications fundamentally change conventional processes and stimulate innovation. Riikkinen et al. (2018). By enhancing productivity, precision, and customer satisfaction, ML is revolutionizing the insurance industry. Although obstacles like data privacy, bias, and interaction with outdated systems persist, the prospective advantages and forthcoming advancements ensure further growth and enhancement in the sector. Accurately utilizing ML can offer insurers a competitive advantage and improve their capacity to address the evolving needs of clients.

16.3.5 Big Data and Insurance

Big data refers to a compilation of organized, unstructured, and semi-structured data that is acquired from disparate sources and applications. Indeed, it has emerged as the most influential buzzword in nearly all industries Ellili, Nobanee, et al. (2023). The application of big data in the insurance industry is developing into a very promising domain for extracting valuable information from extensive data sets and enhancing results while reducing expenses. The concept of big data was originally characterized by three Vs: expanded variety, growing volumes, and increased velocity. Within the context of insurance data, volume pertains to the dimensions, amount, and magnitude. The value of data, including its perceived size, is significantly impacted by the size of the data.

16.4 IMPACT OF AI ON INSURANCE INDUSTRY

Speeding Up the Application Procedures: Before technological reform, insurance product approval took weeks or months. Nowadays, it takes hours or minutes. This rapid progress is driven by AI and mobile apps. Customers can use smartphone apps to submit applications from anywhere using simple forms. AI algorithms can examine this data to determine if an application qualifies for a policy, allowing service providers to serve more clients (Riikkinen et al. 2018).

Underwriting Processes: All insurance companies must undergo underwriting, which can be tedious. Insurtech companies reduce redundancies by automating this process. AI systems can examine client records, reports, and data to identify hazards and generate quotes faster than humans (Arguello, 2021). These options will eliminate outdated, unproductive underwriting methods for customers. Reducing human engagement can help eliminate preconceptions and ensure clients receive fair pricing and benefits.

Expediting the Filing of Claims: Insurtech solutions can accelerate the process of submitting an insurance settlement. Customers may now submit claims using an app with several big insurers, and it often just requires a few minutes (Yan et al., 2018). AI streamlines the process for users while helping the insurer organize crucial data (Pareek et al., 2022). Future insurance technology platforms will be able to incorporate information from Android platforms, satellite photography, and other sources to quickly offer a full picture of the occurrence. Electronic information can also improve the precision of insurance claims.

Processing and Management of Claims: AI can streamline the handling of insurance claims, minimizing human mistakes and speeding up the approval procedure. The detection of fraud is the use of ML algorithms to examine tendencies and abnormalities in claims data to detect possibly illegal phenomena (Doss et al. 2022).

Reduction of Human Error: Particularly in complex circumstances requiring sophisticated knowledge, automated solutions can reduce the possibility of human error. This can lead to more consistent and trustworthy results (Cook and Woods 2018).

Enhanced Risk Assessment: AI technologies enable the processing of complicated data, including free-text descriptions of medical issues (Kaswan et al., 2021). Examples of these technologies include clustering analysis and natural language processing. Compared to conventional techniques that only use structured data, this capability allows for more precise risk assessments.

Predictive Insights: By highlighting characteristics that have a major impact on risk, AI models can offer insightful information about underwriting choices (Sontakke, 2022). With the use of this data, insurers can enhance the overall accuracy of risk classification and streamline their internal procedures.

Cost Reduction: Reduced premiums for customers are one way that insurance companies can pass on large cost savings from the automation of underwriting procedures (Zanke & Sontakke, 2021).

Fraud Identification: In the insurance sector, fraud is a grave issue that costs billions of dollars annually. By analyzing vast volumes of data and seeing trends that point to fraudulent activity, AI can aid insurance companies in detecting and preventing fraud (Riikkinen et al., 2018). AI-powered fraud systems can examine data from a variety of sources, including social media, public records, and claims data (Wilkinson et al., 2024). AI is also capable of learning from previous fraudulent activity, which enhances its capacity to recognize and stop fraud in the future.

Individualized Health Insurance Plans: Chawla and Davis (2013) Based on an individual's past medical history and present health issues, AI can determine and create a health insurance plan for them. By doing this, the insurer will be able to give a proper health insurance plan rather than a package that clients may or may not find useful. Additionally, clients will be urged to select a plan that best suits their needs and avoid paying for medical services they might not use.

Attracting Younger Clients: By addressing the digital demands of a generation that grew up with the internet, technology aids insurers in attracting younger clients. Younger customers can receive help from choosing the best coverage for them rather than following what their parents liked and providing innovative services can help competitors grab their clientele. For millennials and younger clients, convenience and remote access are significant advantages, and both are provided by Insurtech.

Customized Customer Experience: Real-time chatbots and virtual assistants powered by AI can offer immediate assistance, respond to inquiries, and enable insurers to navigate procedures such as submitting claims or comprehending their benefits. The application of AI in prediction analytics enables the analysis of client data to customize insurance policies and provide personalized suggestions according to specific health requirements and choices (Adeoye et al., 2024).

Promoting Health and Well-being: Analyzing collected data from wearable gadgets, AI can keep an eye on health trends and give insurance valuable information for creating individualized Wellness programs (Komalasari, 2024). AI systems can help manage chronic diseases by suggesting preventive treatments and anticipating when symptoms will worsen.

Compliance with Regulations: Data Analysis AI can aid insurers in keeping compliance with regulations by examining and overseeing substantial amounts of regulatory data, therefore guaranteeing that all procedures conform to proper legal norms (Butler & O'Brien, 2019).

AI and Analytics: Behavioral Analysis AI can monitor and evaluate client behavior to enhance engagement methods and provide tailored products and services.

Sentiment Analysis: Through the examination of client comments and interactions, AI can access sentiment and pinpoint areas that need enhancement in the provision of services.

Optimized Risk Evaluation and Control: Payrovnaziri et al. (2020). Personalized risk profiles: AI can examine health records, behavioral facts, and familial traits to generate more precise risk profiles, resulting in improved pricing and risk assessment of insurance policies. Predictive analytics: AI can forecast forthcoming health problems and probable financial claims by examining trends in medical data, enabling underwriters to actively mitigate risks.

Effective Care Management: AI can analyze patient data to give personalized therapies and surveillance, optimizing results for patients. AI can integrate data from numerous sources to improve care coordination and handle all elements of patient treatment.

16.5 THE ADAPTATION OF ARTIFICIAL INTELLIGENCE IN INSURTECH: A CHALLENGE

The presence of inadequate information quality in AI algorithms can result in the introduction of unconscious bias, causing unsuitable conclusions throughout the underwriting and claim process.

Cost: The adoption of AI might incur significant expenses, particularly for SME-sized businesses. Therefore, rely on an AI mobile application firm, whether creating brand-new, AI-powered infrastructure from scratch or trying to improve an already-existing infrastructure. Many companies may be deterred by the upfront expense of investing in the technology.

Privacy of Data and Safety: The use of AI by Insurtech allows for the access and analysis of vast quantities of data, which has generated apprehensions surrounding its worldwide application.

Limited Comprehension: Investors and personnel, fearing job loss resulting from AI deployment, lack a comprehensive understanding of the technology's actual capabilities and are hesitant to undertake its implementation.

Insufficient Proficient Manpower: The implementation of AI needs a cohort of exceptionally competent professionals, encompassing skills in AI, data science, and AI.

16.6 CONCLUSION

AI and adjacent technologies are paving the way for new opportunities, albeit a few challenges within the insurance industry. With the help of technology like AI, ML, big data, IoT, etc., the insurance industry is now offering innovative policies like pay-per-use, responding proactively in identifying probable losses and trying to prevent them, and achieving operational efficiency. Our study revealed that these technologies play a key role in policy generation, calculation of premiums, fraud detection and prevention, and claim settlement, which helps Insurtech companies to save huge costs.

16.7 RECOMMENDATIONS, LIMITATIONS, AND FUTURE RESEARCH

Our study suggests that conventional firms should invest in these technologies to reap the above-mentioned benefits. They may develop these technologies themselves or take the help of a third party or join hands with the technology firms to offer insurance products. Though the study is comprehensive in its coverage, but it lacks an understanding of the perspective of stakeholders. For this, an empirical study may be conducted. Future research may also be conducted to understand the behavior of the insured or their intention to purchase insurance products. These studies will help the insurer to offer better and more innovative products and grow the market.

REFERENCES

Adeoye, O. B., Okoye, C. C., Ofodile, O. C., Odeyemi, O., Addy, W. A., & Ajayi-Nifise, A. O. (2024). Integrating artificial intelligence in personalized insurance products: a pathway to enhanced customer engagement. *International Journal of Management & Entrepreneurship Research*, *6*(3), 502–511.

Agbo, C. C., Mahmoud, Q. H., & Eklund, J. M. (2019, April). Blockchain technology in healthcare: a systematic review. In *Healthcare* (Vol. 7, No. 2, p. 56). MDPI.

Albrecher, H., Bommier, A., Filipović, D., Koch-Medina, P., Loisel, S., & Schmeiser, H. (2019). Insurance: models, digitalization, and data science. *European Actuarial Journal*, *9*(2), 349–360.

Arguello, D. J. (2021). Insurtech In Underwriting and Claims Processing. *The Brief*, *50*(2), 60–65.

Arumugam, S., & Bhargavi, R. (2019). A survey on driving behavior analysis in usage-based insurance using big data. *Journal of Big Data*, *6*(1), 1–21.

Baecke, P., & Bocca, L. (2017). The value of vehicle telematics data in insurance risk selection processes. *Decision Support Systems*, *98*, 69–79.

Barry, L., & Charpentier, A. (2020). Personalization as a promise: Can Big Data change the practice of insurance? *Big Data & Society*, *7*(1), 2053951720935143.

Baudry, M., & Robert, C. Y. (2019). A machine learning approach for individual claims reserving in insurance. *Applied Stochastic Models in Business and Industry*, *35*(5), 1127–1155.

Berthele, E. (2018). Using big data in insurance. *Big Data for Insurance Companies*, *1*, 131–161.

Bhatnagar, N. (2019, March). Role of robotic process automation in pharmaceutical industries. In *International Conference on Advanced Machine Learning Technologies and Applications* (pp. 497–504). Cham: Springer.

Brophy, R. (2019). Blockchain and insurance: a review for operations and regulation. *Journal of Financial Regulation and Compliance*, *28*(2), 215–234.

Butler, T., & O'Brien, L. (2019). Artificial intelligence for regulatory compliance: Are we there yet?. *Journal of Financial Compliance*, *3*(1), 44–59.

Cappiello, A. (2020). The technological disruption of insurance industry: A review. *International Journal of Business and Social Science*, *11*(1), 1–11.

Chawla, N. V., & Davis, D. A. (2013). Bringing big data to personalized healthcare: a patient-centered framework. *Journal of General Internal Medicine*, *28*, 660–665.

Constantinescu, C. C., Stancu, I., & Panait, I. (2018). Impact study of telematics auto insurance. *Review of Financial Studies*, *3*(4), 17–35.

Cook, R. I., & Woods, D. D. (2018). Operating at the sharp end: the complexity of human error. In Marilyn Sue Bogner *Human Error in Medicine* (pp. 255–310). CRC Press.

Cortis, D., Debattista, J., Debono, J., & Farrell, M. (2019). InsurTech. In G. N. Bajpai *Disrupting Finance* (pp. 71–84). Palgrave Pivot, Cham.

Darshan, K. R., & Anandakumar, K. R. (2015, December). A comprehensive review on usage of Internet of Things (IoT) in healthcare system. In *2015 International Conference on Emerging Research in Electronics, Computer Science and Technology (ICERECT)* (pp. 132–136). IEEE.

Doss, S., Pawar, R., & Maddireddy, R. (2022). Intelligent automation in Health Insurance. *Bimaquest*, *22*(1), 67–79.

Eling, M., & Kraft, M. (2020). The impact of telematics on the insurability of risks. *The Journal of Risk Finance*, *21*(2), 77–109.

Eling, M., and M. Lehmann. 2018. The impact of digitalization on the insurance value chain and the insurability of risks. *The Geneva Papers on Risk and Insurance—Issues and Practice*, *43*, 359–396. https://doi.org/10.1057/s41288-017-0073-0

Ellili, N., Nobanee, H., Alsaiari, L., Shanti, H., Hillebrand, B., Hassanain, N., & Elfout, L. (2023). The applications of big data in the insurance industry: A bibliometric and systematic review of relevant literature. *The Journal of Finance and Data Science*, 9, 100102.

Fitzgerald, M., Kruschwitz, N., Bonnet, D., & Welch, M. (2014). Embracing digital technology: A new strategic imperative. *MIT Sloan Management Review*, *55*(2), 1.

Guillen, M., Nielsen, J. P., Ayuso, M., & Pérez-Marín, A. M. (2019). The use of telematics devices to improve automobile insurance rates. *Risk Analysis*, *39*(3), 662–672.

Hamet, P., & Tremblay, J. (2017). Artificial intelligence in medicine. *Metabolism*, *69*, S36–S40.

Hussain, K., & Prieto, E. (2016). Big data in the finance and insurance sectors. In L. Anthony Cox *New horizons for a data-driven economy* (pp. 209–223). Springer, Cham.

Johnson, M., Albizri, A., & Harfouche, A. (2021). Responsible artificial intelligence in healthcare: Predicting and preventing insurance claim denials for economic and social wellbeing. *Information Systems Frontiers*, 1, 1–17.

Kashani, M. H., Madanipour, M., Nikravan, M., Asghari, P., & Mahdipour, E. (2021). A systematic review of IoT in healthcare: Applications, techniques, and trends. *Journal of Network and Computer Applications*, *192*, 103164.

Kaswan, K. S., Gaur, L., Dhatterwal, J. S., & Kumar, R. (2021). AI-based natural language processing for the generation of meaningful information electronic health record (EHR) data. In Loveleen Gaur, Arun Solanki, Samuel Fosso Wamba, Noor Zaman Jhanjhi *Advanced AI techniques and applications in bioinformatics* (pp. 41–86). CRC Press.

Keller, B. (2020). *Promoting responsible artificial intelligence in insurance*. Geneva Association-International Association for the Study of Insurance Economics.

Keller, B., Eling, M., Schmeiser, H., Christen, M., & Loi, M. (2018). *Big data and insurance: Implications for innovation, competition and privacy*. Geneva Association-International Association for the Study of Insurance Economics.

Kenyon, D., & Eloff, J. H. (2017, August). Big data science for predicting insurance claims fraud. In *2017 Information Security for South Africa (ISSA)* (pp. 40–47). IEEE.

Kodali, R. K., Swamy, G., & Lakshmi, B. (2015, December). An implementation of IoT for healthcare. In *2015 IEEE Recent Advances in Intelligent Computational Systems (RAICS)* (pp. 411–416). IEEE.

Komalasari, R. (2024). AI-powered wearables revolutionizing health tracking and personalized wellness management. *Timor Leste Journal of Business and Management*, *6*, 42–50.

Kumar, N., Srivastava, J. D., & Bisht, H. (2019). Artificial intelligence in insurance sector. *Journal of the Gujarat Research Society*, *21*(7), 79–91.

Lamberton, C., Brigo, D., & Hoy, D. (2017). Impact of Robotics, RPA and AI on the insurance industry: challenges and opportunities. *Journal of Financial Perspectives*, *4*(1), 8–20.

Malik, S., Dhall, R., & Tomar, A. S. (2022). InsurTech in insurance: The road ahead for Telematics in India. *International Journal of Health Sciences*, *6*(S3), 5276–5287.

Mokkarala, M. R. (2019). A study on select Indian Insurtech Startups. *Prerana*, *23*, 153–162.

Nayak, B., & Bhattacharyya, S. S. (2020). The changing narrative in the health insurance industry: Wearables technology in health insurance products and services for the COVID-19 world. *Journal of Health Management*, *22*(4), 550–558)

Okada, F. (2018). Business model changes through collaborative dynamic capabilities through insurance company use of IT (InsurTech) in the medical and health sectors. In *Collaborative dynamic capabilities for service innovation* (pp. 153–162). Palgrave Macmillan, Cham.

Pareek, T., Sood, K., & Grima, S. (2022). The impact of big data technology on the advancement of the insurance industry. In Kiran Sood, Balamurugan Balusamy, Simon Grima, Pierpaolo Marano *Big data analytics in the insurance market* (pp. 221–239). Emerald Publishing Limited.

Paruchuri, H. (2020). The impact of machine learning on the future of insurance industry. *American Journal of Trade and Policy*, *7*(3), 85–90.

Payrovnaziri, S. N., Chen, Z., Rengifo-Moreno, P., Miller, T., Bian, J., Chen, J. H., … He, Z. (2020). Explainable artificial intelligence models using real-world electronic health record data: a systematic scoping review. *Journal of the American Medical Informatics Association*, *27*(7), 1173–1185.

Riikkinen, M., Saarijärvi, H., Sarlin, P., & Lähteenmäki, I. (2018). Using artificial intelligence to create value in insurance. *International Journal of Bank Marketing*, *36*(6), 1145–1168.

Saeed, M., Arshed, N., & Zhang, H. (2022). The adaptation of Internet of Things in the Indian Insurance Industry—Reviewing the challenges and potential solutions. *Electronics*, *11*(3), 419.

Sontakke, D. (2022). Automated underwriting systems: Advancements and challenges in the age of AI. *Journal of Computational Intelligence and Robotics*, *2*(1), 33–53.

Spender, A., Bullen, C., Altmann-Richer, L., Cripps, J., Duffy, R., Falkous, C., … & Yeap, W. (2019). Wearables and the internet of things: Considerations for the life and health insurance industry. *British Actuarial Journal*, *24*, 1–31.

Stoeckli, E., C. Dremel, and F. Uebernickel. (2018). Exploring characteristics and transformational capabilities of InsurTech innovations to understand insurance value creation in a digital world. *Electronic Markets*, *28* (3): 287–305.

Wilkinson, D., Christie, A., Tarr, A. A., & Tarr, J. A. (2024). Big Data, Artificial Intelligence and Insurance. In Paul Embrechts *The Global Insurance Market and Change* (pp. 22–46). Informa Law from Routledge.

Xu, Z., & Dukes, A. (2022). Personalization from customer data aggregation using list Price. *Management Science*, *68*(2), 960–980.

Yan, T. C., Schulte, P., & Chuen, D. L. K. (2018). InsurTech and FinTech: banking and insurance enablement. In Durgesh Kumar Mishra, Rashid Sheikh, Sarika Jain *Handbook of Blockchain, Digital Finance, and Inclusion, Volume 1* (pp. 249–281).

Yeole, A. S., & Kalbande, D. R. (2016, March). Use of Internet of Things (IoT) in healthcare: A survey. In *Proceedings of the ACM Symposium on Women in Research 2016* (pp. 71–76).

Zanke, P., & Sontakke, D. (2021). Artificial Intelligence Applications in Predictive Underwriting for Commercial Lines Insurance. *Advances in Deep Learning Techniques*, *1*(1), 23–38.

17 "Prevention is Better Than Cure" *Relevance of mHealth in Prevention Health Care Industry in India*

S. Vijayalakshmi, Ravi Kiran Erra and Kanika Shetty

17.1 INTRODUCTION

The preventive health care industry has been the most dynamic and evolving sector in the world. The sector aims at assuring well-being and detecting potential health risks at an early stage. This forms a critical step in preventing the critical and challenging treatments which impose both productivity and economic loss (Bajwa et al. 2021). However, it is concerning to observe that illnesses which can be prevented (mainly non-communicable diseases) are responsible for 70% of the global deaths, which majority of them occurring in low- and middle-income countries (WHO). Even a report from the World Bank and WHO (2017) estimated that nearly half of the world population do not have access to essential health care services, which aim at preventive services. At this juncture, adoption of evolving technologies in the healthcare sector needs to become imperative. One can observe increasing research in artificial intelligence (predictive models) for the early detection of diseases (Bajwa et al., 2021; Davenport and Kalakota, 2019; Han & Lee, 2018). The predictive models leverage their data from digital devices like mobile phones known as mHealth (Bhatt et al., 2022). It is estimated that adoption of mHealth itself has reduced health costs by approximately \$14billion and \$3.8billion in Brazil and Mexico, respectively (PwC, 2017). As often observed, the application of technology in the healthcare sector has evolved drastically. Apart from detecting the prevailing health issue or providing sophisticated health care services, technology has ventured into playing a key role in preventive strategies. In this regard, mobile health has high potential to emerge as a level-playing industry in the health care sector.

Mobile health (mHealth) solutions are gaining widespread acceptance in advanced nations, leveraging intelligent applications and artificial intelligence (AI) to revolutionize patient care, diagnostics, and treatment organization. In developing countries, for instance, with a market size of \$111.5billion, China leads the adoption of mHealth

DOI: 10.1201/9781003503385-17

in the world. The pace of adoption in third world economies like Ethiopia is much faster than in the other countries (NIH, 2014). According to World Health organization (WHO, 2013) 83% of 112 member states reported the presence of at least one mHealth initiative in their country. This penetration points out that the future of the healthcare industry lies in the adoption of technology at a much faster rate. However, in the case of India, the penetration and adoption of technology in the healthcare sector require immediate attention. It is reported that nearly 30% of the Indian population do not even have access to public healthcare facilities. Shockingly, India accounts for 21% of the global burden of disease (GBD) (PwC, 2015). According to the GBD report, total disability adjusted life years (DALYs) lost are 51.8 million years for the Indian population (PwC, 2015). One pressing healthcare concern in India is the alarming rise in non-communicable diseases (NCD) like cardiovascular disease (CVD), which has become the top cause of mortality in 2022. NCD, according to WHO, encompasses a range of conditions affecting the heart and blood vessels, diabetes, and certain types of cancer. Looking at ADSI NRCB data (Accidental Death and Suicides by National Crime Records Bureau), there is an 18.32% increase in the mortality rate due to NCD from 2010 to 2016. From 2016 to 2021, there is a further 29.83% increase (Table 17.1). These alarming numbers highlight the importance and urgency of the incorporation of technology like mHealth in the preventive health care industry.

The impact of mobile health (mHealth) applications on healthcare outcomes is multifaceted. On one hand, mHealth enhances accessibility and convenience, empowering individuals to manage their health more effectively. Features like remote monitoring and health tracking apps enable early interventions and personalized care, which often result in improved health outcomes. Numerous studies (Wood et al., 2019; Adans-Dester et al., 2020; Zillner et al., 2023; Aldzhyan et al., 2023; Gopalakrishnan et al., 2020) indicate that mHealth apps can help prevent both chronic and acute illnesses. This highlights the potential of mHealth adoption in early detection and prevention, aiding healthcare professionals in providing tailored care plans that further improve outcomes.

The mHealth market is projected to grow at a Compound Annual Growth Rate (CAGR) of 10.11% by 2026 if embraced widely (India mHealth Market, 2021). Integrating AI into healthcare, especially for NCDs, brings significant advantages. AI-powered tools analyze health data to identify risk markers, enabling timely interventions and disease prevention. Wearables and connected apps ensure continuous monitoring, allowing real-time healthcare interventions that can reduce mortality.

TABLE 17.1
Percentage Increase in Mortality Rate Due to NCD

Year	% Increase in NCD Mortality Rate
2010–2016	18.32
2016–2021	29.83

Source: ADSI (NRCB).

Despite government initiatives like the Swasth Bharat mobile app, National Health Portal, and Vaccine Tracker app, many focus more on providing general information than on prevention. The country is on the brink of a digital health revolution, though challenges remain. In India, 71% of the population owns smartphones, and 46% have internet access (World Bank, 2017). India also ranks among the top five countries for search terms related to mHealth, indicating strong interest. However, challenges like data privacy, security, and inadequate infrastructure hinder full adoption. Moreover, identifying reliable apps from over 119,300 available options remains difficult due to a lack of clinical evaluations and concerns about updates and privacy standards.

In this background, the current paper aims for the twin objectives. One is to evaluate the usage and application of mHealth in the prevention of NCD, using both meta-analysis and primary survey. The second objective of the paper is to examine how the data privacy concerns are addressed under the framework of DISHA (Digital Information Security in Healthcare Act) 2018 & Digital Personal Data Protection Act (2023). To address these objectives, the paper is organized into five sections including the introduction. Section 17.2 reviews the extensive literature both on global and Indian health care systems. Section 17.3 details the data and methodology adopted by the study and Section 17.4 discusses the result. Section 17.5 concludes the study with key policy recommendations.

17.2 REVIEW OF LITERATURE

There are extensive research studies and reports which have explored the different dimensions of the application of technology in the healthcare industry. In this section, the paper looks at the studies which have addressed the application and operation of AI in the preventive health care sector. The study explored the theoretical basis for the adoption of mHealth in the preventive care industry. It is observed that, the application of AI is driven by Cognitive Behavior theory (CBT). The CBT is a modified version of Yale Adherence and Competence Scale. AI-CBT practice ensures effective and efficient adaptation of patients' needs on a daily basis than the standard telephone CBT. With AI, the principles from reinforcement learning aid to automatically adapt to patient's unique and changing needs to focus on pain-related outcomes and treatment response (Piette et al., 2016). It is apparent that, CBT model forms the key theoretical basis for our study to explore the role of mHealth in the preventive health care industry. Under the empirical literature, our study has conducted extensive review of both international and Indian studies. The first section will explore the global studies on the relevance of mHealth in the healthcare industry, followed by the Indian studies.

Among the array of studies which discussed the role of technology (Montazeri et al., 2023; Marcolino et al., 2018; Muralidharan et al., 2017; Larburu et al., 2018; Bashingwa et al., 2023; Menictas et al., 2019; Salinari et al., 2023; Martin et al., 2016) (mainly mobile technology) in detecting and preventing the health issues, we have selected a few to elaborate on in detail in this section. A study by Wilmink et al. (2020) finds the AI-driven digital health platform furnishes community staff with actionable insights into the activities and behavior of each resident of the United

States, aiding in the identification of older adults susceptible to health deterioration. Early intervention based on this data mitigates risks of hospitalization-inducing conditions. Wearables and AI-powered platforms show promise in enhancing health outcomes for seniors in assisted living facilities. Al-Azzam (2021) discusses that mHealth endeavors to augment health service quality, diminish clinical errors, and amalgamate resources, thereby enhancing patient well-being. Remote monitoring via communication devices fosters improved patient-provider interaction. This inquiry examined the impact of mobile health applications on patient management by primary healthcare practitioners. Results indicated a favorable reception toward mobile phone utilization across demographics. Notably, mHealth apps positively influenced healthcare effectiveness, educational outreach, notification services, and consultation. This investigation underscores the pivotal role of mHealth applications in refining patient care within primary healthcare contexts. Even a study by Deniz-Garcia et al. (2023), Stein and Brooks (2017), Berrouiguet et al. (2019), El-Sherif et al. (2022), Xiao et al. (2021), Kayyali et al. (2017) and Fiordelli et al. (2013) underlined the importance of mHealth in revolutionizing preventive health care.

Guan et al. (2021) talk about mHealth applications that have proven instrumental in managing the COVID-19 crisis, aiding infection control efforts globally. However, a notable lack of collaboration among countries and authors persists, hindering the advancement of the mHealth field, which necessitates multidisciplinary expertise. Privacy concerns surrounding mHealth persist, underscoring the need for transparent governmental and institutional regulations governing user data usage. Enhanced awareness of digital health's role in facilitating medical care, particularly in transitioning to virtual visits during emergencies, is imperative for ensuring continuity of care. Adans-Dester et al. (2020) concluded that mHealth technology offers a significant potential in monitoring individuals with mild COVID-19 symptoms during self-quarantine, facilitating early detection of exacerbations and timely interventions. The ongoing digital healthcare transformation, accelerated by the pandemic, enhances the integration of mHealth into clinical workflows, ensuring preparedness for future outbreaks and continuity of care services.

A study by Pham et al. (2019) aimed to review the application of analytic indicators of engagement in evaluations of consumer mHealth apps for chronic conditions, aiming to inform future evaluations. A scoping review identified 41 studies meeting inclusion criteria, with the average evaluation being a two-group pre-test and post-test randomized controlled trial of a hybrid-structured mental health self-management app, involving 103 participants over 5 months. Engagement was typically measured using seven analytic indicators, with variations based on app structure. While most studies presented engagement data descriptively, few explored how app engagement related to health outcomes. Enhancing the measurement of analytic indicators of engagement could improve confidence in mHealth app efficacy for chronic health conditions. Wood et al. (2019) in their paper, using meta-analysis, highlights the convergence of mobile phone-based connectivity with infectious disease diagnostics holds promise for enhancing health. However, deployment challenges persist, and regulatory frameworks must address testing, digital access, and data security.

There are extensive studies on the adoption of AI in detecting health illness. For instance, Zhang et al. (2017) used smartphone-based detection of heart disease in

Singapore. Other AI techniques like recurrent neural network analysis attention-based model (Vaswani et al., 2017), chatbot AI in preventive care (Stein & Brooks, 2017), reinforcement learning algorithm of AI in mobile technology (Menictas et al., 2019), and use of wearable biosensors in preventive care (Wong et al., 2020) have been explored in the industry. Further, Zillner et al. (2023) elucidate the potential role of heart rate variability (HRV) and atrial fibrillation (AF) monitoring through wearable health devices as a pivotal diagnostic tool in cardiac surgery (CS) patients. Through screening pertinent databases, the study revealed that continuous monitoring via wearables has significant cardiac event detection. In a pilot study by Lokker et al. (2021), researchers aimed to assess the feasibility of conducting web-based randomized controlled trials (RCTs) of mHealth apps for patients with cardiovascular risk factors using the Trial My App platform, focusing on an app targeting hypertension. The study involved 200 participants with suboptimally controlled hypertension. Primary outcomes include recruitment, retention, and completion rates, alongside app-entered data validation and app effectiveness in improving hypertension control. The study seeks to inform the feasibility of using Trial My App for evaluating mHealth apps, aiding patients in selecting suitable apps and guiding physicians in evidence-based app recommendations for cardiovascular health improvement.

In a narrative review by Ritchie and Turk (2023), the study explored the potential of telehealth in enhancing the accessibility and effectiveness of diabetes prevention programs (DPPs), specifically focusing on older adults. Hong (2024) examined the prevalence of mobile health and behavior tracking (mHBT) adoption among a diverse sample of cancer survivors in the United States. Data from the 2020 to 2021 Health Information National Trends Survey (HINTS), from three cancer registries, was analyzed. The study highlights the potential of patient-generated data for personalized care and monitoring among cancer survivors but underscores the importance of addressing the digital divide to mitigate health disparities.

17.2.1 Studies on Data Privacy

While there are numerous studies on mHealth adoption in preventive healthcare, concerns regarding data privacy and security persist. Mahendrakhan and Nagarathna (2022) highlighted data-related concerns in mobile health applications. Nittari et al. (Nittari et al., 2019) conducted a review of literature from 2010 to 2019, identifying ethical and legal challenges in telemedicine, including gaps in informed consent, data protection, and provider liability. Their findings stress the need for improved standards and legislation to safeguard patient data and ensure accountability in telemedicine services. Kwon (2023) explored how smart devices and big data convergence are transforming healthcare, offering personalized, faster, and more accurate services. The study analyzed 43 articles from 2007 to 2023, demonstrating the potential of smart devices in clinical, preventive, and public health. These technologies enable real-time health monitoring and the promotion of healthy lifestyles through personalized interventions. In Germany, the Digital Healthcare Act mandates evidence-based assessment of digital health apps (DiGA). Dittrich et al. (2023) found that many DiGA apps lacked sufficient evidence of efficacy, raising concerns about patient safety and the need for robust evaluation tools. Overall, while mHealth adoption is impressive globally, significant challenges surrounding data privacy and security must be addressed to ensure widespread and safe use.

17.2.2 Review of Literature – India

A study done by Gopalakrishnan et al. (2020) aimed to examine CHW (Community Health Workers) and beneficiaries' perceptions of a new mHealth intervention (Common Application Software [CAS]) in India. While technology serves as a facilitator for CHWs to enhance service delivery, it may not inherently address social and cultural obstacles hindering CHW-beneficiary interactions needed to foster improvements in knowledge and health behaviors. Future interventions tailored for CHWs, including mHealth initiatives, ought to assess contextual factors in conjunction with assessing acceptability, accessibility, and usability by beneficiaries and community stakeholders.

A study by Feinberg et al. (Feinberg et al., 2016) conducted in Kerala, India, highlights the potential of mHealth interventions in addressing CVD and other NCD. Despite high mobile phone ownership and willingness to receive mHealth advice and medication reminders, preference for voice calls over SMS suggests SMS interventions may not fully reach all patient groups. Most participants trust the confidentiality of mHealth data. While mHealth shows promise, further research is needed to explore its efficacy as a health education tool, with consideration for equitable access across patient demographics. In a similar line, Kumar and Gill, 2020 and Sarangi and Challa (2016) investigate the awareness and usage of mHealth apps among Indians, revealing that age significantly influences perceptions and adoption rates, with younger demographics showing higher usage.

A study by Goswami et al. (2023) assesses the usability of a mobile health app aimed at enhancing type 2 diabetes mellitus (T2DM) health literacy in India. Findings indicate positive user perceptions, particularly among young, educated, urban individuals. The study recommends enhancing app content and providing multilingual options. Overall, results suggest confidence in replicating the app's interface for future health education apps, while identifying areas for improvement, informing the development of more user-friendly health literacy tools. Studies like Murthy et al. (2020) on maternal care, Kaurani (2020) on oral care (Cancer) indicate that the application of mHealth will have a positive impact on the preventive strategy adoption in the health care sector. Even a meta-analysis conducted by Joshi et al. (2023) supports the argument. Gunamany (2022) says that in poor and developing countries, where healthcare costs surpass income levels, the underserved market combined with high mobile phone penetration offers favorable conditions for mHealth adoption. Challenges persist, including the need for training healthcare practitioners and addressing research and investment gaps.

A study by Skaria (2013) underscores the challenge posed by low literacy levels in effectively delivering mHealth information via mobile phones. Subsequently, subscription-based models may deter usage among underprivileged populations. To address this, innovative strategies are necessary to leverage mobile phones as accessible health education tools. Solutions include audible and readable message delivery, integration with health information systems, and automated reminders for appointments and medication. These approaches aim to enhance mHealth adoption and dissemination of vital health information among rural populations.

Amidst these global developments, India, with its colossal population of approximately 1.43 billion people, is experiencing significant strides in technology and healthcare. The healthcare sector remains at the epicenter of both challenges and opportunities in the country. Government initiatives like the BharatNet Udyami Project have connected rural villagers to fiber-optic networks, marking a crucial step forward. The World Bank (2017) reports a notable 46% internet penetration in India. Despite this progress, the integration of technology, particularly mobile health (mHealth), is still in its initial stages.

Despite the advantages of mHealth, like reducing healthcare costs, convenient access to provider, and ability to obtain information, there persist numerous impediments. Poor infrastructure, data concerns, lack of awareness, huge volume and fragmented market, low expectations, manual market, and emergence of non-reliable applications are the key issues to be addressed. Among these various concerns, penetration challenges of mHealth in preventive care industry and the data security concerns are of prime importance. As per a PwC study (PwC, 2012), the top barriers for providers of mHealth are the lack of interest among key users, culture of medical professionals, and lack of information on mHealth. In this background, the current study attempted to fill the research gap identified from the review of literature regarding the awareness level about the importance of mHealth in preventive health care industry. Further, the study also explored the data privacy concerns of mHealth among the users.

17.3 RESEARCH METHODOLOGY AND DATA

To address the objective of the study, the study conducted a primary survey to assess the adoption and awareness of data privacy of mHealth applications. Since, the objective of the study is to assess the usage, the respondents are collected from different age groups of urban population[1] in India. Using Cochran (1977) sample size formula, the study collected a total of 385 samples, out of which 33 responses were non-responses. Hence, to avoid non-response error, the study considered a total of 352 as our total sample size. The responses are collected using a structured questionnaire. Both direct and online interviews were conducted. The survey questionnaire contained three parts, namely, socio-economic profile, mHealth usage, and data privacy concerns. The study has conducted a pilot survey in the month of December 2023 to validate the questionnaire. The main survey was conducted for three months from February 2024 to April 2024. Before pursuing the survey with the respondents, all respondents were informed about the research and the data confidentiality and gave consent for their participation[2].

17.4 DATA RESULT AND DISCUSSION

This section is classified into three sections. Section 17.4.1 provides the socio-economic details of the respondents, Section 17.4.2 details the usage of the app, and

Section 17.4.3 explores the data privacy awareness among the users. At the outset, as the study is conducted to know the adoption of mHealth in preventive healthcare strategies, the respondents are selected randomly across different age groups. Since the first objective of the study is to know the reach and adoption of mHealth, it is hypothesized that, smartphone users might be the active users of mHealth applications. However, contrasting to this, our results rejected the hypothesis stating that not all the smartphone users adopt to mHealth. That is to say, among the total 352 respondents, nearly 61% (i.e. 214) of respondents use the mHealth application, and the remaining 39% (i.e. 138) (Figure 17.1) are either not aware or state that they do not find the requirement of such applications.

In order to investigate the non-adoption of mHealth app among 39%, the study probed the reasons to get deeper insights. Surprisingly, the study found that nearly 34% of respondents are not even aware of the existence of mobile health applications. Further, around 66% stated that they did not find the requirement of such applications. This highlights the lack of awareness and need among the respondents in the adoption of mHealth in preventive healthcare.

17.4.1 Socio-Economic Profile

This section provides details about the socio-economic status of the respondents, namely, age, gender, education, profession, and income. Before providing further analysis, as the study is based on random sample observations, we have targeted those respondents who use smartphones. In the gender profile, it is observed that nearly 55% of the respondents are female, and rest (44%) are male respondents. Though gender variation is not expected to have any relevance in the study (as pointed out by Sarangi and Challa 2016), the same hypothesis has been assumed in the study. From Figure 17.2 we can observe that there is variation of gender across the age group in the use of mHealth applications. This provides an interesting insight that, age-wise gender has crucial implications on the use of mHealth application.

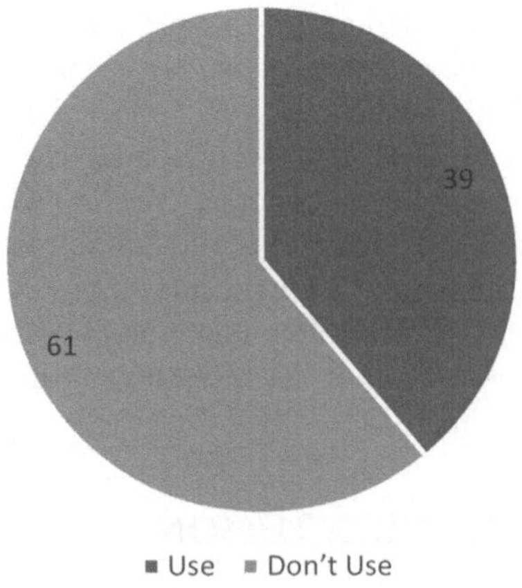

FIGURE 17.1 Percentages of respondents using mHealth applications.

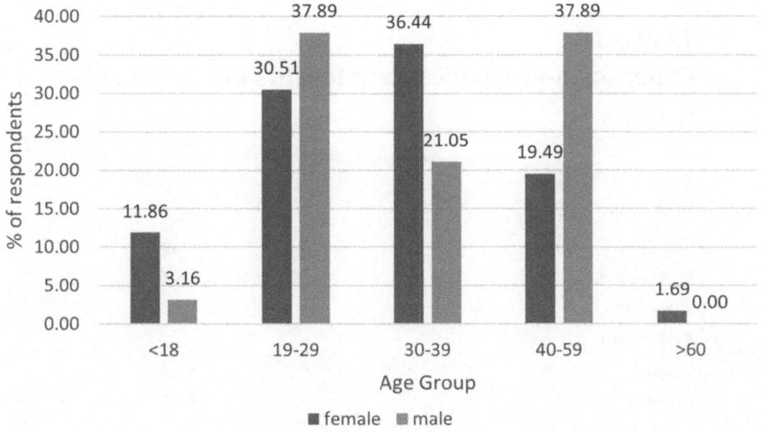

FIGURE 17.2 Variation of gender across the age group using mHealth applications.

For instance, around 37.8% males who belong to younger age group (19–29 years) prefer mHealth application. This can be related to fitness goals among younger males than the counterparts. However, when it comes to the age group of 30–39, female respondents are found to be majority (36.4%). This may be related to the adoption of tracking women-related health issues in the middle age group. Further, male users top in the usage among 40–59 years of age group. This can be related to the adoption for tracking key health indicators like Blood Pressure (BP), Health rates etc., which are common among this age group.

The socio-economic features of the respondents include the education, profession, and income of the respondents which are provided in Table 17.2. We can observe from the data that, as education level is increasing, the use of mHealth applications is also increasing. This indicates that education will have an influence on the use of mHealth applications. The profession of the respondents is classified into three levels[3]. It is observed that level 1 and 2 profession respondents are more adaptive to mHealth app compared to other levels. This might be linked to the type of activity and level of education of the respondents. In the case of income, the respondents belonging to the income level within Rs. 5 lakh (37.6%) and Rs. 5–10 lakh (25.3) per year have higher adoption of the technology. This indicates that, respondents belonging to the middle-income group are more responsive to the mHealth adoption.

17.4.2 Usage and Purpose of mHealth Adoption

The main objective of the study is to explore the nature or purpose of mHealth adoption by the respondents. To investigate this, the study probed the respondents regarding the efficiency of the application in the assumed usage. From the data of 61% of the respondents who reported that they use the mHealth applications, the study elucidated the timeline of adoption. It is important to note here that, as the adoption of mHealth applications has surged after COVID-19 (Singh et al., 2020), the study classified the adoption timeline into three time periods based on COVID-19. It is quite

TABLE 17.2
Other socio-economic characteristics of respondents

Education	**% of respondents**
Primary schooling	0.7
Secondary schooling	1.5
PU/Intermediate	8.4
Graduate/Diploma	54.6
Postgraduate	29.2
Above PG	5.39
Profession	
Level 1	52.3
Level 2	35.3
Level 3	12.3
Annual Income	
No income	11.5
< Rs. 5 lakhs	37.6
Rs. 5-10 lakh	25.3
Rs. 11-20 lakh	8.4
Rs. 21-30 lakh	6.15
Above Rs. 30 lakhs	10.7

Source: Primary Survey, 2024.

interesting to know that nearly 47% of the respondents reported that they started the use of mHealth app before COVID (Figure 17.3). Around 41.5% of the respondents started the use of mHealth app after the COVID period.

Various studies in the literature (Deniz-Garcia et al. 2023; Stein & Brooks, 2017; Berrouiguet et al., 2019; El-Sherif et al., 2022; Meheli et al., 2022; Xiao et al. 2021) indicated that, though there is high potentiality of mHealth apps in preventive health care industry, its adoption might require self-motivation or advice from the medical expert. To examine this in the case of India, the respondents are inquired about the source of recommendation to use the applications. It is quite interesting to note that nearly 70% of the respondents stated that, they are using the mobile health application on their self-interest (Table 17.3). This indicates the self-awareness about the health outcomes is a significant factor in adoption of mHealth among the study respondents. Even the recommendations from friends (11.5%) and fitness coach (10%) hold a significant portion. The more concerning fact is that the recommendations from doctor forms only 4.6%. Even the focused group discussions with medical experts or practitioners revealed that the adoption and the recommendation of the mHealth apps from their community need to be improved significantly. It can be observed that people who do not adopt mHealth (39% in the sample) can be motivated by the medical experts. This not only promotes health tracking but also helps in boosting the preventive care industry.

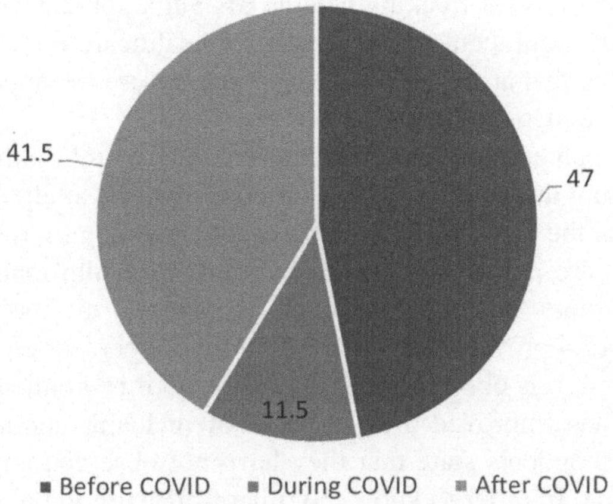

FIGURE 17.3 Percentage of respondents using mHealth applications before, during, and after COVID-19.

TABLE 17.3
Source and purpose of mHealth app recommendations (% of respondents)

Source	**% of respondents**
Doctor	4.6
Friend	11.5
Family/relative	3.8
Fitness coach	10
Self	70
Purpose of the use	
Tracking fitness	58.4
Tracking health (BP, Sugar etc.)	37
Others*	4.6

* Includes menstrual cycle; Source: Primary Survey, 2024.

After the source of recommendation, the study tried to explore the purpose of the usage of mHealth. To facilitate systematic analysis of the purpose of the usage of mHealth application, the study organized a set of predefined categories encompassing common reasons for usage (these categories are based on studies by Han & Lee, 2018 and Pilot survey, 2023). As the health applications are multifunctional, the responses have multiple choices. Respondents aligned their usage intentions with the provided categories and selected the appropriate option accordingly. It is surprising to note that, the majority (around 58.4%) of the respondents use the mHealth application for tracking their fitness in terms of counting steps, calory intake and other physical activities. These tracking are observed to benefit in preventing certain lifestyle-related illnesses. Around 37% of the respondents also reported that they use the mHealth applications for tracking health (BP, Sugar, pO2, respiratory rate, etc.). These adoptions are significant in the preventive healthcare industry. However, it is also important to see that around 4.6% of respondents use the app for tracking other health outcomes like menstrual cycle.

To explore the perceptions regarding the efficacy of mHealth applications and devices in preventing and addressing health concerns, the study examined whether the respondents use the application as the preventive strategies, to ascertain whether these technologies are perceived as proactive aids in health management, encompassing early problem detection, prompt assistance, and potential emergency responses. Figure 17.4 provides the details about these perceptions.

From Figure 17.4, it is observed that the majority of respondents (73%) perceive that, their health has improved after the use of mHealth applications. However, around 27% of respondents state that they have not observed any improvement in their health outcome. In order to know the role of mHealth in preventive healthcare, the respondents are probed to elicit their perception on whether the use of mHealth app has prevented any health issue. It is interesting to know that a majority of 70% of respondents are not sure about the prevention (Figure 17.5). This indicates a lack of information to the users regarding preventive healthcare options from the use of mHealth. A key implication for this is that perception of users has significant influence on the adoption of mHealth. Research studies (Bashingwa et al., 2023; Salinari et al., 2023; Menictas et al., 2019 and many) have extensively indicated the enormous possibility of mHealth apps in preventive healthcare industry.

Though respondents viewing mHealth as preventive health care tool is still emerging in the country, the study tried to explore the type of disease that is being prevented by mHealth apps and devices. Considering the functions of mHealth in preventing illnesses, diseases are categorized into groups such as NCD like respiratory conditions, and cancer and communicable diseases like COVID-19 and other illnesses (gynic-related, healthy diet, etc.). These categories were chosen based on

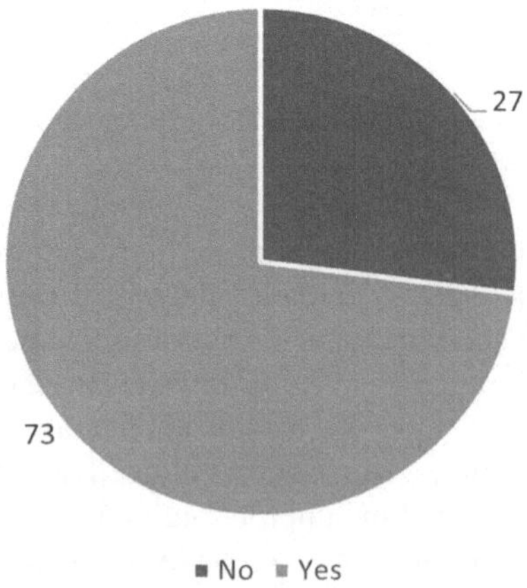

FIGURE 17.4 Percentage of respondents think that their health has improved after using mHealth applications.

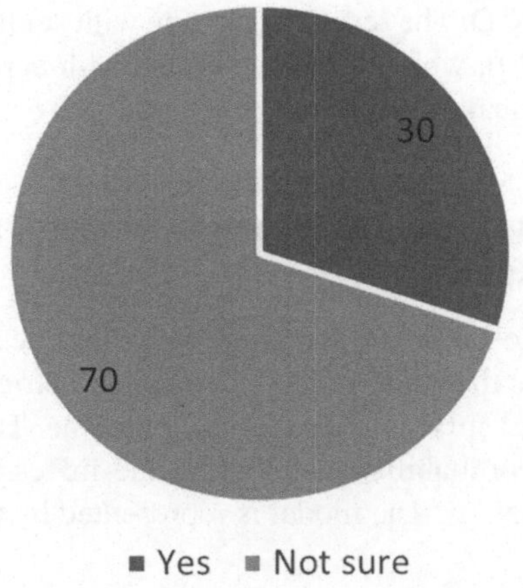

FIGURE 17.5 Percentage of respondents with a perception on whether the use of mHealth app has prevented any health issue.

the predominant areas where mHealth interventions are known to be effective. Figure 17.6 provides valuable insights into how respondents perceive the preventive abilities of mHealth apps and devices across different disease types. Among the respondents who reported that they were able to prevent or detect the health issues (30%), nearly 48% of the respondents opined that they were able to prevent/detect NCD. These NCD includes cardiovascular diseases, diabetes, and others. Around 30% of respondents said they were able to detect communicable diseases like COVID at an early stage. There are around 22% of respondents who opted for other health issues. This finding elucidated the key implication that adoption of mHealth has high

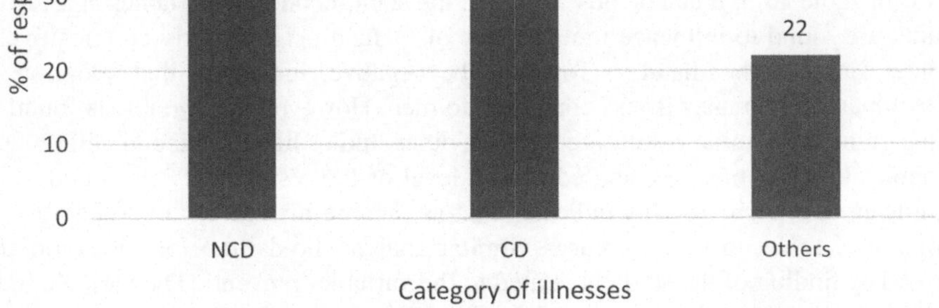

FIGURE 17.6 Percentage of respondents with a specific category of illness.

potential in preventing NCD. The results are in line with studies like El-Sherif (2022), Adans-Dester et al. (2020), which discuss that mHealth apps play a significant role in preventing certain critical health issues.

17.4.3 Factors Influencing the Adoption of mHealth: Binary Logit Regression Results

Further, it is important to know the factors influencing the adoption of mHealth in the case of India. For this the study relied on an econometric approach as the dependent variable (adoption of mHealth) is a binary outcome. The binary logit model is employed to model the probability of adopting the mHealth application based on various independent variables. The model is represented by the formula:

$$P(Y = 1 \backslash X) = \frac{1}{1 + e - (\beta 0 + \beta 1X1 + \beta 2X2 + \cdots + \beta nXn)} \tag{17.1}$$

Here, Y represents the binary outcome, X denotes the independent variables, and β signifies the coefficients. The binary logit regression results are presented in terms of odds ratios and marginal effects. Odds ratios reveal the impact of independent variables on the odds of adoption, while marginal effects denote the change in the probability of adoption due to a unit change in the independent variable.

$$\text{Odds Ratio Formula:} = \text{OR} = e^{\beta} \tag{17.2}$$

$$\text{Marginal Effects Formula : Marginal Effect} = \beta \times P(Y = 1) \times (1 - P(Y = 1)) \tag{17.3}$$

The description of the variables is provided in Table 17.4.

The logit regression results are provided in Table 17.4. The model LR chi2 (14) is 77.31 with p value less than zero indicating that the model is fit. Pseudo R2 is 0.17 and the log likelihood is –187.20. The model result provides key insights into the factors affecting the adoption of mHealth in preventive healthcare in India.

From Table 17.5, it can be observed that the socio-economic variables apart from gender are found to influence the adoption of mHealth significantly and positively. Gender, on the other hand, is found to be negative, indicating that adoption of mHealth among females is less compared to men. However, the variable is found to be insignificant. Similar results are found in other studies like Kumar and Gill (2020). Variables like income, age, and education level of the respondents are found to be significant and positive. This indicates that as income increases, the probability of adoption of mHealth also increases. Similar analysis holds true for education and age. A key finding of the study is related to the variable 'prevent'. The variable indicates the perception of respondents in preventing any health issue due to the use of mHealth. This is found from the model result that; the variable is positive and

TABLE 17.4
Description of variables

Variables	Description
Adp_mhealth (Dependent variable)	0-No; 1-Yes
Gender (Gen)	1-Female (Base Category) 0-Male
Education	Secondary:1; 0=otherwise (Base Category) PUC:1; 0=otherwise Graduate and Higher:1; 0=otherwise
Age	Age1: <21 years:1; 0=otherwise(Base Category) Age2: 22–40 years:1; 0=otherwise Age3: 41–50 years:1; 0=otherwise Age4: 51years and above: 1; 0=otherwise
Income (Y)	Y0: Zero income:1; 0=otherwise (Base Category) Y1: <5LPA:1; 0=otherwise Y2: 5-10LPA:1; 0=otherwise Y3: 11-20 LPA:1; 0=otherwise Y4: 20LPA+:1; 0=otherwise
Professional level	Level 1:1; 0=otherwise Level 2:1; 0=otherwise Level 3:1; 0=otherwise (Base Category)
Prevented any health issue (prevent)	0: No 1: Yes

TABLE 17.5
Binary Logit Regression results

Variables	OR[a]	SE[b]	dy/dx[c]	SE[b]
Gen	-0.16	0.27	-0.03	0.05
PUC	3.28***	0.81	0.66***	0.10
Graduate	3.66***	0.64	0.53***	0.05
Y1	1.42***	0.52	0.29***	0.10
Y2	1.54***	0.59	0.33***	0.12
Y3	1.26***	0.80	0.29***	0.19
Y4	0.51**	0.71	0.91**	0.11
Age2	0.60*	0.57	0.11*	0.10
Age3	0.26**	0.48	0.05**	0.09
Age4	1.02***	0.70	0.22***	0.15
Level1	-0.73	0.52	0.16	0.12
Level2	-0.26	0.37	0.05	0.07
Prevent	8.4***	1.23	0.09***	0.06
constant	5.13***	1.04	-	-

a Odds Ratio.
b Standard Error.
c dy/dx: Marginal effect.

significant. This indicates that respondents who perceive the role of mHealth app in prevention of health issue have higher probability of adoption of the technology by 9%. This makes an important contribution of the study to the existing literature that, perceptions of mHealth app users have significant impact on the preventive health care industry.

17.4.4 Awareness Regarding Data Privacy of mHealth Apps/Devices

The second objective of the study is to understand the awareness regarding the privacy issues of the data being captured by mHealth applications. It has been argued in the literature that the data related to health is not only key information but also serves sensitive information of the person (Mahendrakhan & Nagarathna, 2022). This indicates that the privacy of the information becomes very crucial. The data privacy concerns are well taken by the developed countries like the United States under HIPAA (Health Insurance Portability and Accountability Act, 1996), Data Protection Directive 1995/46/EC, and the e-Privacy Directive 2002/58/EC/IEC 62304 in Europe and many countries. The similar data privacy regulation is provided in India under DISHA (Digital Information Security in Health Care Act, 2018) and Digital Personal Data Protection Act (DPDPA) in 2023. The regulations require that the applications should maintain the utmost level of security regarding the data collected from their database. To understand whether the consumers are aware of these data privacy concerns, the survey has explored whether they are aware of these legalities, and at least do they observe that their data is being protected by the applications. This line of inquiry sheds light on the prevailing level of public knowledge concerning a critical yet often overlooked aspect of the digital data security landscape. There is a common tendency among users to accept terms and conditions without fully comprehending the implications, particularly in the context of health-related technologies. However, given the sensitive nature of health data, individuals may exhibit heightened awareness and scrutiny regarding data capture practices in this domain. The study explored the status of awareness of data privacy in Figure 17.7. It is quite evident that nearly 70% of respondents are aware that their health data is being captured by their mHealth applications. Around 20% of respondents are not sure of it, and the remaining 10% reported that they are not aware of it.

It may be possible that users might be aware of the data being captured by the application, but the more concerning is the trust regarding the data privacy norms by the app providers. To explore this, the study probed the respondents regarding their trust in the mHealth apps, and the result indicates that nearly 52.3% of respondents trust that their data is maintained safely by the app providers. However, around 27% of respondents are not sure of it, and the remaining 20.7% opine that they do not trust the app providers regarding data privacy.

Given this outcome on the trust of data privacy, the study is further motivated to explore the users' awareness regarding the laws governing data privacy called DPDPA (2023). DPDPA provides a pivotal piece of legislation that governs data privacy and security within the healthcare sector, encompassing provisions aimed at safeguarding sensitive health data and ensuring individual privacy rights. Given this legislation in place, it is quite interesting to know whether the users are aware of the

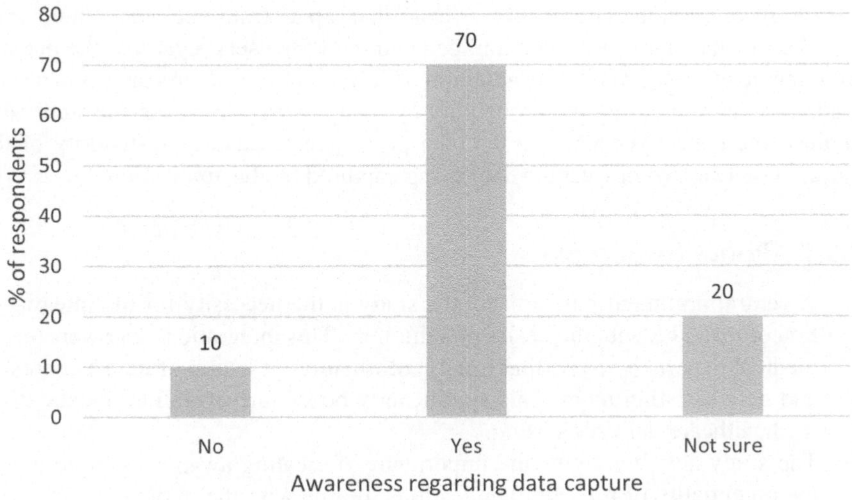

FIGURE 17.7 Percentage of respondents with awareness on data capture.

existence and implications of such laws. To capture this, the study probed the respondents on whether they are aware of such laws. It is quite surprising to know that the majority of respondents (86%) lack such awareness. This forms a key finding of the study, indicating that awareness regarding data privacy should be enhanced in the mHealth aspects.

17.5 SUMMARY AND CONCLUSION

The future of diagnostics is digital, offering transformative potential for healthcare systems. In this regard, mHealth embodies significant potential, especially in the preventive healthcare industry. While mHealth holds a promising step toward transformative healthcare delivery, its success depends on the usage, engagement and mainly the data privacy aspects. In this regard, the present study explored the perceptions of users of mHealth as a preventive tool. It is evident from the literature that, for India, mHealth acts as a game-changer in the healthcare sector. Even this study's findings indicate that mHealth can emerge as a pivotal tool in revolutionizing preventive healthcare industry.

Some of the key findings of the study are pertained to highlight the potentiality and challenges to overcome the adoption of mHealth in the Indian context. The study observes that the majority of the users are aware of the potential of mHealth in improving their health. However, there is non-adoption of mHealth due to the perception that there is no requirement due to lack of awareness. This can be related to the lack of integration between users and the medical sector. Only 4.6% of the users have adopted the mHealth for doctor recommendations. This forms the key gap in the reach of mHealth. Further, those who have adopted mHealth, majority (70%) are not aware of the preventive capabilities of application. However, those who adopted reported that they were able to prevent NCDs from the use of mHealth. The study has extended its scope to explore the factors affecting the adoption of mHealth using binary logit regression. The results indicate that, apart from socio-economic variables like income, age, and education, perception of the users regarding the prevention of the health issue due to the adoption of mHealth has a significant influence on the adoption by increasing the probability by nine percent. However, the study also examined the concerns regarding the data privacy and found that, majority of the users are not aware of or trust the data being captured by the application.

17.5.1 Policy Implications

- A central argument put forth by the study is the necessity for the integration of mHealth with the health practitioners. This integration empowers the medical experts by providing timely information of health of their patients and help assisting them. This significantly boosts the overall efficiency of the healthcare delivery system.
- The study also highlights the importance of creating awareness regarding the potentiality of mHealth applications. In line with the findings of Wood (2019), and Senbekov et al. (2020), awareness of digital health and also privacy concerns of mHealth apps are crucial in the healthcare industry. However, lack of awareness of overall efficacy of mHealth application in the preventive strategy section hinders the comprehensive implications of the technology. It should be noted here that, providing proper and timely guidance regarding the application of mHealth as a preventive strategy tool can provide significant impact on the improvement of health in the Indian domain. It is estimated that mHealth could provide an additional 28.4 million people with access to the healthcare system in Brazil and an additional 15.5 million people with access in Mexico without adding a doctor.
- The Government must allocate the resources and capitalize on the utilization of mHealth, given its substantial potential to contribute to the country's development (PwC, 2017). Though the Government of India, through the website of the National Health portal, created by the Ministry of Health and Family Welfare, took a lot of initiative (even created a body called National e-Health Authority) to showcase several health apps and initiatives to the development of the apps, a proper education regarding the usage is the need of the hour. One such initiative that the Government of India can follow is by adopting MAiHEALTH initiative of a mobile and virtual medical center started in rural Patea. In this initiative, teachers conduct essential health assessments, upload the data to the cloud, and transmit the information to centralized digital health teams. This team can quickly assess the information; clinicians approve treatment plans, and prescriptions are sent to parents or caregivers. With this collected information, the pattern of disease can be extracted and then taught to digital health assessors. This innovative approach holds the potential to reduce emergency visits and hospitalizations, marking a significant step toward more efficient and accessible preventive healthcare delivery.
- Lastly, the study makes a key policy suggestion regarding the data privacy concerns of mHealth applications. As the study found that majority of the

users are not aware of the data privacy and its related legalities, assuring its security should be prime concern. This can be adopted via blockchain technology as suggested by Mahendrakhan and Nagarathna (2022). At the outset, the study makes an important and key policy recommendation to make mHealth as an imperative tool in the preventive health care industry.

The effectiveness of mHealth interventions also depends on factors like user engagement and the integration of these technologies into existing healthcare systems. While mHealth holds promise in transforming healthcare delivery, its success depends on addressing challenges and ensuring widespread acceptance and usability within diverse healthcare settings.

17.5.2 Limitations of the Study

- The study explored the mHealth potentiality in general. Further research can explore the specific application potentiality.
- The study considered urban users of mHealth. However, the rural respondents can be included in the future study.
- The study was limited examining the data privacy norms adopted by the app providers. The study mainly looked at the user perception rather than the provider perception.

NOTES

1 As the penetration of smartphones are high in urban area, we hypothesized that, penetration of mHealth will be adequate.

2 As our study does not involve any criteria as per https://www.bio.cam.ac.uk/psyres/ approval, we proceeded to our survey.

3 First level of employees includes professionals like doctors, chief engineers, professors, general managers, purchase managers, team managers, sales managers, project managers, and chief executives;

Second (middle) level employees include assistant managers, assistant engineers, assistant admin officers, second division clerks, supervisors, assistant HR, Business associates, floor managers, executive engineers, traffic police constables, operational assistants, and senior process managers;

Third (entry) level employees include positions like salespersons, construction workers, carpenters, security guards, street vendors, cleaners, mechanics, petty shop owners, trainees, drivers, and service boys. This level also includes informal sector employees, students, and homemakers.

REFERENCES

Adans-Dester CP et al. (2020) Can mHealth Technology Help Mitigate the Effects of the COVID-19 Pandemic? *IEEE Open Journal of Engineering in Medicine and Biology* 1, 243–248, doi: 10.1109/OJEMB.2020.3015141

Al-Azzam MK (2021). Research on the Impact of mHealth Apps on the Primary Healthcare Professionals in Patient Care. *Appl Bionics Biomech.* 7611686. doi: 10.1155/2021/7611686

Aldzhyan V, Tamamian C, Tabibian JH. (2023) Leveraging telemedicine in gastroenterology and hepatology: a narrative review. *Mhealth.* doi: 10.21037/mhealth-23-27

Bajwa J, Munir U, Nori A, Williams B. (2021) Artificial intelligence in healthcare: transforming the practice of medicine. *Future Healthcare Journal.* 8(2):e188-e194. doi: 10.7861/fhj.2021-0095

Bashingwa J.J.H., Mohan D., Chamberlain S., Scott K., Ummer O., Godfrey A., Mulder N., Moodley D., Lefevre A.E. (2023) Can we design the next generation of digital health communication programs by leveraging the power of artificial intelligence to segment target audiences, bolster impact and deliver differentiated services? A machine learning analysis of survey data from rural India. *BMJ Open* 13(1) doi: 10.1136/bmjopen-2022-063354

Berrouiguet S., Barrigón M.L., Castroman J.L., Courtet P., Artés-Rodríguez A., Baca-García E. Lim H.-A., Vy P.D.T., Choi J. (2019) Combining mobile-health (mHealth) and artificial intelligence (AI) methods to avoid suicide attempts: The Smartcrises study protocol. *BMC Psychiatry* 19 (1). Doi: 10.1186/s12888-019-2260-y

Bhatt P, Liu J, Gong Y, Wang J, Guo Y. (2022). Emerging Artificial Intelligence-Empowered mHealth: Scoping Review. *JMIR Mhealth Uhealth.* 10(6):e35053. doi: 10.2196/35053

Cochran, W.G. (1977) *Sampling Techniques*. 3rd Edition, John Wiley & Sons, New York.

Davenport T, Kalakota R. (2019) The potential for artificial intelligence in healthcare. *Future Healthcare Journal.* 6(2):94–98. doi: 10.7861/futurehosp.6-2-94

Deniz-Garcia A, Fabelo H, Rodriguez-Almeida AJ, Zamora-Zamorano G, Castro-Fernandez M, Alberiche Ruano MDP, Solvoll T, Granja C, Schopf TR, Callico GM, Soguero-Ruiz C, Wägner AM; WARIFA Consortium. (2023) Quality, Usability, and Effectiveness of mHealth Apps and the Role of Artificial Intelligence: Current Scenario and Challenges. *J Med Internet Res.* 4;25:e44030. doi: 10.2196/44030

Dittrich F, Mielitz A, Pustozerov E, Lawin D, von Jan U, Albrecht UV. (2023) Digital health applications from a government-regulated directory of reimbursable health apps in Germany-a systematic review for evidence and bias. *Mhealth.* 9:35. doi: 10.21037/mhealth-23-17

El-Sherif DM, Abouzid M, Elzarif MT, Ahmed AA, Albakri A, Alshehri MM. (2022) Telehealth and Artificial Intelligence Insights into Healthcare during the COVID-19 Pandemic. *Healthcare.* 10(2):385. doi: 10.3390/healthcare10020385

Feinberg L, Menon J, Smith R, Rajeev JG, Kumar RK, Banerjee A. Potential for mobile health (mHealth) prevention of cardiovascular diseases in Kerala: A population-based survey. (2016) *Indian Heart J.* 69(2):182–199. doi: 10.1016/j.ihj.2016.11.004

Fiordelli M, Diviani N, Schulz P (2013) Mapping mHealth Research: A Decade of Evolution. *J Med Internet Res* 15(5):e95; doi:10.2196/jmir.2430

Gopalakrishnan L, Buback L, Fernald L, Walker D, Diamond-Smith N, et al. (2020) Using mHealth to improve health care delivery in India: A qualitative examination of the perspectives of community health workers and beneficiaries. *PLOS ONE*, 15(1): e0227451. Doi: 10.1371/journal.pone.0227451

Goswami, R., Garner, S. L., & George, C. E. (2023). Usability of an mHealth application in India for type 2 diabetes mellitus. *Health Education Journal*, 82(1), 108–116. Doi: 10.1177/00178969221138483

Guan G, Dery Yotam, Yechezkel Matan, Ben-Gal Irad, Yamin Dan, Brandeau Margaret L. (2021) Early detection of COVID-19 outbreaks using human mobility. *PloS One*, *16*(7), e0253865. Doi: 10.1371/journal.pone.0253865

Gunamany, S. (2022). Utility of mHealth initiatives in the Indian context. *International Journal of Community Medicine and Public Health*, 9(5), 2326–2330. Doi: 10.18203/2394-6040.ijcmph20221260

Han, M, Lee, E. (2018) Effectiveness of mobile health application use to improve health behavior changes: A systematic review of randomized controlled trials. *Healthc Inform Res.* 24(3):207–226. doi: 10.4258/hir.2018.24.3.207

Hong, YA. (2024) Mobile health and behavior tracking (mHBT) among cancer survivors: results from a large and diverse sample. *Mhealth.* 2024 Jan 4;10:5. doi: 10.21037/mhealth-23-58

India Mhealth Market (2021) - Forecasts from 2021 to 2026. Accessed from: India Mhealth Market - Forecasts from 2021 to 2026 (researchandmarkets.com)

Joshi V, Joshi N, Bhardwaj P, Singh K, Ojha D, Jain Y. (2023) The Health Impact of mHealth Interventions in India: Systematic Review and Meta-Analysis. *Online J Public Health Inform* 15:e50927. https://ojphi.jmir.org/2023/1/e50927; DOI: 10.2196/50927

Kaurani, Pragati. (2020). Oral cancer and mHealth in India: An overview. International Journal of Scientific Research ((PDF) Oral cancer and mHealth in India: An overview (researchgate.net))

Kayyali R, Peletidi A, Ismail M, Hashim Z, Bandeira P, Bonnah J. (2017) Awareness and Use of mHealth Apps: A Study from England. *Pharmacy*. 5(2):33. Doi: 10.3390/pharmacy5020033

Kumar, Sanjiv & Gill, Shikha. (2020). Awareness, Usage of mHealth Apps and Consequent Health-Seeking Behaviour Changes Amongst Smartphone Users in India https://www.researchgate.net/publication/344362474_Awareness_Usage_of_mHealth_Apps_and_Consequent_Health_Seeking_Behaviour_Changes_Amongst_Smartphone_Users_in_India

Kwon KH (2023). Utilization of smart devices and the evolution of customized healthcare services focusing on big data: a systematic review. *Mhealth*. 10:7. doi: 10.21037/mhealth-23-24

Larburu N., Artetxe A., Escolar V., Lozano A., Kerexeta J. (2018) Artificial intelligence to prevent mobile heart failure patients decompensation in real time: Monitoring-based predictive model. *Mobile Information Systems*. Doi: 10.1155/2018/1546210

Lokker C, Jezrawi R, Gabizon I, Varughese J, Brown M, Trottier D, Alvarez E, Schwalm J, McGillion M, Ma J, Bhagirath V (2021) Feasibility of a Web-Based Platform (Trial My App) to Efficiently Conduct Randomized Controlled Trials of mHealth Apps For Patients With Cardiovascular Risk Factors: Protocol For Evaluating an mHealth App for Hypertension. *JMIR Res Protoc* 10(2):e26155. DOI: 10.2196/26155

Mahendrakhan K., Nagarathna P. (2022) Cyber Security in Healthcare with Artificial Intelligence. *MysuruCon 2022 – 2022 IEEE 2nd Mysore Sub Section International Conference*. Doi: 10.1109/MysuruCon55714.2022.9972597

Marcolino MS, Oliveira JAQ, D'Agostino M, Ribeiro AL, Alkmim MBM, Novillo-Ortiz D (2018) The Impact of mHealth Interventions: Systematic Review of Systematic Reviews. *JMIR Mhealth Uhealth*. 6(1):e23. doi: 10.2196/mhealth.8873

Martin CK, Gilmore LA, Apolzan JW, Myers CA, Thomas DM, Redman LM. (2016) Smartloss: A Personalized Mobile Health Intervention for Weight Management and Health Promotion. *JMIR Mhealth Uhealth*. 4(1):e18. doi: 10.2196/mhealth.5027

Meheli S., Sinha C., Kadaba M. (2022) Understanding People With Chronic Pain Who Use a Cognitive Behavioral Therapy-Based Artificial Intelligence Mental Health App (Wysa): Mixed Methods Retrospective Observational Study. *JMIR Human Factors*. 9(2) doi: 10.2196/35671

Menictas M., Rabbi M., Klasnja P., Murphy S. (2019) Artificial intelligence decision-making in mobile health. Biochemist 41(5). Doi: 10.1042/bio04105020

Montazeri M, Galavi Z, Ahmadian L. The role of mobile health in prevention, diagnosis, treatment and self-care of COVID-19 from the healthcare professionals' perspectives. *Digit Health*. 2023 May 2;9:20552076231171969. doi: 10.1177/20552076231171969

Muralidharan, S., Ranjani, H., Anjana, R. M., Allender, S., & Mohan, V. (2017). Mobile health technology in the prevention and management of type 2 diabetes. *Indian journal of endocrinology and metabolism, 21*(2), 334–340. DOI: 10.4103/ijem.IJEM_407_16

Murthy N, Chandrasekharan S, Prakash MP, Ganju A, Peter J, Kaonga N, Mechael P. (2020) Effects of an mHealth voice message service (mMitra) on maternal health knowledge and practices of low-income women in India: findings from a pseudo-randomized controlled trial. *BMC Public Health*. 20(1):820. doi: 10.1186/s12889-020-08965-2

NIH (2014): Mobile-Health Approach: A Critical Look at Its Capacity to Augment Health Systems of Developing Countries. Accessed from: Mobile-Health Approach: A Critical Look on Its Capacity to Augment Health System of Developing Countries - PMC (nih.gov)

Nittari, G, Khuman Ravjyot, Baldoni Simone, Pallotta Graziano, Battineni Gopi, Sirignano Ascanio, Amenta Francesco, and Ricci Giovanna (2019) Telemedicine Practice: Review of the Current Ethical and Legal Challenges. *Telemedicine and e-Health.* Dec 2020. 1427–1437. http://doi.org/10.1089/tmj.2019.0158

Pham Q, Graham G, Carrion C, Morita PP, Seto E, Stinson JN, Cafazzo JA. A Library of Analytic Indicators to Evaluate Effective Engagement with Consumer mHealth Apps for Chronic Conditions: Scoping Review. *JMIR Mhealth Uhealth.* 2019 Jan 18;7(1):e11941. doi: 10.2196/11941

Piette J.D., Krein S.L., Striplin D., Marinec N., Kerns R.D., Farris K.B., Singh S., An L., Heapy A.A. (2016) Patient-Centered Pain Care Using Artificial Intelligence and Mobile Health Tools: Protocol for a Randomized Study Funded by the US Department of Veterans Affairs Health Services Research and Development Program. *JMIR Research Protocols.* 5 (2). doi:10.2196/resprot.4995

PwC (2012) Consumers Are Ready to Adopt Mobile Health Faster than the Health Industry is Prepared to Adapt, Finds PwC Study on Global mHealth Adoption. Accessed from: India ranks high on mHealth maturity: Press Release - PwC India

PwC (2015): Emerging mHealth: Paths for growth. Accessed from: https://www.pwc.com/gx/en/healthcare/mhealth/assets/pwc-emerging-mhealth-full.pdf

PwC (2017): How mHealth can revolutionise the Indian healthcare industry. Accessed from: how-mhealth-can-revolutionise-the-indian-healthcare-industry.pdf (pwc.in)

Ritchie ND, Turk MT. Enhancing access and impact of the Medicare Diabetes Prevention Program using telehealth: a narrative review. *Mhealth.* 2023 Dec 11;10:10. doi: 10.21037/mhealth-23-37

Salinari A., Machì M., Armas Diaz Y., Cianciosi D., Qi Z., Yang B., Ferreiro Cotorruelo M.S., Villar S.G., Dzul Lopez L.A., Battino M., Giampieri F. (2023) The Application of Digital Technologies and Artificial Intelligence in Healthcare: An Overview on Nutrition Assessment. *Diseases.* 11 (3), 97. Doi: 10.3390/diseases11030097

Sarangi, M, Radhakumari Challa (2016). Role of mHealth Apps in Accelerating the Health Care Services in Indian Scenario- A Study of Citizen Perspective; *Int.J.Curr.Res.Aca. Rev.* 2016; 4(12): 27–46; http://doi.org/10.20546/ijcrar.2016.412.003

Senbekov M, Saliev T, Bukeyeva Z, Almabayeva A, Zhanaliyeva M, Aitenova N, Toishibekov Y, Fakhradiyev I. The Recent Progress and Applications of Digital Technologies in Healthcare: A Review. *Int J Telemed Appl.* 2020 Dec 3;2020:8830200. doi: 10.1155/2020/8830200

Singh H, Couch D, Yap K. 2020. Mobile health apps that help with COVID-19 management: scoping review. *JMIR Nursing*, *3*(1), e20596. doi: 10.2196/20596

Skaria, G. (2013) mHealth in Health Information Delivery; The Indian Scenario; *Journal MTM.* 2:1:26–29, 2013; DOI:10.7309/jmtm.2.1.5

Stein N., Brooks K. (2017) A fully automated conversational artificial intelligence for weight loss: Longitudinal observational study among overweight and obese adults. *JMIR Diabetes.* 5(2). doi:10.2196/diabetes.8590

Vaswani, A., Shazeer, N., Parmar, N., Uszkoreit, J., Jones, L., Gomez, A. N., … & Polosukhin, I. (2017). Attention is all you need. *Advances in neural information processing systems, 30.*

WHO (2013) Cardiovascular diseases. Accessed from: https://www.who.int/health-topics/cardiovascular-diseases#tab=tab_3

WHO (2017) World Bank and WHO: Half the world lacks access to essential health services, 100 million still pushed into extreme poverty because of health expenses. Accessed from https://www.who.int/news/item/13-12-2017-world-bank-and-who-half-the-world-lacks-access-to-essential-health-services-100-million-still-pushed-into-extreme-poverty-because-of-health-expenses

Wilmink G, Dupey K, Alkire S, Grote J, Zobel G, Fillit HM, Movva S. Artificial Intelligence-Powered Digital Health Platform and Wearable Devices Improve Outcomes for Older Adults in Assisted Living Communities: Pilot Intervention Study. *JMIR Aging*. 2020 Sep 10;3(2):e19554. doi: 10.2196/19554

Wong C.K., Ho D.T.Y., Tam A.R., Zhou M., Lau Y.M., Tang M.O.Y., Tong R.C.F., Rajput K.S., Chen G., Chan S.C., Siu C.W., Hung I.F.N. (2020) Artificial intelligence mobile health platform for early detection of COVID-19 in quarantine subjects using a wearable biosensor: Protocol for a randomised controlled trial. *BMJ Open*. 10(7). doi: 10.1136/bmjopen-2020-038555

Wood, C.S., Thomas, M.R., Budd, J. et al. (2019) Taking connected mobile-health diagnostics of infectious diseases to the field. *Nature*. 566:467–474. Doi: 10.1038/s41586-019-0956-2

World Bank (2017): Individuals using the Internet (% of population) – India. Accessed from: Individuals using the Internet (% of population) - India | Data (worldbank.org)

Xiao J., Luo J., Mapes O.L., Wu T.T., Dye T., Jallad N.A., Hao P., Ruan J., Bullock S., Fiscella K. (2021) Assessing a smartphone app (aicaries) that uses artificial intelligence to detect dental caries in children and provides interactive oral health education: Protocol for a design and usability testing study. *JMIR Research Protocols*. 10(10). doi: 10.2196/32921

Zhang H, Jiang Y, Nguyen HD, Poo DC, Wang W. (2017) The effect of a smartphone-based coronary heart disease prevention (SBCHDP) programme on awareness and knowledge of CHD, stress, and cardiac-related lifestyle behaviours among the working population in Singapore: a pilot randomised controlled trial. *Health Qual Life Outcomes*. 15(1):49. doi: 10.1186/s12955-017-0623-y

Zillner L, Andreas M, Mach M. (2023) Wearable heart rate variability and atrial fibrillation monitoring to improve clinically relevant endpoints in cardiac surgery-a systematic review. *Mhealth*. 10:8. doi: 10.21037/mhealth-23-19

18 AI in Medicine

Addressing Advancements, Personhood Status and Liability Concerns for AI-Related Errors

Ditipriya Dutta Chowdhury and Sangeeta Roy Maitra

18.1 INTRODUCTION

Judge Posner stated, "*Computers can only issue mandatory instructions- they are not programmed to exercise discretion*" (Pompeii Estates, Inc. v. Consolidated Edison Co, 1977). Today, five decades down the road, the statement is no longer strictly accurate. Artificial Intelligence ("**AI**") is now a reality, and it stands as an advancing field, capable of reproducing human thought processes. With the rapid rise in innovation and pharmaceutical research and development, there is a surge in patenting AI medical applications and devices.

It has been observed that both healthcare providers and patients are relying more frequently on AI-based medical platforms and systems to prevent, detect, and manage medical conditions (Duffourc & Gerke, 2024). Physicians may use AI-based medical systems to answer clinical questions or generate treatment documentation (Brumfiel, 2023). Patients and several other consumers have turned to AI for quick, cost-effective solutions to their medical concerns. A recent study even found that when compared with human physicians, "*Chatbot responses were [also] rated significantly more empathetic than physician responses*" (Ayers et al., 2023, p. E1). In addition to the generic AI platforms, AI-based healthcare platforms have been developed to answer questions related to healthcare and medicine. For instance, Microsoft Cloud for Healthcare is designed to "*[a]ccelerate innovation and improve healthcare experiences with AI-powered solutions*", and it further uses AI algorithms to assist healthcare providers "*make data-driven decisions*" (Microsoft Cloud for Healthcare, para. 1; McGuinness, 2023, para. 2). While AI algorithms can be trained to interpret medical data and images, "*it also produces inaccurate medical information and recommendations, endangering patient safety. For example, the accuracy of an AI's output is highly dependent on the quality of its training data, which can be limited or biased*" (Duffourc, & Gerke, 2024, p. 6). There have been instances where AI-based medical

 DOI: 10.1201/9781003503385-18

applications have provided incorrect clinical diagnosis or decisions. Incorrect clinical diagnosis or faulty treatments can lead to injury claims and raise questions of liability. The legal framework for medical AI in medicine is still underdeveloped, and to address such liability concerns, the existing legal framework of AI must be understood.

AI *per se* lacks the legal capacity for patent rights since Section 3(k) of the Indian Patents Act, 1970 ("**Patents Act, 1970**") does not allow for patenting of a software or computer program *per se* unless integrated with hardware as integral components. The current legislation only recognizes "*human inventors*" (Stephen L Thaler v. Comptroller General of Patents, Design and Trade Mark, 2020) and thus AI lacks legal "*personhood*". In the absence of a framework that answers the "*personhood*" question of AI, the primary question that arises is "*who is liable*" for AI-driven erroneous decisions. One way to answer is to carefully examine whether it is: (a) the software developer or (b) the company which has commercialized the product or (c) the hospital that has adopted the AI or (d) the doctor, who has relied upon the AI to treat patients. This article analyses the promising contributions of AI in medicine along with its perplexities and attempts to comprehend the liability of each stakeholder applying principles of tort law.

Therefore, in a nutshell, the major contributions here are that the article:

- Provides an analysis of the evolution and advancements of AI in medicine, both worldwide and in India.
- Discusses the challenges associated with using AI in medicine, including the issue of liability in cases of injury caused by AI-based medical applications.
- Citing relevant case laws and liability principles under tort law, establishes a comprehensive roadmap for addressing the liability of each human stakeholder involved in the use of such AI-based medical applications in India.

18.2 EVOLUTION OF AI IN MEDICINE

Medicine was already an established sector when AI was first introduced in this field in the 1970s. In 1984, Clancey and Shortliffe observed that

> Medical artificial intelligence is primarily concerned with the construction of AI programs that perform diagnosis and make therapy recommendations and unlike medical applications based on other programming methods, such as purely statistical and probabilistic methods, medical AI programs are based on symbolic models of disease entities and their relationship to patient factors and clinical manifestations
>
> *(Coiera, 1996, p. 363).*

MYCIN, INTERNIST and CASNET were a few of the first expert AI systems in medicine developed by Standford University, University of Pittsburgh, and Rutgers Research Resource, respectively (Sharma & Manchikanti, 2020). AI had begun as a 'if/ then rules' abstract series, but over the years its development has been such that at present AI is capable of functioning in a manner like the human brain. Figure 18.1 represents the projected growth of the AI-based healthcare market which was "*valued at USD 10.4 billion in 2021 and expected to expand at a compound annual growth rate of 38.4 % from 2022 to 2030*" (Williams, 2023, para. 2).

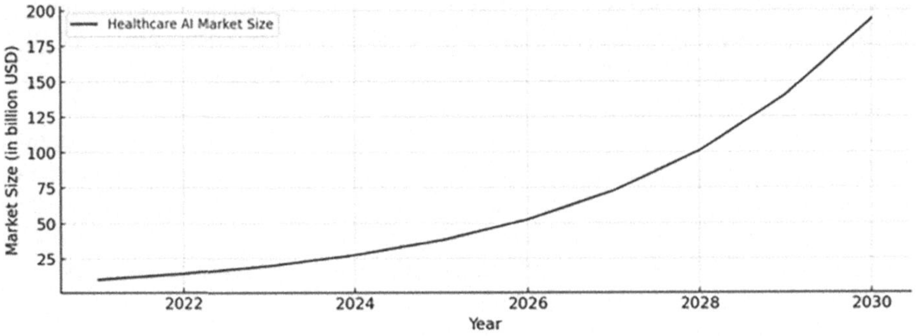

FIGURE 18.1 Global AI healthcare market size (2021–2030).

Adapted from Williams, 2023.

AI has been successfully employed by various healthcare companies, namely, Atomwise, Berg, IBM, Insilico Medicine, TwoXAR, Google, etc. to obtain certain desired results with the help of machine learning ("**ML**") and deep linking ("**DL**").

18.3 ADVANCEMENTS OF AI IN MEDICINE

The medical sector, at present, is witnessing a shift towards a more machine-centric arrangement. The contribution of AI in medicine extends beyond research by assessing huge amounts of data.

18.3.1 Diagnostic Tools

The field of diagnostics has witnessed remarkable development in terms of AI. In 2015, Capitol Health Limited, an Australian radiology service company, and Enlitic, announced their inaugural collaboration to revolutionize diagnostics using deep learning technologies for radiologists and healthcare providers (Enlitic, 2015; Sharma & Manchikanti, 2020). In 2017, Stockholm3 test, a blood-based prostate cancer diagnostic test, was launched by a team at Karolinska Institutet and it is being clinically practiced in Nordic countries (Eddy, 2020; Sharma & Manchikanti, 2020). Further, in 2018, NITI Aayog entered into an agreement with Microsoft and Forus Health to leverage AI solutions to develop healthcare system for detecting diabetic retinopathy (NITI Aayog, 2018). Forus Health has developed the 3Nethra series for evaluation and diagnosis of visual health, including 3Nethra Neo, for detection of ocular diseases in infants. Table 18.1 represents AI systems developed in the recent past in the field of medicine and healthcare.

18.3.2 Surgical Robots

Robots backed by AI serve as invaluable tools in different surgical disciplines, namely, urology, gynaecology, orthopaedics, and cardiothoracic surgery, amongst many others.

The da Vinci Surgical System, developed by Intuitive Surgical in 1999, is one of the revolutionary systems that enables surgeons to perform minimal invasive

TABLE 18.1
Examples of AI-based Diagnostic Tools in Medicine and Healthcare

Company	Name & Year of Development of the AI System	Target Solution(s)
IBM	IBM Watson (2010)	Data support
Microsoft	Microsoft Azure (2010)	Health cloud platform
Aidoc	Aidoc aiOS™ (2016)	AI platform for identifying abnormalities in radiology, cardiovascular, and neuro scans
Google Health	Medical Brain (2018)	AI algorithms for tasks such as predicting patient outcomes and assisting with clinical decision-making
Tempus	Tempus|TO (2023)	Precision medicine for cancer patients

Data collected from respective company websites.

procedures with enhanced agility and visualization, faster recuperation time, and less postoperative complications. Another notable example is Globus Medical's ExcelsiusGPS® robotic navigation platform, which provides real-time image guidance to surgeons to execute complex spinal surgeries. Further, Zimmer Biomet's ROSA® Robotics, provides neurosurgeons with "*objective soft tissue feedback and accurate bone resections*" in order to restore knees and hips of patients based on their unique anatomy (Zimmer Biomet, n.d.).

18.3.3 Remote Monitoring

AI applications can remotely track the vital signs and other health metrics of patients and provide timely alerts and insights to health providers. Several pharmaceutical organizations have successfully developed wearables such as smartwatches and smartphone applications which can track heart rate, rhythm irregularities, and even detect potential signs of heart attack (Nahavandi et al., 2021). In 2023, a 29-year-old woman was diagnosed with blood clot in her lungs, and she underwent life-saving surgery at the hospital after her "*Apple Watch alerted her that her heart rate had been too high for over 10 minutes. Her heart rate had spiked to 178 beats per minute…*" (Singh, 2023, para. 3). Figure 18.2 indicates the increase in number of smartwatch users from 2021 to the end of 2023—-from 202.58 million to 216.43 million (Williams, 2023, para. 3).

Chronic diseases like diabetes are also managed remotely through Continuous Glucose Monitors ("**CGM**") which collect real-time blood glucose levels and analyse the glucose trend in the patient's body. CGM has helped several diabetic patients to regulate and take measures against imminent hypo- and hyperglycemia attacks (American Diabetes Association, 2024).

18.3.4 Discovery and Development of Drugs

AI algorithms are potent tools for drug discovery and development processes, as traditional methods are often time-consuming and costly, risking high rates of failures.

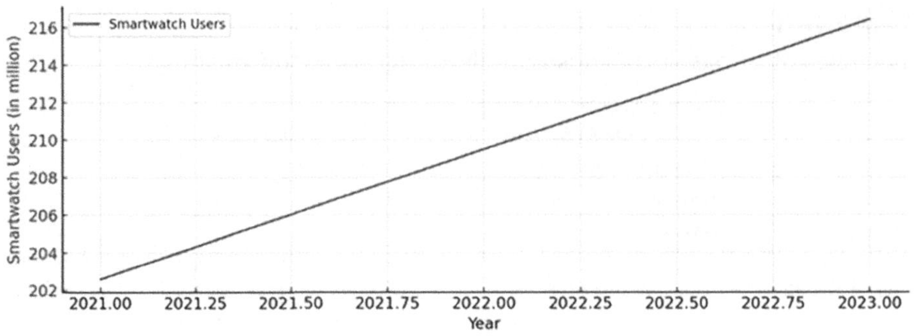

FIGURE 18.2 Number of smartwatch users (2021–2023).

Adapted from Williams, 2023.

ML systems gather, processes and analyses large quantity medical data and stores it securely in a centralized storage cloud or system called the Electronic Medical Records ("**EMR**"). Based on such EMR, specific genetic traits, potential drug candidates, and effect of and response to certain medicines and treatments are identified (Shameer et al., 2018). Cleveland Clinic researchers developed "*Deep Profiler, a multitask deep neural network*" that analyses EMRs like CT images to determine the most effective "*radiotherapy dose*" (Lou et al., 2019, p. e137). In 2019, Eisai Co. Ltd. received the approval for use of anticancer agent Halaven® (eribulin mesylate) for the treatment of patients with locally advanced or metastatic breast cancer. Eisai had used AI algorithm to analyse cancer cell images and predict the efficacy of potential drug compounds, leading to the discovery of Eribulin. Recently, in 2022, Atomwise has entered into "*strategic and exclusive research collaboration*" with Sanofi to use its AtomNet® platform for data processing and discovery of up to five drug targets (Atomwise, 2022, para. 1).

18.4 AI IN THE INDIAN MEDICAL SECTOR

In the last few years, numerous Indian medical start-ups have leveraged AI algorithms to develop solutions and platforms to deliver quality healthcare to patients. Companies like Tricog Health and Sigtuple Technologies are using AI algorithms to enhance diagnostic accuracy and efficiency, particularly in areas such as cardiology and smart diagnostic solutions, respectively.

In 2016, Geeta Manjunath founded Niramai Health Analytix that uses AI to scan thermography images to detect breast cancer. The company has developed a "*low cost, accurate, automated, portable, radiation-free, non-touch and non-painful cancer screening tool that can be operated in any clinic*" (Niramai Health Analytix Private Limited, para. 2, n.d.).

In the field of radiology, Qure.ai has grown significantly. It has developed qXR and qTrack to scan chest X-rays for detection and management of tuberculosis (Qure.ai, para. 1, n.d.). Figure 18.3 represents Qure.ai's qXR report on chest X-rays.

Therefore, it can be observed AI algorithms have the full potential to revolutionize healthcare delivery in India by making it more effective, affordable, and most importantly accessible for millions of people across the diverse country.

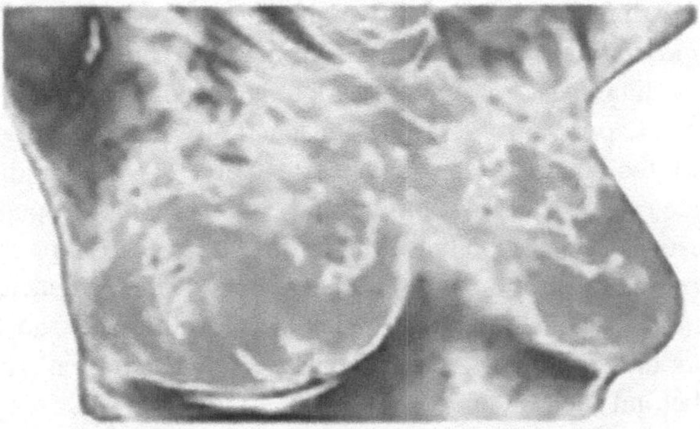

FIGURE 18.3 Chest X-ray report using qXR to detect tuberculosis.
Source: https://qure.ai/.

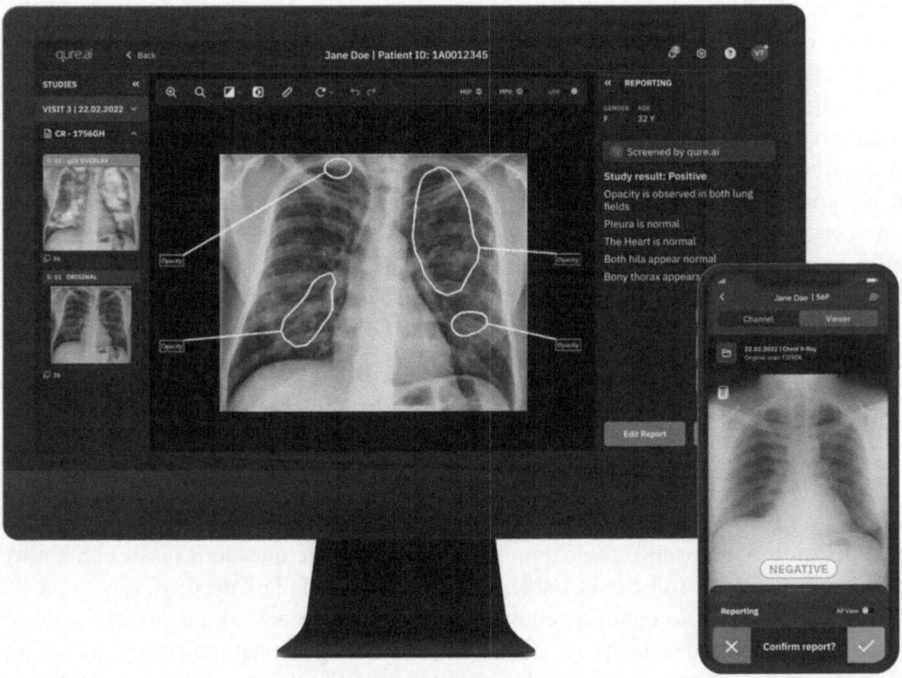

FIGURE 18.4 Chest X-ray report taken from Qure.AI.

18.5 CHALLENGES IN AI'S ROLE IN MEDICINE

Amidst the commendable contributions of AI in medicine, there are several challenges involved when it comes to the involvement of AI in the medical sector. While an AI system can make *"real-time inferences from a large patient population..."* (Neill, 2013, p. 92), one major hurdle is guaranteeing its precision and dependability in case of predictive diagnosis. The quality of data is paramount when it comes to data analysis by AI, and any kind of bias or error in the data can amount to false predictions and incorrect diagnosis. For example, there is a smartphone app where patients can upload images of apprehensive skin lesions, and the AI algorithm advice whether a consultation with the doctor is required (Freeman et al., 2020). Studies have shown that the occurrence of skin cancer is based on the skin colour of a person (Bradford, 2009), and as a result, AI can retain biases regarding skin tones (Hardesty, 2018). Over 1200 images were analysed in a study by researchers of the Massachusetts Institute of Technology and it was observed that the facial-recognition AI had an error rate of 34% in classifying darker skin tones, particularly amongst women (Hardesty, 2018). The main cause behind such incongruity was due to the use of uneven patient data of "*77 % male and 83% white*" by the AI algorithm for its evaluation (Dueno, 2020).

Moreover, a study has shown that the incorporation of surgical robots into patient treatment can be challenging because a lot of times robotic surgery results in prolonged operating time, increase in hospital costs, and maintenance costs as compared to laparoscopic surgery (Jeong et al., 2017). In the case of robot-controlled surgeries, instances of robotic malfunctions have been reported to be 3.7% (Rajih et al., 2017), and therefore, mistakes by autonomous surgical robots will possibly be one of the safety and liability issues in this field.

Further, while preparing an EMR, if there is any "*under-representation*" of data of a certain section of the population, it may "*hide population differences in disease risk or treatment efficacy*" (Lawry et al., 2018, p. 6). If data is collected from wearables, it automatically represents a richer population which has access to such devices, internet connectivity, and cloud services (Lawry et al., 2018). The lack of transparency regarding the data collection and decision-making process of the AI raises questions on the authenticity of the EMR. To remedy such situations, the extent of liability that may be attached to the respective AI-related errors needs to be analysed.

18.6 AI-RELATED ERRORS IN MEDICINE: WHO IS LIABLE?

18.6.1 Defining "Personhood": Legal Status of AI

AI holds immense power in reforming the medical sector, but whenever it is integrated into decision-making and surgical interventions, there are questions of accountability and liability. For AI to be held liable for its mistakes, the law needs to recognize AI as a person eligible to claim inventorship. Though there are arguments in favour of granting personhood status to AI, patent systems only grant natural persons inventorship of patents. For instance, in the United States ("**US**"), Section 100 (f) of the Patent Act recognizes "*individual(s)*" as inventors, and not corporations or machines (Patent Act, 1952). Similarly, the Supreme Court of the United Kingdom ("**UK**") in the DABUS case (Thaler v. Comptroller-General of Patents, Designs and Trade Marks, 2023) held that an AI system cannot be an inventor since the scope of an inventor under Sections 7 and 13 of the UK Patents Act, 1977 is mandatorily limited to a natural person. In India, the Controller General of Patents cited Sections 2 and 6 of the Patents Act, 1970, while recording objections in granting inventorship to the AI in the examination report of the DABUS application (Rampal & Raghuwanshi, 2024).

Therefore, to date, leading jurisdictions have refused to grant "*personhood*" status to AI under the current patent law regime, and only natural persons are considered to be "*persons*" while attributing inventorship rights. Since AI lacks "*personhood*", it is legally not possible to hold an AI application accountable for any of its mistakes.

18.6.2 Liability under Tort Law for AI-Related Errors

The question that transpires is, "*If AI cannot be held liable, then who is responsible for the AI-related errors?*" There is no straightforward answer to this question. There are several stakeholders attached to an AI system, and it is challenging to decide who should be held liable. A software developer first develops an algorithm, and the same is patented by pharmaceutical companies. Thereafter, AI-based pharmaceutical companies "*work*" the invention by selling or licensing the invention to hospitals. Finally, doctors rely on AI-based medical devices to deliver treatment to patients.

In the absence of an established legal framework, assigning accountability is challenging. The most prudent evaluation is to assess the involvement and duties of each stakeholder and apply the same to liability principles available under the law. However, the issue of assigning liability for AI-related errors has not been addressed under any codified laws at present. Tort laws, though uncodified, are well-established in India through multiple precedents in compensating individuals who have suffered legal injury because of others' acts or omissions. "*Tort laws have a history of evolving to adapt to technological changes- and it will here too*" (Mello & Guha, 2024, p. 2).

18.6.2.1 Liability of Manufacturers

Software developers develop AI algorithms as part of their employment for pharmaceutical companies. While they remain the inventors, the ownership rights lie with the manufacturing companies. It is the duty of these companies to provide adequate instructions and warnings regarding the shortcomings of the AI-based devices. The Supreme Court of Washington had held that it is the "*manufacturers' duty to warn*" and it is "*their liability to ensure the product safety*" (Taylor v. Intuitive Surgical, Inc., 2017). "*Typically, when a product injures a patient, courts look to well-established rules to determine how to allocate liability between the party using the product and the company that made it*" (Mello & Guha, 2024, p. 2).

Applying the "neighbor principle" in such cases, the manufacturers would be held liable in case of any default of the AI system since manufacturers can reasonably foresee the injury or harm that may be caused to patients due to their negligence or failure to warn regarding the limitations of their AI system (Donoghue v. Stevenson, 1932). Further, the European Union's Artificial Intelligence Act, 2024 (the "**AI Act**") considers AI-based medical devices to be products. The AI Act has assumed a risk-based approach, and Article 6 of the AI Act identifies "*medical devices and in vitro diagnostic medical devices*" as "*High Risk AI*". If there is a defect in such products, the Product Liability Directive, 1985, shall apply, wherein providers of such products, i.e., the manufacturers, are held strictly liable. Thus, if manufacturing companies fail to inform of such defects to their consumers, these companies may also attract strict liability for such default (Boston Scientific MedizintechnikC, 2015), with the burden of proof lying with the company.

18.6.2.2 Liability of Hospitals

To keep pace with technological advancements, all major hospitals and clinics either take licenses or buy AI-based medical devices from pharmaceutical companies. Hospitals must ensure the following before implementing AI systems: a) proper integration of the AI system into their existing infrastructure, b) adequate training for their doctors, and c) appropriate safeguard mechanisms to avoid adverse outcomes. If the hospitals fail to observe their duties, they can be held liable for negligence. In several cases, the Hon'ble Supreme Court of India has held the hospital vicariously liable for the acts of its doctors and awarded significant damages to a deceased patient's family who had died due to medical negligence at a private hospital (Dr. B. Prasad v. Dr. K. Saha, 2014; Maharaja Agrasen Hospital v. Master Rishabh Sharma, 2020).

18.6.2.3 Liability of Doctors

The Hon'ble Supreme Court of India observed that "*a medical practitioner has various duties towards his patient and he must act with a reasonable degree of skill and knowledge and must exercise a reasonable degree of care. This is the least which a patient expects from a doctor*" (Achutrao Haribhau Khodwa v. St. of Maharashtra, 1996). While relying upon AI systems, like EMR or surgical robots, doctors must understand that the "*key step [is] separating prediction from action and recommendation*" (Casciola, 2022, p. 32). If a doctor is using robotic assistance in a surgery, he may surrender some control to the robots, but he needs to be generally in charge of the robots to lessen any injury risks (Roe, 2019) and ensure a reasonable standard of care is observed. The UK Supreme Court stressed upon patient-centric care and observed that it is the duty of the doctors to give the patients sufficient information for them to make informed decisions regarding their treatment (Montgomery v. Lanarkshire Health Board, 2015). The same should be applied when AI is used for treatment processes, as proof of negligence may attract criminal liability for medical negligence (Dr. B. Prasad v. Dr. K. Saha, 2014). Therefore, responsibility lies with the doctors to consider important factors before diagnosing and treating patients with the help of AI, such as the medical history of the patient, laboratory tests, and physical examination (Tokio Matsuzaki, 2018).

18.7 CONCLUSION

The era of digitization has helped AI become a predominant tool of assistance in medicine. India has several disruptive start-ups engaged in AI-based diagnostics which provide AI solutions for various forms of healthcare. However, there have been incidents of AI bias and AI-related mistakes in medicine and medical devices resulting in erroneous diagnosis. Since AI cannot be held liable for its mistakes, a human in the loop is required to be identified to make him/her responsible for such mistakes. But in the case of AI-based medical devices, identifying one single person poses a significant challenge.

This article has thus determined the liability of each stakeholder and established principles of liability under tort laws. First, companies commercializing AI devices should be strictly liable for failing to warn the hospitals or consumers of any defects in their products. Second, hospitals should be held vicariously liable for medical negligence of their doctors caused by reliance upon AI assistance. Further, doctors owe a reasonable standard of care towards all patients, and it is imperative that they ensure that the EMR or the predictive diagnosis relied upon is free from bias. Failure to do so may result in criminal liability for their medical negligence.

India, like the European Union, may perhaps formulate a uniform legal framework committed to AI to define concepts like personhood and regulate AI-based medical devices and inventions to mitigate risks and ensure patient safety. In the absence of a dedicated legal framework for AI, the comprehensive approach provided by this article may be undertaken to answer the question "*who is liable*?" in addressing AI-generated error claims.

REFERENCES

Achutrao Haribhau Khodwa v. State of Maharashtra, 1996 SCC (2) 634.

American Diabetes Association. (2024). Continuous glucose monitors. https://diabetes.org/advocacy/cgm-continuous-glucose-monitors

Atomwise. (2022). Atomwise Signs Strategic Multi-Target Research Collaboration with Sanofi for AI-Powered Drug Discovery. https://www.atomwise.com/2022/08/17/atomwise-signs-strategic-multi-target-research-collaboration-with-sanofi-for-ai-powered-drug-discovery/

Ayers, J.W., et al. (2023). Comparing Physician and Artificial Intelligence Chatbot Responses to Patient Questions Posted to a Public Social Media Forum. *JAMA Internal Medicine*, *183*(6), 589–596. doi:10.1001/jamainternmed.2023.1838

Bradford, P.T. (2009). Skin Cancer in Skin of Color. *Dermatology Nursing*. https://www.ncbi.nlm.nih.gov/pmc/articles/PMC2757062/

Brumfiel, G. (2023). Doctors Are Drowning in Paperwork. Some Companies Claim AI Can Help. *NPR*. https://www.npr.org/sections/health-shots/2023/04/05/1167993888/chatgpt-medicine-artificial-intelligence-healthcare

Casciola, C. (2022). Artificial Intelligence and Health Care: Reviewing The Algorithmic Accountability Act in Light of The European Artificial Intelligence Act. *Vermont Law Review*, *47*(1), 127–155.

CJEU, Boston Scientific MedizintechnikC GmbH v. AOK Sachsen-Anhalt – Die Gesundheitskasse, Betriebskrankenkasse RWE, (Joined cases C-5o0/13 and C-5o0/13), 5 March 2015.

Coiera, E. W. (1996). Artificial intelligence in medicine: The challenges ahead. *Journal of the American Medical Informatics Association*, *3*(6), 363–366. https://academic.oup.com/jamia/article/3/6/363/823662

Donoghue v Stevenson, [1932] AC 562 (HL).

Dr. Balaram Prasad v. Dr. Kunal Saha & Ors., (2014) 1 SCC 384.

Dueno, T. (2020). Racist Robots and the Lack of Legal Remedies in the Use of Artificial Intelligence in Healthcare. *Connecticut Insurance Law Journal*, *27*, 337.

Duffourc, M., & Gerke, S. (2024). Decoding U.S. Tort Liability in Healthcare's Black-Box AI Era: Lessons from the European Union. *Stanford Technology Law Review*, *27*(1). https://law.stanford.edu/wp-content/uploads/2024/02/Publish_27-STLR-1-2024_Decoding-U.S.-Tort-Liability-in-Healthcares-Black-Box-AI-Era.pdf

Eddy, N. (2020). AI platform helps diagnose prostate cancer, Lancet report shows. *Healthcare IT News*. https://www.healthcareitnews.com/news/ai-platform-helps-diagnose-prostate-cancer-lancet-report-shows

Enlitic. (2015). Enlitic and Capitol Health announce global partnership. *EnliticTM News*. https://www.enlitic.com/enlitic-and-capitol-health-announce

Freeman, et al. (2020). Algorithm Based Smartphone Apps to Assess Risk of Skin Cancer in Adults: Systematic Review of Diagnostic Accuracy Studies. *BMJ*. https://www.bmj.com/content/368/bmj.m127

Hardesty, L. (2018). Study Finds Gender and Skin-Type Bias in Commercial Artificial-Intelligence Systems. https://news.mit.edu/2018/study-finds-gender-skin-type-bias-artificial-intelligence-systems-0212

Jeong, G., et al. (2017). Association of Robotic-Assisted vs Laparoscopic Radical Nephrectomy with Perioperative Outcomes and Health Care Costs, 2003 to 2015. *Journal of the American Medical Association (JAMA)*, *318*(16), 1561–1568. https://doi.org/10.1001/jama.2017.14586

Lawry, T., et al. (2018). Realizing the Potential for AI in Precision Health. *The SciTech Lawyer*, *15*(1). https://www.americanbar.org/groups/science_technology/publications/scitech_lawyer/2019/fall/realizing-potential-ai-precision-health/

Lou, B., et al. (2019). An image-based deep learning framework for individualising radiotherapy dose: A retrospective analysis of outcome prediction. *The Lancet Digital Health*, *1*(1), e136–e147. https://doi.org/10.1016/S2589-7500(19)30058-5

Maharaja Agrasen Hospital v. Master Rishabh Sharma, (2020) 6 SCC 501.

Mello, M.M., & Guha, N. (2024). Understanding Liability Risk from Healthcare AI. *Stanford University HAI Policy and Society* 2. https://hai.stanford.edu/sites/default/files/2024-02/Liability-Risk-Healthcare-AI.pdf

Microsoft Cloud for Healthcare. *Microsoft*. https://www.microsoft.com/th-th/industry/health/microsoft.cloud-for-healthcare; McGuinness, T. (2023, April 12). Microsoft Cloud for Healthcare: Empowering healthcare to deliver meaningful outcomes. *Microsoft*. https://www.microsoft.com/en-us/industry/blog/healthcare/2023/04/12/microsoft.cloud-for-healthcare-empowering-healthcare-to-deliver-meaningful-outcomes/

Montgomery v. Lanarkshire Health Board, [2015] UKSC 11.

Nahavandi, D., et al. (2021). Application of artificial intelligence in wearable devices: Opportunities and challenges. *Computer Methods and Programs in Biomedicine, 213*. https://doi.org/10.1016/j.cmpb.2021.106541

Neill, D.B. (2013). Using artificial intelligence to improve hospital Inpatient care. *IEEE Computer Society*, *92*. http://www.cs.cmu.edu/~./neill/papers/ieee-is2013.pdf

Niramai Health Analytix Private Limited. https://www.niramai.com/

NITI Aayog. (2018). National strategy for artificial intelligence. https://indiaai.gov.in/documents/pdf/NationalStrategy-for-AI-Discussion-Paper.pdf

Patent Act, 35 U.S.C. § 100(f) (1952).

Pompeii Estates, Inc. v. Consolidated Edison Co., 91 Misc. 2d 233, 237 (N.Y. Civ. Ct. 1977).

Qure.ai. https://www.qure.ai/global-health

Rajih, E., et al. (2017). Error Reporting from the Da Vinci Surgical System in Robotic Surgery: A Canadian Multispecialty Experience at a Single Academic Centre. *Canadian Urological Association Journal 11*(5). http://doi.org/10.5489/cuaj.4116

Rampal, R.B. & Raghuwanshi, S.S. (2024). Demystifying Rights of AI Generated Inventions. *Live Law*. https://www.livelaw.in/law-firms/law-firm-articles-/ai-generated-inventions-chatgpt-indian-patent-act-dabus-united-states-patent-trademark-office-european-patent-office-226394?infinitescroll=1

Roe, M. (2019). Who's Driving That Car?: An Analysis of Regulatory and Potential Liability Frameworks for Driverless Cars. *Boston College Law Review 60*, 317, 337. https://bclawreview.bc.edu/articles/278

Shameer, K., et al. (2018). Machine learning in cardiovascular medicine: Are we there yet? *Heart (British Cardiac Society)*, *104*(14), 1156–1164. https://doi.org/10.1136/heartjnl-2017-311198

Sharma, K., & Manchikanti, P. (2020). Regulation of artificial intelligence in drug discovery and healthcare. *Biotechnology Law Report*, *39*(5), 371–380. http://doi.org/10.1089/blr.2020.29183.ks

Singh, S. (2023). Apple Watch alerts high heart rate, saves 29-year-old woman's life from fatal blood clot. *Business Today*. https://www.businesstoday.in/latest/trends/story/apple-watch-alerts-high-heart-rate-saves-29-year-old-womans-life-from-fatal-blood-clot-386381-2023-06-20

Stephen L Thaler v. Comptroller General of Patents, Design and Trade Mark, [2020] EWHC 2412 (Pat).

Taylor v. Intuitive Surgical, Inc., 187 Wash. 2d 743,389 P.3d 517 [2017].

Thaler v. Comptroller-General of Patents, Designs and Trade Marks, [2023] UKSC 49.

The Patents Act, 1970, No. 39, Acts of Parliament, 1970 (India).

Tokio Matsuzaki, T. (2018). Ethical Issues of Artificial Intelligence in Medicine. *California Western Law Review*, *55*, 255.

Williams, D. (2023). Losses from AI in Healthcare: Who is Liable? *Parker Smith & Feek.* https://www.psfinc.com/articles/losses-from-ai-in-healthcare-who-is-liable/

Zimmer Biomet. ROSA® Robotic Surgery. https://www.zimmerbiomet.com/en/products-and-solutions/specialties/knee/rosa--knee-system.html

19 Adoption and Implementation Challenges of Artificial Intelligence in Healthcare Settings

John T. Abraham, Swapna K. Cherian, Blessing T. John and Angel T. John

19.1 INTRODUCTION

Artificial intelligence (AI) is the term for technologies that permit computers to perform cognitive tasks comparable to those of humans, such as neural networks, natural language processing, machine learning, and computer vision. All these several decades, AI has demonstrated incredible feats, such as piloting self-driving automobiles and even upsetting the world go champion. In fact, AI has the capacity to reform health care by enhancing clinical judgment, boosting productivity, and cutting expenses. However, there are plenty of issues that essential to be fixed before AI can be adopted and used in healthcare settings. In order to assist in addressing long-standing issues like rising prices, physician fatigue, medical errors, lack of accessibility to care, and disparities in quality of care, the healthcare industry is placing great hopes on AI.

Applications of AI are already showing promise for enhancing the provision of healthcare. Large-scale patient data can be analyzed using machine learning to find patterns that help doctors diagnose patients and forecast their health (Topol, 2019). Initial patient interviews and triage services can be performed by chatbots and virtual assistants that use natural language processing (Davalbhakta et al., 2020). Radiologists can detect anomalies and monitor the course of diseases with the use of computer vision (Liu et al., 2019).

Thanks to developments in machine learning and data analytics, the application of AI in healthcare has accelerated recently (Smith, 2022). Nevertheless, despite its revolutionary potential, there are a number of obstacles to overcome before AI can be widely used in healthcare settings, including ethical, legal, and technological issues (Johnson & Lee, 2023). Understanding these obstacles is essential for successful

 DOI: 10.1201/9781003503385-19

integration and optimization as institutions work to incorporate AI solutions (Miller et al., 2024).

The core contributions of the chapter:

- This chapter examines the various obstacles to the widespread use of AI in healthcare, using case studies and current research to give a thorough picture of the situation as it is today.
- Notwithstanding this promise, considerable obstacles have prevented AI technology from being widely adopted and used in actual clinical settings.
- This essay looks at the main obstacles and offers suggestions for getting beyond them.

19.2 STATEMENT OF THE PROBLEM: CHALLENGES HINDERING ADOPTION AND IMPLEMENTATION

Let's examine the issues that are preventing AI from being widely used and implemented in healthcare settings:

19.2.1 Technological Limitations

- Complexity of AI algorithms: Developing, implementing, and maintaining sophisticated algorithms that demand a large amount of processing power and knowledge is a common feature of healthcare AI. For healthcare institutions with limited technological resources, the intricacy can present difficulties.
- Integration with current systems: A lot of healthcare institutions use outdated technology, which can make AI solutions incompatible with them. It can be difficult to smoothly integrate AI into these systems without upsetting current workflows.
- Issues with scalability and reliability: It is imperative to guarantee that AI algorithms are scalable to manage substantial data sets and function dependably in actual healthcare environments. Problems like algorithm drift—a gradual deterioration in performance—and insufficient resilience may make implementation difficult.

19.2.2 Data Privacy Concerns

- Security of data related to patients: Sensitive data, counting health accounts and pictorial scans, is a major component of healthcare AI. Really, crucial to ensuring the safety and privacy of the information to halt misuse, cracks, and unsolicited admission.
- Regulation adherence: AI solutions for healthcare should obey acts like Health Insurance Portability and Accountability Act (HIPAA) of US and the General Data Protection Regulation (GDPR) of Europe. Due to the complicated legal environment, achieving compliance while using data for AI applications might be difficult.

- Ethical implications of data usage: Informed consent for data usage, algorithmic decision-making fairness, and avoiding algorithmic bias are a few of the moral issues that should be considered when using Artificial Intelligence in healthcare weighing possible advantages of AI against privacy-related ethical considerations.

19.2.3 Regulatory Hurdles

- FDA approval procedure: Before being sold and utilized in clinical settings in the United States, healthcare AI products may need to receive approval from the Food and Drug Administration (FDA). The process of navigating the regulatory approval system can be quite costly and time-consuming, which frequently entails stringent testing and validation requirements.
- Adherence to healthcare standards: In order to guarantee patient safety, interoperability, and data accuracy, healthcare AI solutions must abide by industry standards and norms. It can be difficult for healthcare firms to innovate with AI technologies and still meet these criteria.
- Legal ambiguities and liabilities: The legal environment around AI in healthcare, including who is responsible for mistakes or unfavorable results, is still developing. Establishing clear legal obligations and liabilities for AI systems in healthcare environments is crucial to promoting acceptance and confidence.

19.2.4 Moral Issues to Take Into Account

Bias and fairness in AI systems: AI systems that have been trained on incomplete or biased data sets run the risk of escalating or maintaining inequities in healthcare outcomes. It is a difficult task to safeguard justice and impartiality in algorithmic decision-making; meticulous data curation, algorithm design, and continuous monitoring are necessary.

- Interpretability and transparency: Healthcare AI structures often keep role as "black boxes," making it challenging to comprehend the decision-making process. Increasing interpretability and AI algorithm transparency is crucial to winning over patients, regulators, and medical professionals.
- Effect on patient-provider relationship: The use of AI in healthcare settings may change the dynamics of the patient-provider relationship. Adoption success depends on preserving patient trust and making sure AI enhances rather than replaces human competence.

19.2.5 Resistance to Change

- Cultural hurdles in healthcare organizations: Due to cultural norms, cynicism about technology, or fear of losing their jobs, healthcare personnel may be reluctant to adopt AI. Overcoming resistance to change requires effective communication, education, and stakeholder participation in the adoption process.

- Workforce preparedness and training requirements: In order to employ AI tools in clinical practice effectively, healthcare professionals must pick up new skills and competencies. For the successful use and integration of AI, healthcare workers must receive thorough training programs and assistance.
- Fear of job displacement: Adoption may be hampered by worries that AI may replace human workers, particularly in positions that healthcare professionals have historically undertaken. Gaining acceptance requires addressing these concerns and highlighting AI's function as a helpful tool rather than a substitute.

Healthcare organizations, legislators, and technology developers can obtain a deeper comprehension of the challenges related to the adoption and deploying AI in healthcare settings and devise effective methods to get over these specific problems by tackling them.

19.3 CHALLENGES IN AI ADOPTION AND IMPLEMENTATION

19.3.1 Lack of Trust in AI

Patients' and healthcare practitioners' mistrust of AI systems is a significant barrier (Bhjhvani et al., 2021). Clinicians are reluctant to rely on AI for diagnosis and treatment recommendations due to worries about performance, transparency, and potential biases. The technology's reputation has been further damaged by past missteps such as IBM's Watson for Oncology (Ross & Swetlitz, 2018). Additionally, patients can be leery of AI making decisions or helping with clinical judgments. More proof of AI's superior results is required, as are initiatives to increase its transparency and dependability.

19.3.2 Difficulties Integrating AI into Workflows

Clinical workflows are intricate procedures that have developed over an extended length of time. AI integration into current electronic health record (EHR) systems, diagnostic tools, and provider workflows poses obstacles (Krittanawong, 2020). Adoption of AI depends on seamless integration; if not, it runs the risk of becoming simply another isolated technology that bothers clinicians. Solutions that are created without enough feedback from end users frequently fall flat. It is crucial to co-design systems with important stakeholders.

19.3.3 Lack of Training and Expertise

According to Jiang et al. (2017), a large number of healthcare personnel lack the necessary data literacy and AI skills to use these technologies effectively. To supplement their decision-making with AI without depending too much or too little on its predictions, clinicians need to be trained in how to use and interpret the technology properly. For the purpose of fostering adoption and developing the requisite skills, health systems must fund the creation of specialist teams and cross-training programs.

19.3.4 Ethical and Legal Uncertainty

There are serious moral and legal concerns with using patient data to build and use AI (Morley & Floridi, 2020). Difficult regulatory gaps arise from issues including informed consent for data use, accountability for AI decisions affecting patient outcomes, potential biases in data and algorithms, and privacy/security concerns. To offer direction and mitigate hazards, more transparent laws, procedures, and industry standards are required.

19.4 STRATEGIES FOR OVERCOMING CHALLENGES

Let's explore strategies for overcoming the challenges in connection with adoption and application of AI in healthcare situations in detail.

19.4.1 Technological Limitations

- Make research and development investments: Allocate resources toward research and development to address technological challenges such as improving the scalability, reliability, and efficiency of AI algorithms. Working together with academic institutions and business associates can accelerate innovation in AI technologies.
- Standardize Interfaces and Protocols: Establish standardized interfaces and protocols to enable smooth integration of AI solutions with prevailing healthcare structures. Developing interoperable AI platforms that can communicate with multiple types of EHR structures and health policies will simplify implementation.
- Emphasis on User-Centered Design: Give top priority to the concepts of user-centered design in order to create AI solutions that are easy to use, intuitive, and compatible with healthcare professionals' workflow requirements. Involving end users in the process of designing and developing AI solutions helps guarantee that they fulfill their needs and improve usability.

19.4.2 Data Privacy Concerns

- Implement Robust Security Measures: Implement cutting-edge access controls, authentication procedures, and encryption to protect patient data against breaches and unwanted access. To find and fix possible security holes in AI systems, conduct routine security audits and assessments.
- Adhere to Regulatory Compliance: Keep abreast of legal standards like GDPR and HIPAA, and make sure AI solutions abide by laws protecting data privacy. To preserve patient privacy when using sensitive healthcare data to train AI models, use privacy-enhancing technologies like federated learning and differential privacy.
- Enhance Transparency and Accountability: Provide transparency to patients regarding how their data will be used for AI applications and obtain informed

consent. Establish clear accountability mechanisms for data handling and processing within healthcare organizations to build trust and confidence among patients and stakeholders.

19.4.3 Regulatory Hurdles

- Engage with Regulatory Authorities: Foster collaboration and communication with regulatory agencies such as the FDA to navigate the regulatory approval process for AI-driven healthcare products. Proactively seek guidance from regulatory authorities to ensure compliance with applicable regulations and streamline the approval pathway.
- Advocate for Regulatory Reform: Advocate for regulatory reforms that promote innovation while ensuring patient safety and efficacy of AI technologies. Work with policymakers and industry associations to develop regulatory frameworks tailored to the unique characteristics of healthcare AI, such as risk-based regulatory approaches.
- Establish Regulatory Sandboxes: Create regulatory sandboxes or pilot programs where healthcare organizations can test and validate AI applications in a controlled environment with regulatory oversight. This approach allows for iterative development and refinement of AI solutions while addressing regulatory concerns.

19.4.4 Ethical Considerations

- Address Bias and Fairness: Use techniques like algorithmic audits, biased detection tools, and diverse and representative training data to reduce bias in AI algorithms. Incorporate fairness metrics and transparency mechanisms to ensure equitable outcomes and enhance trust in AI systems.
- Promote Ethical AI Governance: Establish interdisciplinary ethics committees or advisory boards within healthcare organizations to oversee the ethical use of AI in clinical practice. Develop ethical guidelines and frameworks for AI deployment that prioritize patient welfare, autonomy, and privacy.
- Engage in Public Dialogue: Foster open dialogue with patients, healthcare professionals, ethicists, and policymakers to discuss the ethical implications of AI in healthcare. Encourage participation in moral deliberations and policy-making processes to ensure that AI deployments align with societal values and norms.

19.4.5 Resistance to Change

- Provide Education and Training: Provide healthcare workers with extensive training programs and chances for ongoing education to improve their technical and AI literacy. Give frontline employees the skills and self-assurance they need to successfully implement and use AI tools in their work.
- Create a Culture of Innovation: Foster culture of innovation inside healthcare organizations that embraces experimentation, training from failures, and

constant enhancement. Recognize and reward innovation initiatives that successfully integrate AI into clinical workflows and improve patient outcomes.
- Address Job Displacement Concerns: Proactively address concerns about job displacement by emphasizing the complementary role of AI in healthcare delivery.

Emphasize how AI has the ability to complement human expertise rather than replace it, giving healthcare workers more time to concentrate on high-value duties like patient care and decision-making.

Healthcare organizations can overcome the obstacles involved in adopting and deploying AI, realize the full potential of AI technology, and ultimately enhance patient outcomes and healthcare delivery by putting these tactics into practice together.

19.5 LIMITATIONS ON CURRENT AI KNOW-HOWS

While great progress has been made, AI remains imperfect and narrowly focused (Topol, 2019). Near-term expectations must be tempered. AI can augment human intelligence but cannot fully replace the knowledge and critical thinking of clinicians. AI's reliance on large training datasets also limits deployment of cutting-edge techniques in many health systems. Sufficient high-quality data required to train AI is lacking in some contexts. Work is needed to improve generalizability and build shared data repositories.

Let's explore the limitations of current AI technologies in healthcare in detail.

19.5.1 Data Quality and Availability

- Restricted Access to High-Quality Data: For training and validation, AI systems need a large quantity of high-quality data. The effectiveness of AI models, however, can be hampered by the fragmented, inadequate, and inconsistent quality of healthcare data.
- Data Bias and Imbalance: Biases and imbalances in healthcare data, such as underrepresentation of certain demographic groups or clinical conditions, can lead to biased AI predictions and exacerbate disparities in healthcare outcomes.
- Data Silos and Interoperability Challenges: Since healthcare data is frequently kept in multiple systems and formats, integrating and harmonizing data from many sources can be difficult. Lack of interoperability hinders the development of comprehensive AI solutions that leverage diverse data types.

19.5.2 Interpretability and Explainability

- Black-Box Nature of AI Models: A lot of artificial intelligence algorithms, especially deep learning models, function as "blackboxes" with opaque and challenging-to-understand decision-making processes. Inadequate interpretability has the potential to erode confidence in AI-supported clinical decision-making and restrict healthcare practitioners' use of AI tools.

- Limited Explainability in Complex Models: As AI models advance in sophistication and complexity, explaining their decisions in a comprehensible manner becomes increasingly challenging. The inability to provide meaningful explanations for AI predictions hampers transparency and accountability in healthcare settings.

19.5.3 Generalization and Robustness

- Limited Generalizability: AI models may find it difficult to generalize to new or unexplored data if they were trained on particular datasets or healthcare contexts., leading to poor performance in real-world clinical scenarios. Generalization challenges pose barriers to the widespread adoption of AI technologies across diverse patient populations and healthcare contexts.
- Vulnerability to Adversarial Attacks: Adversarial attacks, in which input data is purposefully altered, might affect AI models to cause misclassification or erroneous predictions. Confrontational occurrences can compromise the trustworthiness and safety of AI-driven healthcare systems, particularly in security-critical applications.

19.5.4 Regulatory and Legal Encounters

- Complicated Regulatory Environment: Strict regulations apply to healthcare AI technologies, including approval processes by regulatory agencies such as the FDA. Navigating the regulatory landscape, ensuring compliance with standards, and gaining regulatory certification for AI products might require a significant investment of time and resources.
- Liability and Legal Uncertainties: The legal framework surrounding AI in healthcare is still evolving, leading to uncertainties regarding liability for mistakes or unfavorable effects brought about by AI-driven actions. Clarifying legal responsibilities and liabilities for AI developers, healthcare providers, and regulatory bodies is crucial to alleviate legal hazards and foster conviction in AI skills.

19.5.5 Ethical Considerations

- Algorithmic Fairness and Bias: AI systems may unintentionally reinforce or magnify biases seen in medical records, which may result in discriminatory practices or unjust treatment. Fairness metrics and bias reduction strategies must be carefully considered in order to ensure parity and fairness in AI-driven decision-making.
- Patient Privacy and Consent: Sensitive patient data is frequently analyzed in AI applications, which raises questions regarding data security, permission, and privacy. Protecting patient privacy rights and obtaining informed consent for data usage are paramount to upholding patient confidence while adhering to legal obligations.

19.5.6 Combining Clinical Workflow Integration

- Workflow Disruption: Introducing AI technologies to clinical workflow can disrupt established practices and workflows, leading to resistance from healthcare professionals. Integration challenges, such as workflow compatibility, user interface design, and training requirements, must be addressed to ensure seamless adoption and acceptance of AI tools by healthcare providers.
- User Acceptance and Adoption: Healthcare professionals may lack confidence in AI technologies due to unfamiliarity with AI concepts, concerns about job displacement, or skepticism about AI's clinical utility. Engaging stakeholders, providing education and training, and demonstrating the value of AI in improving patient outcomes are essential for fostering user acceptance and adoption.

All parties involved in the healthcare ecosystem, researchers, clinicians, legislators, and tech developers—must work together to find solutions to these constraints. Stakeholders may leverage the revolutionary potential of AI to improve patient outcomes, enhance clinical decision-making, and advance the delivery of healthcare services by recognizing and minimizing the limitations associated with current AI technologies in healthcare.

19.6 ADOPTION OF AI IN HEALTH CARE IS NOT A MYTH

Absolutely, the adoption of AI in healthcare is not a myth but a reality that is rapidly transforming the way healthcare is carried out, managed, and experienced.

19.6.1 Improved Diagnostic Accuracy and Clinical Decision Support

AI-driven diagnostic tools, like natural language processing (NLP) systems and image recognition algorithms, have shown impressive accuracy in diagnosing diseases using clinical notes, pathology slides, and medical photographs.

AI-powered clinical decision support systems (CDSS) give medical professionals real-time insights, evidence-based suggestions, and predictive analytics to help with patient management, treatment planning, and diagnosis.

19.6.2 Treatment Optimization and Personalized Medicine

AI algorithms examine a plethora of patient data, such as genetic data, medical histories, and clinical results, to customize interventions and treatment regimens according to the unique traits and preferences of each patient.

Precision medicine approaches leverage AI to identify biomarkers, predict treatment response, and stratify patient populations for targeted therapies, resulting in improved efficacy and reduced adverse effects.

19.6.3 Enhanced Patient Engagement and Care Coordination

AI-driven chatbots and virtual assistants facilitate individualized patient interaction, remote monitoring, and self-management assistance, resulting in better patient outcomes, treatment compliance, and patient satisfaction.

AI-powered care coordination platforms make it easier for healthcare practitioners to collaborate, communicate, and exchange information, which improves the effectiveness of care delivery across various contexts.

19.6.4 Streamlined Healthcare Operations and Administrative Efficiency

AI solutions reduce administrative load, minimize errors, and optimize resource allocation in healthcare companies by automating typical administrative operations like billing coding, scheduling appointments, and processing claims.

Predictive analytics models powered by AI optimize hospital operations, resource utilization, and capacity planning, leading to reduced wait times, improved patient flow, and better allocation of healthcare resources.

19.6.5 Early Disease Detection and Prevention

Proactive interventions, lifestyle changes, and preventive care tactics are made possible by AI-driven predictive modeling and risk stratification tools, which identify people who are more susceptible to chronic diseases or their complications. These measures slow the progression of disease and enhance patient outcomes.

AI-enabled wearable sensors and remote monitoring devices allow for continuous tracking of vital signs, symptoms, and behavioral patterns, which makes it easier to identify health issues early and take appropriate action.

19.6.6 Research and Drug Discovery Advancements

By analyzing large datasets, modeling molecular interactions, and identifying promising drug candidates with higher success rates and lower development costs, AI speeds up the process of finding and developing new drugs. AI-driven drug repurposing platforms utilize current drug databases and biomedical literature to find new therapeutic applications for current pharmaceuticals, accelerating the development of new treatments for a range of illnesses.

19.6.7 Addressing Healthcare Disparities and Access to Care

By offering scalable, affordable solutions for marginalized populations, distant communities, and environments with limited resources, AI technologies have the potential to increase access to care and lessen healthcare inequities.

AI-powered telehealth solutions facilitate remote monitoring, virtual consultations, and telemedicine services, therefore reducing geographic obstacles and increasing access to specialist treatment and knowledge.

AI technologies have the ability to improve access to care and reduce healthcare disparities by providing scalable, cost-effective solutions for underserved populations, remote communities, and resource-constrained areas.

Telehealth technologies driven by AI make remote monitoring, virtual consultations, and telemedicine services possible. This lowers geographical barriers and expands access to specialized care and information.

19.7 FUTURE DIRECTIONS

Let's take a closer look at the possible developments and future paths for the acceptance and application of AI in healthcare settings:

19.7.1 Advanced AI Algorithms

Deep Learning Evolution: More complex AI algorithms for healthcare applications will be made possible by ongoing developments in deep learning approaches, such as convolutional neural networks (CNNs) and recurrent neural networks (RNNs). EHRs, imaging, genetics, and other complex medical data types will all be handled more accurately and efficiently by these algorithms.

Explainable AI (XAI): By shedding light on how AI algorithms decide, explainable AI models will help overcome the interpretability conundrum. Artificial intelligence (XAI) methods include interpretable machine learning models and attention processes that will improve openness and confidence in AI-driven clinical decision-making.

19.7.2 Personalized Medicine and Precision Health

Genomic medicine: Genomic analysis tools powered by AI will enable personalized treatment recommendations based on the unique genetic profile of each patient. Precision medicine techniques for the diagnosis and treatment of complicated diseases, including cancer and uncommon genetic abnormalities, will be made easier by the integration of genomic and clinical data.

Predictive analytics: Using long-term patient data, AI systems will forecast adverse occurrences, the course of a disease, and how well a treatment will work. AI-powered predictive analytics models will make proactive patient specific therapies and personalized healthcare interventions possible.

19.7.3 Augmented Intelligence and Human-AI Collaboration

- Augmented Diagnostic Tools: With the help of AI, medical practitioners will be able to read pathology slides, medical photographs, and other diagnostic procedures more quickly and accurately. These instruments will supplement human knowledge by offering guidance and lowering errors in diagnosis.
- Clinical Decision Support Systems (CDS): To assist healthcare professionals in making evidence-based decisions, AI-driven CDSS will incorporate patient data, clinical guidelines, and medical literature. In a variety of healthcare settings, CDSS will improve patient outcomes, optimize treatment strategies, and strengthen care coordination.

19.7.4 Remote Monitoring and Telehealth

- Remote Patient Monitoring: Wearable sensors and AI-enabled remote monitoring devices will make it possible to continuously track patients' health parameters outside of conventional hospital settings. Real-time streaming data analysis will be performed by AI algorithms in order to anticipate health occurrences, identify early indicators of deterioration, and enable prompt interventions.

- Telehealth Optimization: By automating administrative processes, enhancing diagnostic accuracy through virtual consultations, and customizing patient interaction, AI-driven telehealth platforms will improve the delivery of virtual care. AI-powered telehealth services will increase underprivileged and distant populations' access to healthcare and enhance care coordination.

19.7.5 Ethical and Regulatory Considerations

Ethical AI Governance Frameworks: The creation of thorough ethical AI governance frameworks will guarantee the ethical and responsible application of AI technology in the medical field. The ethical issues of patient privacy, algorithmic bias, informed consent, and openness in AI-powered decision-making will all be covered by these frameworks.

Harmonization of Regulations: Ensuring patient safety and data privacy while promoting the worldwide use of AI in healthcare can be achieved through harmonizing regulatory standards and guidelines across jurisdictions. Regulatory agencies, industry participants, and legislators working together will expedite the regulatory approval process for AI-powered medical software and equipment.

19.7.6 Continuous Learning and Adaptation

Continual Model Improvement: AI models will evolve through continual learning and adaptation based on feedback from real-world clinical data and user interactions. Adaptive learning algorithms will enhance model performance, generalizability, and robustness over time, enabling AI systems to keep pace with evolving healthcare challenges.

Federated Learning: While maintaining data security and privacy, federated learning techniques will allow cooperative model training across dispersed healthcare data sources. Without the need for centralized data aggregation, federated learning will make it easier for healthcare organizations to share knowledge and improve their models.

19.7.7 Socioeconomic Impact and Equity

- Addressing Healthcare Disparities: AI-driven interventions will prioritize addressing healthcare disparities and improving health equity across diverse populations. Targeted interventions, community-based outreach programs, and culturally sensitive AI applications will reduce disparities in healthcare access, outcomes, and quality of care.
- Affordable and Accessible AI Solutions: Efforts to develop affordable and accessible AI solutions will ensure widespread adoption and equitable access to AI-driven healthcare innovations. Collaborations between public

and private sectors, technology developers, and healthcare providers will drive the affordability and scalability of AI technologies in resource-limited settings.

19.7.8 Interdisciplinary Collaboration and Education

- Cross-Disciplinary Collaboration: Interdisciplinary collaboration among healthcare professionals, data scientists, engineers, ethicists, and policymakers will drive innovation and adoption of AI in healthcare. Collaborative research initiatives, interdisciplinary training programs, and knowledge exchange platforms will foster a culture of innovation and collaboration across diverse disciplines.
- AI Literacy and Training: The goal of educational programs is to raise patients', healthcare providers', and the public's awareness of AI. Stakeholders will be equipped with the knowledge and abilities to comprehend, assess, and apply AI technology in healthcare decision-making and practice through training courses, workshops, and online resources.

The healthcare sector can overcome current obstacles, enhance patient outcomes, spur innovation in healthcare delivery, and advance customized medicine by adopting these future directions and utilizing AI's disruptive potential. The future of AI in healthcare will be shaped by ongoing investments in research, technology development, regulatory frameworks, and interdisciplinary collaboration. These efforts will also open the door to a healthcare system that is more patient-centered, equitable, and efficient.

19.8 RECOMMENDATIONS

Implementing AI successfully in healthcare will require a concerted effort to address the challenges outlined above. Specific recommendations include:

Launch educational initiatives for healthcare professionals on AI capabilities, appropriate uses, and limitations. Provide concrete training on integrating AI insights into clinical practice.

Early and often involve all stakeholders (providers, patients, IT) in co-designing AI solutions that are suited to end-user needs and clinical workflows.

Establish regulations and voluntary best practices guiding transparent development, rigorous validation, and ethical use of health care AI, including methods to identify and address biases.

Select AI techniques such as rule-based systems that provide interpretable explanations alongside predictions rather than "black box" methods.

Start with focused use cases where AI can augment clinician decisions without fully replacing them. Allow clinicians to vet AI recommendations.

Build shared data repositories to facilitate the development of more robust and generalizable healthcare AI models.

19.9 CONCLUSION

AI adoption in healthcare holds tremendous potential but faces substantial barriers around trust, integration challenges, lack of expertise, ethical concerns, and immature technology. This chapter examines the key barriers to AI adoption and implementation in healthcare, including lack of trust in AI, difficulties in integrating AI into clinical workflows, lack of training for healthcare professionals, concerns about ethical and legal implications, and limitations of current AI technologies. Recommendations are provided for overcoming these challenges through education, developing regulations and best practices, choosing transparent and interpretable AI methods, involving key stakeholders in development and deployment, and starting with focused applications of AI that augment rather than replace human judgment. In order to minimize hazards and maximize the benefits of AI in healthcare, a careful strategy will be needed. A thoughtful, targeted approach focused on augmenting clinicians will be critical to overcoming these hurdles and realizing benefits for patients. With proper governance and training, AI can be implemented successfully to enhance clinical decision-making and improve healthcare outcomes.

BIBLIOGRAPHY

Adams, J., & Patel, L. (2023). Navigating Ethical Dilemmas in AI-Enhanced Healthcare. *Bioethics and AI*, 15(2), 89–102.

Baker, M., & Thompson, P. (2020). AI and Patient Privacy: Balancing Innovation with Confidentiality. *Journal of Privacy and Security*, 19(4), 345–360.

Bhjhvani, Z.P., Watanabe, A., Lopez, R.J., Melo, J., Regan, L., & Fatemi, M.(2021). Machine learning in healthcare: A systematic literature review. *DigitalMedicine*, 4(1), 1–16.

Carter, J., & Davis, L. (2021). Machine Learning Algorithms in Predictive Healthcare: A Systematic Review. *AI in Medicine*, 28(2), 77–95.

Chen, Y., & Zhang, T. (2021). The Impact of AI on Clinical Decision-Making: Opportunities and Challenges. Medical AI Review, 18(3), 97–112.

Davalbhakta, S., Advani, S., Kumar, S., Bhoyar, S., Fedirko, E., Bhoyar, P., … Agarwal, V.(2020). A Systematic Review of Application of Artificial Intelligence in Telemedicine during COVID-19Pandemic. *Journal of Medical Systems*, 44(9), 1–8.

Elliott, S., & Green, M. (2022). Challenges in AI Data Integration for Electronic Health Records. *Health Informatics Journal*, 26(3), 204–221.

Foster, R., & Walker, J. (2023). AI in Radiology: Advancements and Implementation Hurdles. *Radiology Today*, 47(1), 12–25.

Garcia, M., & Roberts, D. (2022). Implementation Strategies for AI Technologies in Medical Settings. *Healthcare Technology & Innovations*, 9(1), 56–74.

Garcia, N., & Johnson, T. (2020). Understanding the Ethical Implications of AI in Healthcare. *Journal of Medical Ethics*, 46(6), 393–400.

Harris, P., & Clarke, R. (2021). AI for Predictive Analytics in Healthcare: Opportunities and Risks. *Journal of Health Data Science*, 11(2), 60–74.

Ibrahim, S., & Lee, J. (2024). Legal Challenges in Implementing AI-Based Healthcare Solutions. *Health Law Review*, 39(1), 89–105.

Jiang, F., Jiang, Y., Zhi, H., Dong, Y., Li, H., Ma, S., … Wang, Y. (2017). Artificial intelligence in healthcare: past, present and future. *Stroke and Vascular Neurology*, 2(4), 230–243.

Johnson, M., & Lee, K. (2023). Ethical and Regulatory Challenges in AI-Driven Healthcare. *Journal of Health Informatics*, 34(2), 145–159.

Jones, A., & Edwards, C. (2023). Adopting AI in Clinical Practice: A Review of Best Practices and Barriers. *Clinical Decision Support Journal*, 33(4), 145–160.

Kim, D., & Nguyen, H. (2022). AI and Patient Safety: A Review of Potential Risks and Mitigation Strategies. *Patient Safety Journal*, 17(3), 210–226.

Krittanawong, C.(2020). The rise of artificial intelligence and the uncertain future for physicians. *European Journal of Internal Medicine*, 76, 13–14.

Lee, M., & Anderson, B. (2020). Evaluating AI Technologies for Healthcare: Methodological Considerations. *AI Research and Applications*, 24(2), 92–108.

Liu, X., Faes, L., Kale, A. U., Wagner, S. K., Fu, D. J., Bruynseels, A., … Shamdas, M. (2019). A comparison of deep learning performance against health-care professionals in detecting diseases from medical imaging: a systematic review and meta-analysis. *The Lancet Digital Health*, 1(6), e271–e297.

Miller, R., Patel, S., & Gomez, A. (2024). Barriers to AI Integration in Healthcare Systems: A Comprehensive Review. *Health Technology Journal*, 29(1), 22–38.

Morley, J., & Floridi, L. 2020). The limits of empowerment: How to reframe the role ofm-Healthtoolsinthehealthcareecosystem. *Scienceandengineeringethics*, 26(5), 2759–2779.

Morris, L., & Green, R. (2021). Strategies for Effective AI Integration in Healthcare Organizations. *Journal of Healthcare Management*, 66(3), 199–212.

Norton, J., & Patel, K. (2022). AI-Driven Diagnostic Tools: Adoption Challenges and Future Directions. *Diagnostic Technology Review*, 20(2), 118–134.

O'Connor, P., & Ramirez, L. (2023). Navigating the Regulatory Landscape for AI in Healthcare. *Compliance and Regulation Journal*, 31(1), 43–57.

Patel, V., & Brown, S. (2024). AI in Personalized Medicine: Opportunities and Implementation Issues. *Personalized Medicine Journal*, 19(1), 76–89.

Qin, J., & Zhang, Y. (2021). The Role of AI in Transforming Healthcare Delivery Models. *Health Systems and Policy Journal*, 29(3), 150–167.

Roberts, M., & Lee, T. (2020). Ethical and Social Implications of AI in Healthcare. *Bioethics Review*, 22(4), 205–218.

Ross, C., & Swetlitz, I. (2018). IBM's Watson supercomputer recommended 'unsafe and incorrect' cancer treatments, internal documents show. STAT News. Retrieved from https://www.statnews.com/2018/07/25/ibm-watson-recommended-unsafe-incorrect-treatments/

Smith, A. (2022). *Advancements in AI and Machine Learning for Healthcare Applications*. Springer.

Sullivan, E., & West, H. (2023). Adoption Challenges of AI in Healthcare Settings: Insights from Recent Case Studies. *Journal of Medical Systems*, 47(2), 123–137.

Taylor, S., & Wilson, J. (2022). Data Security Concerns in AI-Enhanced Healthcare Systems. *Information Security Journal*, 14(3), 170–184.

Topol, E. J. (2019). High-performance medicine: the convergence of human and artificial intelligence. *Nature Medicine*, 25(1), 44–56.

Usher, R., & Fox, A. (2024). AI Implementation in Healthcare: Lessons Learned from Pilot Programs. *Innovations in Health Technology*, 11(1), 45–60.

Vargas, D., & Young, K. (2021). AI and Patient Outcomes: Assessing the Impact and Challenges. *Journal of Healthcare Outcomes*, 12(4), 88–102.

Wilson, E., & Thompson, H. (2020). Regulatory Frameworks for AI in Healthcare: An Analysis of Current Policies. *International Journal of Healthcare Management*, 13(4), 210–225.

Index

Pages in *italics* refer to figures and pages in **bold** refer to tables.

A

artificial intelligence (AI), 1, 21, 23–24, 33, 61, 72, 77, 82, 86–88, 95, 122, 138, 140, 143, 156, 170–173
artificial neural networks, 156

B

big data, 23–25, 33–34, **174**, 201, 228–229, 231, **233**, 234, 237, 245
biomedical, 25, 28, 46–49, 52–53, 55, 57, 94, 99, **175**, 218, 224, 285

C

chatbots, 86, 172, 184, 187, 232, **233**, 235, 276, 284
computer-aided diagnostics (CAD), 156–157, 160–163, 165
conventional neural networks (CNN), 25, 49, 86, 89–90, 94, 102–104, 122–124, 138, 141, 145, *147*, 148–152, 157, 160–163, 286

D

deep learning, 21, 25, 47–50, 61–62, 65, 81, 86, 100–101, 122, 141, 145, 157–158, 171, 209–210, 212, 216–217, 222, 224, 266, 282, 286
digitalization, 199, 201–202, 229, 231

E

explainable artificial intelligence (XAI), 80–82, 87–89, 92–95, 286

G

generative AI, 60–62, 65, 69–70, 184–185, 187–189, 194–195

H

healthcare, 1–11, 16–17, 19–21, 23–25, 27–30, 32–42, 47–48, 60–66, 69–70, 72–75, 77–82, 86–87, 90, 94–95, 137, 141, 145, 153, 156, 158, 164–165, 170–180, 184–185, 189–191, 193–196, 209, 211–213, 215–225, 241–248, 252, 254, 256–259

I

InsurTech, 228–230, 232, 234–237
IoT, 14, 19–30, 33–34, 61, 217, 225, 228–232, **233**, 237

M

machine learning (ML), 21, 23, 25, 33, 46–48, 50–51, 54–57, 60–61, 65, 72, 79, 86–87, 141, 145, 156–157, 171, **174**, **176**, 177, 184, 190, 209–210, 214, 217–218, 228, 232, **233**
MIoT, 20–21, 23–24

N

natural language processing (NLP), 45–48, 52–53, 57, 65, 184, *186*, 187, 195, 209–210, 212, 215–219, 222, 276, 284
neurology, 3, 160

R

radiology, 45–46, 50, 156, 158–159, 162, 165, 211, 266–268
radiomics, 24–26, 158–159
robotic process automation, 172, 179, 232, **233**
robotics, 1–4, 10, 16–17, 73, 232, 267

T

telehealth, 212, 216–217, 223–224, 245, 285–287
telemedicine, 9, 20–21, 24, 28, 30, 60, 62, 156, 159, 180, 203–205, 217–218, 245, 285